Medical Intelligence Unit

Oral Tolerance:
The Response of the Intestinal Mucosa to Dietary Antigens

Olivier Morteau, Ph.D.

Department of Biomedical Sciences
Division of Infectious Diseases
Tufts University School of Veterinary Medicine
North Grafton, Massachusetts, U.S.A.

Landes Bioscience / Eurekah.com
Georgetown, Texas
U.S.A.

Kluwer Academic / Plenum Publishers
New York, New York
U.S.A.

ORAL TOLERANCE:
THE RESPONSE OF THE INTESTINAL MUCOSA TO DIETARY ANTIGENS

Medical Intelligence Unit

Eurekah.com / Landes Bioscience
Kluwer Academic / Plenum Publishers

Copyright © 2010 Eurekah.com and Kluwer Academic / Plenum Publishers

Printed in the U.S.A.

Kluwer Academic / Plenum Publishers, 233 Spring Street, New York, New York, U.S.A. 10013
http://www.wkap.nl/

Please address all inquiries to the Publishers:
Eurekah.com / Landes Bioscience, 810 South Church Street
Georgetown, Texas, U.S.A. 78626
Phone: 512/ 863 7762; FAX: 512/ 863 0081
www.Eurekah.com
www.landesbioscience.com

Oral Tolerance: The Response of the Intestinal Mucosa to Dietary Antigens edited by Olivier Morteau, Landes / Kluwer dual imprint / Landes series: Medical Intelligence Unit

While the authors, editors and publisher believe that drug selection and dosage and the specifications and usage of equipment and devices, as set forth in this book, are in accord with current recommendations and practice at the time of publication, they make no warranty, expressed or implied, with respect to material described in this book. In view of the ongoing research, equipment development, changes in governmental regulations and the rapid accumulation of information relating to the biomedical sciences, the reader is urged to carefully review and evaluate the information provided herein.

Library of Congress Cataloging-in-Publication Data

Morteau, Olivier.
   Oral tolerance : the response of the intestinal mucosa to dietary antigens / Olivier Morteau.
      p. ; cm. -- (Medical intelligence unit)
Includes bibliographical references and index.
ISBN 978-1-4419-3425-3
   1. Mucous membrane. 2. Intestinal mucosa. 3. Antigens. 4. Immunity.
I. Title. II. Series: Medical intelligence unit (Unnumbered : 2003)
   [DNLM: 1. Immunity, Mucosal--physiology. 2. Intestinal
Mucosa--immunology. WI 400 M887o 2003]
RC802.9.M675 2003
616.07'9--dc22
                              2003021854

CONTENTS

EDITOR

Olivier Morteau, Ph.D.
Department of Biomedical Sciences
Division of Infectious Diseases
Tufts University School of Veterinary Medicine
North Grafton, Massachusetts, U.S.A.
olivier.morteau@tufts.edu
Chapter 5

CONTRIBUTORS

Mona Bajaj-Elliott
Department of Adult and Paediatric
  Gastroenterology
St Bartholomew's and The Royal
  London School of Medicine
  and Dentistry
University of London
London, U.K.
mbelliott@mds.qmw.ac.uk
Chapter 1

Pekka Collin
Coeliac Disease Study Group
Institute of Medical Technology
University of Tampere
Tampere, Finland
pekka.collin@uta.fi
Chapter 9

Kohtaro Fujihashi
Immunobiology Vaccine Center
Departments of Oral Biology
  and Microbiology
The University of Alabama
  at Birmingham
Birmingham, Alabama, U.S.A.
kohtarof@uab.edu
Chapter 3

Dirk Haller
Department of Medicine and the Center
  for Gastrointestinal Biology
  and Disease
Division of Digestive Disease
  and Nutrition
University of North Carolina
Chapel Hill, North Carolina, U.S.A.
Chapter 7

Martine Heyman
INSERM EMI0212
Faculté Necker-Enfants Malades
Paris, France
heyman@necker.fr
Chapter 8

Steffen Husby
Department of Pediatrics
Odense University Hospital
Odense, Denmark
Steffen.Husby@ouh.fyns-amt.dk
Chapter 6

Hirotomo Kato
Immunobiology Vaccine Center
Departments of Oral Biology
  and Microbiology
The University of Alabama
  at Birmingham
Birmingham, Alabama, U.S.A.
Chapter 3

Katri Kaukinen
Coeliac Disease Study Group
Institute of Medical Technology
University of Tampere
Tampere, Finland
katri.kaukinen@uta.fi
Chapter 9

Thomas T. MacDonald
Division of Infection, Inflammation
   and Repair
School of Medicine
University of Southampton
Southampton General Hospital
Southampton, U.K.
t.t.macdonald@soton.ac.uk
Chapter 4

Markku Mäki
Coeliac Disease Study Group
Institute of Medical Technology
University of Tampere
Tampere, Finland
markku.maki@uta.fi
Chapter 9

Jerry R. McGhee
Immunobiology Vaccine Center
Departments of Oral Biology
   and Microbiology
The University of Alabama
   at Birmingham
Birmingham, Alabama, U.S.A.
mcghee@uab.edu
Chapter 3

Giovanni Monteleone
Cattedra di Gastroenterologia
Dipartimento di Medicina Interna
Universita tor Vergata
Rome, Italy
Chapter 4

Allan McI Mowat
Department of Immunology
   and Bacteriology
University of Glasgow
Western Infirmary
Glasgow, Scotland
a.m.mowat@clinmed.gla.ac.uk
Chapter 2

Mary H. Perdue
Intestinal Research Disease Programme
McMaster University
Hamilton, Ontario, Canada
perdue@mcmaster.ca
Chapter 8

Jesper Reinholdt
Department of Oral Biology
Royal Dental College
University of Aarhus
Aarhus, Denmark
jr@microbiology.au.dk
Chapter 6

Ian R. Sanderson
Department of Adult & Paediatric
   Gastroenterology
St Bartholomew's & The Royal London
   School of Medicine & Dentistry
University of London
London, U.K.
irsanderson@mds.qmw.ac.uk
Chapter 1

R. Balfour Sartor
Department of Medicine and the Center
   for Gastrointestinal Biology
   and Disease
Division of Digestive Disease and
   Nutrition
University of North Carolina
Chapel Hill, North Carolina, U.S.A.
rbs@med.unc.edu
Chapter 7

Howard L. Weiner
Center for Neurologic Diseases
Brigham and Women's Hospital
Harvard Medical School
Boston, Massachusetts, USA
Chapter 10

PREFACE

Oral tolerance, a major property of the gastrointestinal mucosa, is classically defined as a state of hyporesponsiveness to fed antigens. Extensive studies have increased our understanding of this mechanism, first described by H.G. Wells in 1911 and led the way to potential clinical applications in the most recent years.

Oral Tolerance: The Response of the Intestinal Mucosa to Dietary Antigens has been designed as a concise yet comprehensive overview of the newest advances in the field of mucosal tolerance.

In Chapter 1, Mona Bajaj-Elliott and Ian R. Sanderson describe the unique structure, physical and immunological functions of the gastrointestinal mucosa. Their chapter emphasizes the role of the mucosa in allowing metabolic exchanges with luminal nutrients while maintaining the host's immune integrity.

Allan McI Mowat offers in Chapter 2 a synthetic view of oral tolerance. His review includes the immunological impact of oral tolerance, the factors involved in its development (antigen dose and frequency, host age and immune status), the role of intestinal absorption and antigen uptake and the modulation of oral tolerance.

In Chapter 3, Kohtaro Kujihashi, Hirotomo Kato, and Jerry R. McGhee explore the new concept that oral tolerance can translate into both systemic and mucosal immune unresponsiveness. They revisit the roles of T cell populations and Peyer's patches in mucosal immunity.

Chapter 4, written by Giovanni Monteleone and Thomas T. MacDonald, focuses on the key function of T cells in maintaining the integrity of the healthy mucosa and in mediating the mucosal inflammatory response of the injured mucosa.

The roles of cytokines and prostaglandins in oral tolerance and intestinal inflammation are presented in Chapter 5.

Jesper Reinholdt and Steffen Husby give in Chapter 6 a comprehensive presentation of the IgA response. They review the structure, source and functions of IgA antibodies and offer new insights on their role in mucosal tolerance.

In Chapter 7, Dirk Haller and R. Balfour Sartor reflect on the importance of bacterial antigens in the induction of tolerogenic versus pathogenic mucosal responses. They defend the theory that commensal enteric bacteria are key factors, along with the host genetic susceptibility, in the establishment of chronic intestinal inflammation.

Written by Mary H. Perdue and Martine Heyman, Chapter 8 is an extensive review of food and milk allergies as direct consequences of the breakdown of oral tolerance in susceptible individuals. Their chapter includes the clinical and mechanistic aspects of food allergies, with an emphasis on the role of epithelial cells in these pathologies.

One of the most important types of food allergies, celiac disease, is the topic of Chapter 9, by Katri Kaukinen, Markku Mäki, and Pekka Collin. The clinical, genetic, immunological and pathogenetic aspects of the disease are presented in this comprehensive chapter.

Chapter 10, by Howard L. Weiner, is devoted to the clinical applications of oral tolerance. Based on promising studies in various inflammatory models, this review explores the potential of oral antigens as a therapeutic tool in the treatment of autoimmune diseases.

I want to thank the authors for their outstanding contributions and their patience in working with me to bring this volume to a most successful conclusion. I am grateful to Ron Landes for offering me the opportunity to design and edit this book and to Balfour Sartor for his enthusiastic guidance in the field of intestinal inflammation. I also express my gratitude to Cynthia Conomos and the production staff at Landes Bioscience.

Olivier Morteau

CHAPTER 1

Structure and Function of the Gastrointestinal Mucosa

Mona Bajaj-Elliott and Ian R. Sanderson

Introduction

The large mucosal surface of the gastrointestinal tract faces many challenges while maintaining overall body metabolic integrity.[1,2] The primary function of the small intestine is to digest and absorb essential nutrients from the complex milieu of the gut lumen into the circulation.[3] The mucosal surface extends to the largest area of the body in direct contact with the external environment, which leads to greater exposure to potential noxious stimuli (digestive enzymes, bile salts, acids, pathogenic bacteria). The gut also harbours a wide range of commensal nonpathogenic microflora, some of which are vital for the development of the intestine.[4] The vast array of ingested antigens and the gut flora form the major constituents of the gut lumen. This is particularly true for the distal ileum and the colon where the resident anaerobic bacteria exist in very high (10^8 to 10^{12} bacteria/gram of luminal contents) concentrations.[5] To deal with this continuous and diverse antigenic exposure, a unique immune system exists at the surface of the gastrointestinal tract, which is distinct from the systemic immune system.[6] Normal tissue homeostasis in the small intestine is maintained by exquisite interplay between the contents of the gut lumen, the surface epithelium and the immune cells in the lamina propria. The structure and the function of these various cellular constituents that provide dynamic cross-talk between the gut luminal environment and the appropriate host response are the subject of this review.

Organization of the Intestinal Epithelium

The intestinal epithelium consists of a single layer of epithelial cells that undergo a rapid and continuous renewal, an essential process for the digestion and absorption of nutrients that also reduces potential colonisation by microorganisms.[7,8] The epithelial layer has a complex but defined anatomical structure. In the small intestine, the epithelium displays finger-shaped projections or villi, which measure 0.5 to 1.5 mm in length and tend to be broader and shorter in the ileum than in the jejunum. Regularly spaced in the troughs between the villi are the crypts of Lieberkühn, which are straight, tubular intestinal glands that secrete fluid and electrolytes. There are about 5-10 crypts/villus with a 6:1 average ratio of villus height to crypt depth in the jejunum. Each crypt is monoclonal, derived from a single stem cell.[9] The anatomical distribution of the various cell types in the crypt/villus axis is depicted in Figure 1.

Oral Tolerance: The Response of the Intestinal Mucosa to Dietary Antigens,
edited by Olivier Morteau. ©2004 Eurekah.com and Kluwer Academic / Plenum Publishers.

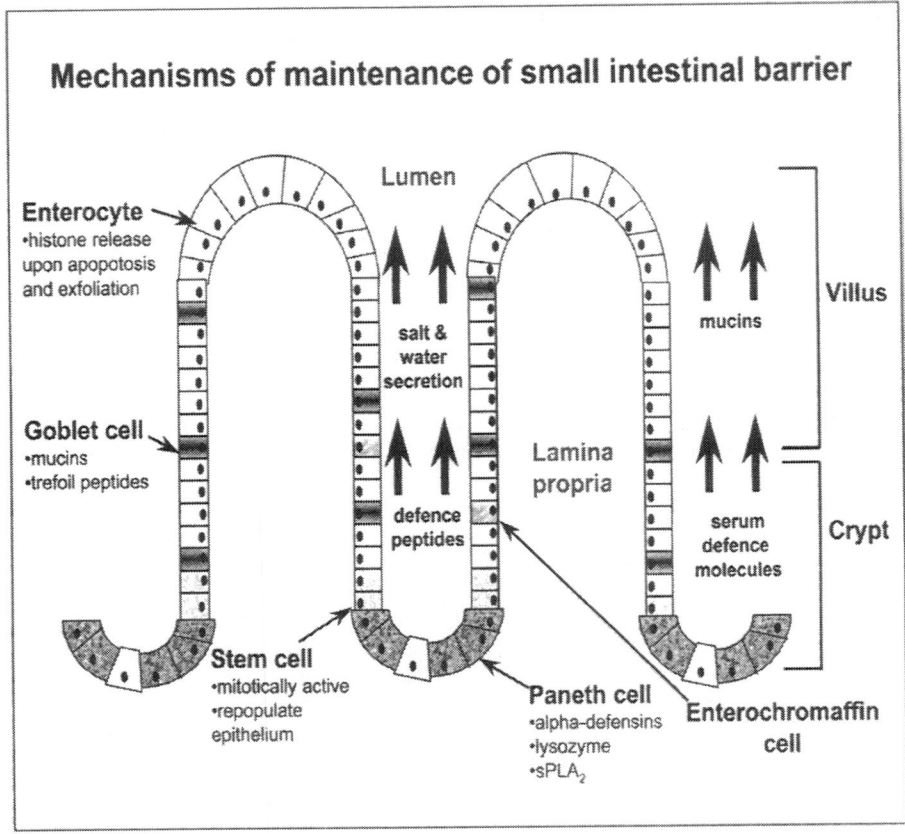

Figure 1. Schematic representation of a crypt and villus showing the anatomical distribution of the major cell types that reside in the lamina propria and the epithelium of the small intestine.

Pluripotent stem cells reside in these crypts and give rise to proliferating daughter cells that differentiate during migration onto the villus or to the base of the crypt. The four major terminally differentiated cell types in the intestine are: a, absorptive columnar enterocytes; b, mucus secreting goblet cells; c, enteroendocrine cells, which secrete specific hormones; and d, Paneth cells, which synthesise peptides and proteins that play a major role in the host innate immune response. Despite the high rate of cell renewal in the crypt, proliferation ceases in the upper third of the crypt and only fully differentiated cells are observed in the villus tip. The absorptive enterocytes represent 90-95% of the cells on the villus surface. A spatially complex epithelium is maintained from crypt to villus tip and from duodenum to colon (reviewed in detail by Madara and Trier[10]).

Barrier Function of the Surface Epithelium

The surface epithelium represents a highly selective barrier between the underlying lamina propria and the external environment.[1] This barrier allows a selective uptake of macromolecules from the gut lumen, via the epithelial cell itself (transcellular route) or through the spaces between the cells (paracellular route). All intestinal epithelial cells have extensive junctional complexes located at the apical margin of the lateral membrane.[11] Three types of cellular junctions localised along the apical to basolateral margin have been identified: zonula occludens (tight junction), zonula adherens (belt desmosome) and macula adherens (spot desmosome). The rate-limiting barrier to diffusion between cells is provided by the tight junctions.[12] Tight junctions consist of protein complexes that provide a highly regulated intercellular barrier allowing paracellular transport when required. The maintenance of the barrier function is essential for normal gut homeostasis as the breakdown of its integrity has been implicated in various inflammatory diseases.[13] This mucosal barrier is a key element of the mucosal defence system, in addition to nonimmunological physiological barriers including motility, mucus secretion and cell turnover. The mutually competitive interactions of the commensal gut flora also provide a critical protective role.[14]

The normal mucosa is protected by a lubricating mucus layer secreted by the epithelium and the underlying glands. The mucus lining is composed of high molecular weight glycoproteins (mucins) that form polymers and create a viscous, sticky gel. The exact composition of the mucus varies greatly during development and between species.[15] The mucus coat offers protection in a number of ways. The sticky quality of the mucus is an important factor preventing the penetration of organisms, as it has been observed with *Entameoba histolytica* trophozoites.[16] The carbohydrate moeities on the mucin molecules could also act as competitors to the binding of microorganisms at the enterocyte surface thus inhibiting invasion of potential pathogens.

A major contribution of the mucosal immune system to increased epithelial barrier function is the presence of antibodies. Immunoglobulins (Ig) A present in mucosal secretions are able to interact directly with noxious antigens still 'external' to the host. This immune exclusion or barrier function of IgA has been known for several decades.[17] Secretory IgA and IgM are generated by the interaction between J chain-expressing plasma cells that produce polymeric IgA and pentameric IgM, and secretory epithelial cells that express the polymeric Ig receptor (pIgR) involved in the active transport of the antibodies to the lumen.[18,19] The Fab portions of the IgA can also be occupied by antigens during the transport to the mucosal surface; IgA and IgM neutralise viruses intracellularly and carry the pathogens and their products back to the lumen, functioning as an excretory antibody that helps eliminate antigens from the body.[20]

Phenotype of the Intestinal Epithelium

Absorptive Epithelia

During migration along the crypt-villus axis, the crypt cell differentiates from a secretory cell into an absorptive enterocyte, a predominant cell type. This change is reflected anatomically by the formation of tiny microvilli on the luminal plasma membrane, the interface that interacts directly with the external environment. As revealed by light microscopy, the presence of microvilli gives the apical surface of the epithelia the appearance of a 'brush', leading to the term 'brush-border.'[21] Differentiated absorptive enterocytes are highly polarised, tall columnar cells resembling other cell types (e.g., colonic and gall-bladder epithelia) that specialise in transport. In addition to their barrier function, these cells also regulate a variety of asymmetrical transport processes that are necessary for normal fluid and nutritional homeostasis.[22] Several gene products are characteristic of the differentiated enterocyte and are first expressed in the upper crypt region of the crypt-villus junction. As an example, studies on the regulation of sucrase-isomaltase gene expression have shed light on events that regulate development and differentiation of the enterocyte.[23] The enzyme is first expressed in the upper third of the crypt and crypt-villus junction, then at high levels in the mid-villus, and then its expression decreases at the villus tips. Transcriptional regulation of the sucrase-isomaltase gene is intimately associated with the cessation of cell proliferation in the upper third of the crypt.

Goblet Cell

Small intestine goblet cells are highly polarised mucus-secreting cells present in both the crypt and the villous epithelium; their number increase progressively from the mid-jejunum to the terminal ileum.[24] Mucus-producing goblet cells, which are readily identified using periodic acid-Schiff staining, are less frequent near the villus tip. The apical two-thirds of the cell is distended by the presence of mucin granules, giving it the appearance of a brandy goblet. The goblet cell matures as it migrates up the crypt, and the structural changes include mucin granule formation; these mature cells are observed in the upper crypt.[25] The morphology of the goblet cell is similar throughout the small intestine. Mucus production is a well established marker of goblet cell differentiation.[7] The mucus acts as a barrier against potentially noxious intraluminal agents.[26] Studies have shown direct stimulation and increase of mucin secretion by pathogens such as *E. coli* and *V. cholera*.[27] Furthermore, both rat and human mucins can directly bind and inhibit the adherence of *E. histolytica* lectins, suggesting an active role for these glycoproteins in host defence. Goblet cells also secrete lectin-like molecules. Although their function is unknown, they may cross-link the mucin glycoproteins and stabilise the mucus gel.

Paneth Cell

Paneth cells contribute to the mucosal barrier function by synthesising and secreting proteins associated with innate immunity and host defence, into the lumen of the crypts of Lieberkühn in the small intestine.[2,28] Unlike other epithelial cells, Paneth cells mature below the proliferative zone, differentiate as they migrate downward and occasionally extend up the lateral walls of the crypt.[29] Histologically, Paneth cells have prominent eosinophilic granules and intense basophilia of the remaining cytoplasm, suggesting their secretory nature. Paneth cells are found in most mammalian species with the exception of cats, dogs and pigs. Interestingly, this species difference does not seem to correlate with any dietary and environmental factors. Until recently, research has focused mainly on the characterisation of Paneth cell protein secretions. Murine intestinal cell fractions enriched with Paneth cell granules contain high levels of lysozyme, an enzyme that hydrolyses bacterial cell wall peptidoglycan, which suggests that Paneth cells are involved in host defence.[30] Other anti-microbial agents, such as secretory phospholipase A2,[31] anti-trypsin[32] and antimicrobial peptides of the α-defensin family,[33] have been identified as major components of the Paneth cell secretory granules. Two members of the alpha-defensin family of antimicrobial peptides, human defensin (HD)-5 and HD-6, are constitutively expressed in Paneth cells. The genes encoding HD-5 and HD-6 are detectable by RT-PCR in the developing foetus as early as 13.5 weeks of gestation. These expressions coincide with the appearance of Paneth cells in early ontogeny.[34] There is immuno-histochemical evidence of intracellular HD-5 peptide in Paneth cells at 24 weeks gestation.[35] The physiological significance of defensin expression in the sterile environment of the developing foetus remains unclear.

Enterochromaffin Cell

Enterochromaffin (EC) cells are not limited to the epithelium of the small intestine but are distributed throughout the digestive tract. Endocrine cells first appear in human foetal small intestine between 10 and 12 weeks of gestation, as the crypt and the villi begin to form.[36] In the adult small intestine, EC cells are most abundant in the crypt and decrease in number towards the villus tip. These cells are columnar but narrower than the absorptive cells. Their apical microvilli are more irregular and sparse than those of absorptive cells. Endocrine cells are generally classified based on the shape and content of their secretory granules. Many different peptides are produced by these cells, including motilin and somatostatin, which are involved in the control of fasting motor activity. There are at least eight different subclasses of enteroendocrine cells identified to date. They include serotonin, peptide YY, cholecystokinin, gastrin, glucagon-like peptide 1, neurotensin and secretin-like immunoreactive cells.

Mucosal Immune System

The integrity of the gastrointestinal tract is maintained via both innate and adaptive mucosal immune mechanisms.[2,37] Primary mucosal immune responses are believed to be elicited mainly in organised gut associated lymphoid tissue (GALT). The GALT is the ring of lymphoid tissue circling the oropharynx, Peyer's patches in the small intestine, lymphoid nodules lining the appendix, and isolated follicles in the rectum. The GALT is divided into two anatomically and functionally distinct compartments. The first compartment includes the small intestinal Peyer's patches, the isolated lymphoid follicles and the mesenteric lymph nodes. The second compartment consists of immune cells diffused throughout the lamina propria and interspersed within the epithelium.

Peyer's Patches

Peyer's patches (PPs), first described by J.C. Peyer in 1667, are essentially made up of noncapsulated clusters of lymphoid cells. In the human foetus, clusters of lymphoid cells appear at about 11-12 weeks of gestation when subepithelial accumulation of CD4[+], CD3[-], HLA-DR[+] and DP[+], but not DQ[+] accessory cells, are present.[38] By 16 weeks of gestation, loosely defined T and B cell areas can be observed. IgM and IgD expressing B cells and CD3[+] and CD4[+] T cells predominate. The first organised PPs emerge around 19 weeks of gestation, when distinct zonation of T and B cells areas can be observed. Macrophages are also detectable at this stage.[39] The average number of PPs increases to about 50 at 24-29 week of gestation. PPs are well developed by the fifth month of foetal life and progressively increase in size and number as gestation proceeds, and after birth. Their number increases up to about 250 by age 12 and then decreases progressively with age.[40,41]

In the human small intestine, PPs are located on the antimesenteric wall of the small bowel with the highest density in the ileum. Anatomically, lymphoid follicles appear as dome-like swellings arising from the mucosal surface of the gut. The lymphoid cells of such an aggregate are separated from the intestinal lumen only by the overlying specialised follicle associated-epithelium (FAE). FAE is characterised by a decrease in goblet cells and mucin, and the presence of M (membranous or microfold) cells. M cells play a key role in mucosal immunity through their capacity to sample and transport macromolecules via transepithelial vesicular transport mechanisms.[42-44] The apical surface of M cells differs from that of neighbouring absorptive enterocytes, since it lacks the typical brush border and is associated with glycocalix, a structure likely to facilitate access and adherence of particles and micro-organisms to the cell surface.[45,46] The basolateral surface of M cells is in close association with the underlying mucosal immune system.[45,46] Unlike absorptive enterocytes, M cells have a reduced or no expression of the poly-Ig receptor on their basolateral surface.[47] The cytoplasm of M cells is rich in vesicles involved in the antigen transport from the lumen to the underlying lymphoid tissue. M cells have a thin apical cytoplasm and a basaly located nucleus. Membranous indentations on the basolateral surface allow the formation of a large intraepithelial pocket. The ontogeny and origin of M cells remains unclear, although there is increasing evidence for an 'epithelial' origin.[48]

Adherence of Antigen to M Cells

The structure of the M cells is finely adapted to its role in antigen sampling. The endocytotic activity of the M cell far exceeds that of the absorptive cell. Between the short, irregular microvilli or microfolds on the apical surfaces are many microdomains from which endocytosis can occur.[49] The antigen uptake at these sites may be nonspecific. However, the apical surface of M cells has abundant glyco conjugates that may serve as binding sites for cationic and lectin-like microbial surface molecules.[50,51] M cells can take up particles, macromolecules or organisms by endocytosis or phagocytosis, involving extensive membrane rearrangement. All these pathways allow the transport of foreign material into endosome-like tubules and vesicles located in the apical cytoplasmic layer. The M cell has exquisitively shortened its transcytotic pathway by drawing its basolateral membrane towards the apical surface, as well as by directing apical endosomes directly to the specialised basolateral pocket domain. A range of protein antigens such as lectins, wheat germ agglutinin, gram-negative bacteria (*Salmonella typhi*,[52] *Vibrio cholerae*[53]) and viruses (polio,[54] reovirus,[55]) use the M cells as a route of entry in the gastrointestinal tract.

Between the epithelium and the follicle-region is a dome-shaped lymphocyte-rich region referred to as the corona, where aggregated follicles are separated by interfollicular areas.[56,57] High endothelial venules, sites of extravasation of circulating lymphocytes, are situated in the interfollicular areas of lymphoid organ tissues. In this area lies an extensive network of dendritic cells, macrophages intermingled with CD4⁺ T cells and B cells from the underlying follicle.[58] The general organisation of a lymphoid follicle in a PP (a dark, lymphocyte-rich peripheral zone with an inner lighter germinal centre) is depicted in Figure 2. Follicular dendritic cells within the germinal centre are involved in the affinity maturation of antibody-expressing cells and the generation of memory cells. Most B cells in the periphery of the mucosal follicle and the corona express IgM surface receptors, whereas B cells in the germinal centre have switched to the IgA type.[59]

Lamina Propria T Cells

According to the current paradigm of mucosal immunity, initial antigen-driven activation, proliferation and partial differentiation occur primarily in the GALT. As shown in Figure 2, partially activated T cells migrate via the mesenteric lymph nodes and thoracic duct where they undergo further differentiation, into the peripheral circulation before homing to the appropriate cellular compartment in the intestinal mucosa.[6,60,61]

Messenger RNA expression for the rearranged T cell receptor (TCR) and loci is detectable early in gestation.[62,63] However, the total number of T cells remains low[64] and the follicles undergo very little development until birth, when the gut is exposed to dietary and bacterial antigens. Germinal centres do not appear within lymphoid follicles in the human small intestine until after birth.[65]

In healthy adults, T cells are present in both the lamina propria and the epithelium. Adult lamina propria lymphocytes (LPLs) are predominantly CD4⁺ T cells expressing the TCR[66] and peripheral blood lymphocytes (PBLs) exhibit a similar (2:1) ratio of CD4⁺ to CD8⁺ T cells.[67,68] LPLs and PBLs share several common phenotypic features, but differ in their apparent maturation state. LPL CD4⁺ T cells bear the hallmarks of 'activated' cells, since they express specific activation markers on their surface. 70-95% of LPLs express the effector CD45RO form of the CD45 molecule and therefore bears little or no L-selectin.[57] Approximately half the CD8⁺ lamina propria cells express the CD28 molecule associated with cytolytic function.[68] The increased association of the activated (memory/cytolytic) phenotype with LPLs is most likely due to continuous challenge in the intestinal environment.

One major functional consequence of LPL activation is a marked IgA production, which provides crucial immunity at the mucosal surface.[69] Most LPL actions are mediated via the production of soluble and membrane-bound factors (cytokines). These cytokines are divided into two subgroups: Th1 (IL-2, IFNγ, TNFα) and Th2 (IL-4, IL-5, IL-10) cytokines, which are associated with cell mediated immunity and humoral immunity, respectively. As one might predict, a Th2 cytokine environment predominates in the healthy bowel, facilitating IgA production. Since the early 1990's, there has been increasing evidence for an imbalance

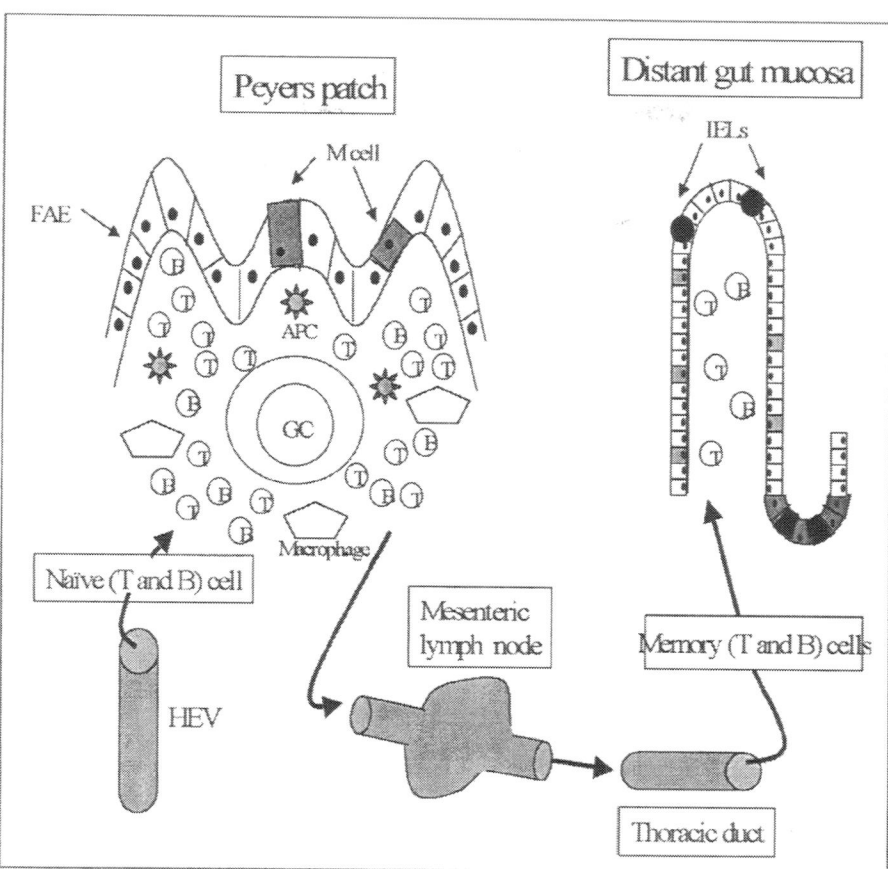

Figure 2. Schematic representation of the components of the human mucosal immune system. Naive lymphocytes are recruited from the peripheral blood to the GALT where antigen sampling occurs. Antigen-primed T and B cells then move via the efferent lymph and peripheral blood and the thoracic duct, before finally homing to the appropriate distant effector sites (lamina propria and the epithelium).

in the Th1/Th2 host response at the source of various gastrointestinal inflammatory diseases.[70,71]

CD8[+] T cells accomplish their immunological functions by either secreting cytokines, such as IFNγ and TNFα, or by lysing infected cells via the perforin or Fas/FasL pathways (for review, see Slifka and Whitton[72]). Interestingly, a third mechanism by which cytotoxic T cells may control microbial infection has recently come to light. Ernst, Krensky and colleagues have identified and characterised a protein (Granulsyin) from T cells that exhibits antimicrobial activity against a range of pathogens.[73]

Intraepithelial Lymphocytes (IELs)

As the name suggests, IELs of the small and the large intestine reside interspersed with the surface epithelium bearing both αβ and γδ TCR-positive lymphocytes. One CD3[+] T cell can be found for every six epithelial cells.[74] IELs are located in the basal part of the epithelium lying on the basement membrane below the inter-epithelial tight junctions. Although IELs were first described nearly a century ago, it is mostly the discovery of their rearranged genes in the last decade, rather than the knowledge of their biological function that has helped elucidate their functional characteristics.

IELs constitute 10-20% of the total GALT with decreasing numbers in the distal gut, and particularly in the colon. Adult small and large intestine IELs exhibit the resting phenotype not expressing markers associated with cytolytic activity, such as granzyme B, perforin, Fas ligand and TNFα.[75]

A unique anatomical feature of the IEL compartment is the occurrence of high numbers of γδ T cells when compared to other organised systemic lymphoid tissues.[76] Although mucosal γδ T cells possess unique features, the immunobiology of this subset remains unclear.[77] A majority (~80%) of these cells are CD8[+] and the distribution of TCR usage differs between mouse and man. IELs from adult mice are 40 to 70% αβ TCRs and 30 to 60% γδ TCRs compared with only 10-15% γδ TCR usage in humans.[78] In mice, most γδ TCR IELs and many αβ TCR IELs use the CD8αα homodimer instead of CD8αβ expressed in blood-borne T cells.[79] Unlike peripheral γδ T cells, CD8αα IELs have a population of CD5⁻ Thy⁻ cells, which supports the hypothesis that IELs may have an extra thymic origin.[80] Saito and colleagues recently identified 'regions' of the murine intestinal mucosa referred to as 'cryptopatches'.[81] These patches consisted primarily of primarily consisted of immature T cells (c-kit[+], IL7R[+]). The authors removed these regions and areas of lymph nodes and injected them into the blood system of immunodeficient mice lacking T cells. As predicted, the recipient mice with the cryptopatches developed T cells in their gut unlike the latter group.[81]

There is increasing evidence that γδ T cells may play a vital role in host defence at the time of birth when the load of dietary and bacterial antigens is markedly increased. In spite of a restricted receptor usage, γδ T cells may have important functions in host defence. MICA and MICB, two surface molecules that share homology with the MHC family members are known to be upregulated on epithelial cells during stress (e.g., in an infectious episode). Tom Spies and colleagues have shown that under these conditions γδ T cells have the ability to recognise MICA and MICB and to kill the cells displaying these molecules.[82] This study provides evidence for a dual role for γδ T cells in the intestine: γδ act as the front line of defence by protecting the mucosa against infectious agents, and play an important role in the subsequent immune regulation in the gut.

Summary

The gastrointestinal mucosa regulates nutrient and water absorption from the lumen while protecting the tissue integrity against a vast array of agents. Our aim was to highlight the structure and function of the various cells that allow the intestinal mucosa to fulfil its function. Breakdown in either structure (e.g., epithelial barrier) or function (exaggerated immune response) of the mucosa is now known to contribute to disease, highlighting the importance of maintaining host tissue integrity. Future studies are likely to identify the molecular mechanisms that allow further cross-talk between the various cell types in 'sensing' the external environment to its advantage.

References

1. Sanderson IR, Walker WA. Mucosal barrier. In: Ogra R, Mestecky J, McGhee J et al, eds. Handbook of Mucosal Immunology. 2nd ed. San Diego: Acadaemic Press, 1999:5-17.

2. Bevins CL, Martin-Porter E, Ganz T. Defensins and innate host defence of the gastrointestinal tract. Gut 1999; 271:14038-14045.

3. Field M, Frizzel RA. Intestinal absorption and secretion. In: Schultz SG, ed. The Gastrointestinal System. Vol. IV. Bethesda: American Physiology Society, 1991.

4. Bengmark S. Ecological control of the gastrointestinal tract. The role of probiotic flora. Gut 1998; 42:2-7.

5. Donaldson RM Jr. Normal bacterial population of the intestine and their relation to intestinal function. N Eng J Med 1981; 270:938-943.

6. Brandtzaeg P, Farstad IN, Helgeland L. Phenotypes of T cells in the gut. Chem Immunol 1998; 71:1-26.

7. Cheng H, Leblond C. Origin, differentiation and renewal of the four main epithelial cell types in the mouse small intestine. Am J Anat 1974; 141:461-479.

8. Quaroni A, Isselbacher KJ. Study of intestinal cell differentiation with monoclonal antibodies to intestinal cell surface components. J Dev Biol 1985; 111:267-279.

9. Ponder BAJ, Schmidt GH, Wilkerson MM et al. Derivation of mouse intestinal crypt from a single progenitor cell. Nature 1985; 313:689-691.

10. Madara JL, Trier JS. The functional morphology of the mucosa of the small intestine. In: Johnson LR, ed. Physiology of the Gastrointestinal Tract. 3rd ed. New York: Raven Press, 1994:1577-1622.

11. Farquhar MG, Palade GE. Junctional complexes in various epithelia. J Cell Biol 1963; 17:375-412.

12. Stevenson BR, Keon BH. The tight junction: Morphology to molecules. Ann Rev Cell Biol 1998; 14:89-109.

13. Sanderson IR, Walker WA. Uptake and transport of macromolecules by the intestine: Possible role in clinical disorders. Gastroenterology 1993; 104:622-639.

14. Alderberth I, Hanson LA, Wold AE. Ontogeny of the intestinal flora. In: Ogra R, Mestecky J, McGhee J et al, eds. Handbook of Mucosal Immunology. 2nd ed. San Diego:Academic Press, 1999:279-292.

15. Shub MD, Pang KY, Swann DA et al. Age-related changes in chemical composition and physical properties of mucus glycoproteins from rat small intestine. Biochem J 1983; 215:405-411.

16. Leitch GJ, Dickey AD, Udezuler IA et al. Entameoba histolytica trophozoites in the lumen and mucus blanket of rat colons studied in vivo. Infect Immun 1985; 47:68-73

17. Stokes CR, Soothill JF, Turner MW. Immune exclusion is a function of IgA. Nature 1975; 255:745-746.

18. Brandtzarg P, Prydz H. Direct evidence for an integrated function of J chain and secretory component in epithelial transport of immunoglobulins. Nature 1984; 311:71-73.

19. Mostov KE. Transepithelial transport of immunoglobulins. Ann Rev Immunol 1994; 12:63-84.

20. Mazanec MB, Coudret CL, Fletcher DR. Intracellular neutralisation of influenza virus by immunoglobulin A anti-hemagglutini monclonal antibodies. J Virol 1995; 69:1339-1343.

21. Moosker MS. Organisation, chemistry and assembly of the cytoskeletal apparatus of the intestinal brush border. Ann Rev Cell Dev Biol 1985; 1:209-241.

22. Ferraris RP, Buddington RK, David ES. Ontogeny of nutrient transporters. In: Sanderson IR, Walker WA, eds. Development of the Gastrointestinal Tract. Ontario: Decker BC Inc., 1999:123-146.

23. Traber PG, Yu L, Wu G et al. Regulation of sucrase-isomaltase gene expression along the crypt-villus axis of human small intestine is regulated at the level of mRNA abundance. Am J Physiol 1992; 262:G123-G130.

24. Moe H. On goblet cells, especially of the intestine of some mammalian species. Intern. Rev Cytol 1955; 4:299-334.

25. Merzel J, Leblond CP. Origin and renewal of goblet cells in the epithelium of the mouse small intestine. Am J Anat 1969; 124:281-306.

26. Bansil R, Stanley E, Lamont JT. Mucin biophysics. Ann Rev Physiol 1995; 57:635-657.

27. Moon HW, Whipp SC, Baetz AL. Comparative effects of enterotoxins from E.coli and V.cholera on rabbit and swine small intestine. Lab Invest 1971; 25:133-140.

28. Ouellette AJ. Mucosal immunity and inflammation. IV. Paneth cell antimicrobial peptides and the biology of the mucosal barrier. Am J Physiol 1999; 40:G257-G261.

29. Bjerknes M, Cheng H. The stem-cell zone of the small intestine epithelium. IV. Effects of resecting 30% of the small intestine. Am J Anat 1981; 160:93-103.

30. Ghoos Y, Vantrappen G. The cytochemical localisation of lysozyme in Paneth cell granules. Histochem J 1971; 3:175-178.

31. Mulherkar R, Rao RS, Wagle AS et al. Enhancing factor, a Paneth cell specific protein from mouse small intestines: Predicted amino acid sequences from RT-PCR amplified cDNA and its expression. Biochem Biophys Res Commun 1993; 195:1254-1263.

32. Molmenti EP, Perlmutter DH, Rubin DC. Cell specific expression of anti-trysin in human intestinal epithelium. J Clin Invest 1993; 92:2022-2034.

33. Jones DE, Bevins CL. Paneth cells of the human small intestine express an antimicrobial peptide gene. J Biol Chem 1992; 267:23216-2322.

34. Mallow EB, Harris A, Salzman N et al. Human enteric defensins-gene structure and developmental expression. J Biol Chem 1996; 271:4038-4045.

35. Salzman NH, Polin RA, Harris MC et al. Enteric defensin expression in necrotising enterocolitis. Paed Res 1998; 44:20-26.

36. Moxey PC, Trier JS. Endocrine cells in the human fetal small intestine. Cell Tissue Res 1977; 183:33-50.

37. Kraehenbuhl JP, Neutra MR. Defence of mucosal surfaces: Pathogenicity immunity and vaccines. Curr Top Microbiol Immunol 1999; 236:1-296.

38. Spencer J, MacDonald TT, Finn T et al. Development of Peyer's patches in human fetal terminal ileum. Clin Exp Immunol 1986; 64:536-543 39.

39. Spencer J, MacDonald TT, Isaacson PG. Heterogeneity of non lymphoid cells expressing HLA-D region in human fetal gut. Clin Exp Immunol 1987; 67:415-424.

40. Cornes JJ. Number, size and distribution of Peyer's patches in the human small intestine. Gut 1965; 6:225-229.

41. Owen RL, Jones AL. Epithelial cell specialisation within human Peyer's patches. An ultrastructural study of intestinal lymphoid follicles. Gastroenterology 1974; 66:189-203.

42. Neutra MR, Philips TL, Mayer EL et al. Transport of membrane-bound macromolecules by M cells in follicle-associated epithelium of rabbit Peyer's patch. Cell Tissue Res 1987; 247:537-546.

43. Neutra MR, Pringault E, Kraechenbuhl JP. Antigen sampling across epithelial barriers and infection of mucosal immune responses. Ann Rev Immunol 1996; 14:275-300.

44. Kraehenbuhl JP, Neutra MR. Epithelial M cells: Structure and function. Ann Rev Cell Dev Biol 2000; 16:301-332.

45. Bhalla DK, Owen RL. Migration of B and T lymphocytes to M cells in Peyer's patch follicle epithelium: An autoradiographic and immunocytochemical study in mice. Cell Immunol 1983; 81:105-117.

46. Kerneis S, Bogdanova A, Colucci-Guyon E et al. Cytosolic distribution of villin M cells from Peyer's patches with the absence of a brush border. Gastroenterology 1996; 110:515-521.

47. Pappo J, Owen RL. Absence of secretory component expression by epithelial cells overlying rabbit gut-associated lymphoid tissue. Gastroenterology 1988; 95:1173-1177.

48. Kerneis S, Bogdanova, A, Kraehenbuhl JP et al. Conversion by Peyer's patch lymphoctes of human enterocytes into M cells that transport bacteria. Science 1997; 277:948-952.

49. Neutra MR, Wilson JM, Weltzin RA et al. Membrane domains and macromolecular transport in intestinal epithelial cells. Ann Rev Respir Dis 1988; 138:S10-S16.

50. Clark MA, Jepson MA, Simmons NL et al. Differential expression of lectin-binding sites defines mouse intestinal M cells. J Histochem Cytochem 1993; 41:1679-168.

51. Falk P, Roth KA, Gordon JI. Lectins are sensitive tools for defining the differentiation programs of epithelial cell lineages in the developing and adult mouse gastrointestinal tract. Am J Physiol 1994; 266:G987-G1003.

52. Kobhata S, Yokobata H, Yabuuchi E. Cytopathogenic effect of Salmonella typhi GIFU 10007 on M cells of murine ileal Peyer's patches in ligated ileal loops: An ultrastructural study. Microbiol Immunol 1986; 30:1225-1237.

53. Owen RL, Pierce NF, Apple RT et al. M cell transport of Vibrio cholerae from the intestinal lumen into Peyer's patches: A mechanism for antigen sampling and for microbial transepithelial migration. J Infect Dis 1986; 153:1108-1118.

54. Sicinski P, Rowinski J, Warchol JB et al. Polivirus type 1 enters the human host through intestinal M cells. Gastroenterology 1990; 98:56-58.

55. Amerongen HM, Wilson GAR, Fields BN et al. Proteolytic processing of reovirus is required for adherence to intestinal M cells. J Virol 1994; 68:8428-8432.

56. Ermak TH, Owen RL. Differential distribution of lymphocytes and accessory cells in mouse Peyer's patches. Anat Rec 1986; 215:144-152.

57. Farstad IN, Halstensen TS, Fausa O et al. Heterogeneity of M cell-associated B and T cells in human Peyer's patches. Immunology 1994; 83:457-464.

58. Bjerke K, Halstensen TS, Jahnsen F et al. Distribution of macrophages and granulocytes expressing L1 protein (calprotectin) in human Peyer's patches compared with normal ileal lamina propria and mesenteric lymph nodes. Gut 1993; 34:1357-1363.

59. Lebman DA, Griffin PM, Cebra JJ. Relationship between expression of IgA by Peyer's patch cells and functional IgA memory cells. J Exp Med 1987; 166:1405-1418.

60. Jalkanen S, Nash GS, Toyos DL et al. Human lamina propria lymphocytes bear homing receptors and bind selectively to mucosal lymphoid high endothelium. Eur J Immunol 1989; 19:63-68.

61. Zeitz M, Schieferdecker HL, Ullrich R et al. Phenotype and function of lamina propria T lymphocytes. Immunol Res 1991; 10:199-206.

62. Koninsberger JC, Chott A, Logtenberg T et al. TCR expression in human fetal intestine and identification of an early T cell receptor-transcript. J Immunol 1997; 159:17775-17782.

63. Howie D, Spencer J, DeLord D et al. Extrathymic T cell differentiation in the human intestine early in life. J Immunol 1998; 161:5862-5872.

64. Spencer J, Dhillion SB, Isaacson PG et al. T cell subclasses in human fetal ileum. Clin Exp Immunol 1986; 65:553-558.

65. Perkkio M, Savilhati E. Time and appearance of immunoglobulin-containing cells in the mucosa of the neonatal intestine. Paed Res 1980; 14:953-955.

66. Brandtzaeg P, Bosnes V, Halstensen TS et al. T lymphocytes in human gut epithelium preferentially express the antigen receptor and are often CD45/UCHL1-positive. Scan J Immunol 1989; 30:123-128.

67. Selby WS, Janossy G, Bofill M et al. Lymphocyte subpopulations in the human small intestine. The findings in normal mucosa and in the mucosa of patients with adult celiac disease. Clin Exp Immunol 1983; 52:219-228.

68. James SP, Fiocchi C, Graeff AS et al. Phenotypic analysis of lamina propria lymphocytes. Predominance of helper-inducer and cytolytic T cell phenotypes and deficiency of suppressor-inducer phenotypes in Crohn's disease and control patients. Gastroenterology 1986; 91:1483-1489.

69. Smart CJ, Trejdosiewicz LK, Badr-el-Din S et al. T lymphocytes of the human colonic mucosa: functional and phenotypic analysis. Clin Exp Immunol 1988; 73:63-69.

70. MacDonald TT, Bajaj-Elliott M, Pender SLF. T cells orchestrate intestinal mucosal shape and integrity. Immunol Today 1999; 20:505-510.

71. McDonald V. Host cell-mediated responses to infection with Crytosporidium. Parasite Immunol 2000; 22:597-604.

72. Slifka MK, Whitton JL. Anitgen-specific regulation of T cell mediated cytokine production. Immunity 2000; 12:451-457.

73. Ernst WA, Thoma-Uszynski S, Teitelbaum R et al. Granulysin, a T cell product, kills bacteria by altering membrane permeability. J Immunol 2000; 165:7102-7108.

74. Ferguson A, Parrott DM. The effect of antigen deprivation on thymus-dependent and thymus-independent lymphocytes in the small intestine of the mouse. Clin Exp Immunol 1972; 12:477-488.

75. Chott A, Gerdes D, Spooner A et al. Intraepithelial lymphocytes in normal human intestine do not express proteins associated with cytolytic function. Am J Path 1997; 151:435-442.

76. Goodman T, Lefrancois L. Expression of the T-cell receptor on intestinal CD8+ intraepithelial lymphocytes. Nature 1988; 333:855-858.

77. Kiyono H, McGhee JR. Mucosal immunology: Intraepithelial lymphocytes. Adv Host Def Mech 1994: 9:1-204.

78. Spencer J, Diss TC, Isaacson PG et al. Expression of disulphide and nondisulphide linked forms of gamma/delta T cells in the human small intestinal epithelium. Eur J Immunol 1989; 19:1335-1338.

79. Guy-Grand D, Cerf-Bensussan N, Malissen B et al. Two gut intraepithelial CD8+ lymphocyte populations with different T cell receptors: A role for gut epithelium in T cell differentiation. J Exp Med 1991; 173:471.

80. Guy-Grand D, Vassalli P. Gut intraepithelial T lymphocytes. Curr Opin Immunol 1993; 5:247.

81. Saito H, Kanamori Y, Takemori T et al. Generation of intestinal T cells from progenitors residing in gut cryptopatches. Science 1998; 280:275-278.

82. Groh V, Steinle A, Bauer S, Spies T. Recognition of stress-induced MHC molecules by intestinal epithelial-T cells. Science 1998; 279:1737-1740.

CHAPTER 2

Oral Tolerance: An Overview

Allan McI Mowat

Introduction

The diet of all animals contains a wide variety of proteins of animal and vegetable origin, most of which are potentially antigenic. Contrary to much popular belief, a significant proportion of this material is absorbed in an immunologically intact form, generating intact protein and/or protein fragments that would be capable of stimulating immune responses if administered by other routes.[1-5] The gut-associated lymphoid tissues (GALT) are the largest in the body, comprising a battery of potent effector mechanisms whose purpose is to defend this essential organ against invasion by pathogens. Mobilization of these responses against food antigens would be undesirable, not only because it would limit their uptake and metabolic usefulness, but also because hypersensitivity to foods can produce intestinal pathology, as typified by coeliac disease and other food sensitive enteropathies (FSE). These conditions are rare because the intestinal immune system can discriminate between antigens which are harmless and those which are of pathogenic importance. This ability is responsible for the phenomenon of oral tolerance, in which administration of soluble antigens by the oral route can prevent subsequent systemic immune responses to the same antigen given in an immunogenic form. A similar mechanism is now believed to prevent hypersensitivity responses to the normal bacterial flora of the intestine, which are also essential for life and are a source of harmless antigens. A breakdown in the physiological state of tolerance to these antigens appears to underlie inflammatory bowel diseases such as Crohn's disease and ulcerative colitis.[6] In addition to these physiological roles of oral tolerance, it can also be exploited to deliver specific immunotherapy against autoimmune and inflammatory conditions[7] and it constitutes an important obstacle to the development of orally active vaccines containing purified or recombinant protein antigens. Thus an understanding of the immunoregulatory mechanisms that determine the induction and expression of oral tolerance is important for several aspects of gastroenterology and immunology. An analogous phenomenon can be induced by intranasal or aerosol exposure of animals to soluble antigen[8] and also by injection of antigen into the anterior chamber of the eye,[9] indicating that the mucosal surfaces may share common immunoregulatory mechanisms to ensure that nonresponsiveness is the default response to non-invasive antigens.

Here we will describe the fundamental features of oral tolerance, while later chapters in this volume will review the immunoregulatory mechanisms involved, as well as its potential use as a therapy. For a more detailed treatment of the biology and historical perspectives of the phenomenon, the reader is referred to previous reviews.[10-12]

Oral Tolerance: The Response of the Intestinal Mucosa to Dietary Antigens,
edited by Olivier Morteau. ©2004 Eurekah.com and Kluwer Academic / Plenum Publishers.

Scope of Oral Tolerance

Oral tolerance can be demonstrated most readily by feeding a protein such as ovalbumin (OVA) to laboratory rodents and then challenging the animal by a parenteral route with the same antigen together with an adjuvant. The phenomenon has also been described in several other animal species, including pigs,[13,14] dogs,[15,16] guinea pigs,[17] rabbits[18] and man.[19-25] However rabbits or guinea pigs may be less susceptible,[26,27] while adult ruminants[28] and chickens[29] may not develop significant oral tolerance at all.

Systemic tolerance can be induced by feeding a wide variety of different nonreplicating antigens, including many proteins (including autoantigens), contact sensitizing agents, haptenated self proteins, superantigens, heterologous red blood cells, allogeneic leukocytes, extracts of pollen or Dermatophagoides mites and inactivated viruses or bacteria.[12] Although it is also possible to induce oral tolerance of T cell responses, antibody production and autoimmune disease by feeding appropriate epitope peptides,[30-37] more variable results have been reported, perhaps reflecting a lack of knowledge about the best doses to use and of the factors that regulate the uptake and handling of short peptides in the gut.

Not all antigens induce tolerance via the gut. Organisms such as invasive viruses or bacteria can stimulate active immunity by this route[38,39] and in general, particulate antigens are more immunogenic than soluble material. Thus, inclusion of proteins in particulate carriers often allows them to stimulate active immunity by the oral route, especially if the carriers are formed from polymers which help protein to resist digestion in the intestine.[40,41] Such carriers may even be sufficiently immunogenic to induce systemic immunity when administered orally to animals with existing oral tolerance.[42] The relative immunogenicity of particulate materials may reflect their ability to be taken up by M cells in Peyer's patches, the route taken by several pathogenic organisms which induce protective immunity.[43-46] Alternatively, their size may allow them to gain access to different populations of antigen-presenting cells (APC) than those which normally take up orally administered proteins (see below). The priming effect of simple particles may not be an absolute phenomenon, but may merely reflect a shift in the dose response, as others have reported that particulate vectors such as microspheres or multiple emulsions can induce tolerance very efficiently to doses of antigen much smaller (>1000 fold less) than those which are effective when using the intact protein.[47] In one of these studies, higher doses of β lactoglobulin in poly(lactide-co-glycolide) microspheres could not induce tolerance.[48] Therefore the apparent priming effect found in other studies using particulate antigens may reflect the fact that these agents protect associated protein from proteolytic digestion so that they may deliver higher effective amounts of antigen to the immune system and subvert the usual regulatory mechanisms.

For a particle to be inherently immunogenic by the oral route, it may also require to represent itself as a "danger" to the immune system by inducing inflammation. This is supported by the fact that viable or invasive micro-organisms induce active immunity via the intestine, but the same organism in killed or inactivated form is tolerogenic.[39,49] Importantly for vaccine development, this rule also applies to antigens which would normally induce tolerance when given in native form, but which become immunogenic when expressed in invasive organisms. This idea may also help explain why commensal bacteria appear to induce specific tolerance.[50,51] Thymus-independent antigens such as those found in large quantities on many intestinal pathogens also do not induce oral tolerance, even if administered in association with a thymus-dependent antigen.[38,52] Indeed thymus-dependent K antigens mice on *E. coli* induce tolerance, whereas the thymus-independent O antigen on the same organism stimulates active local and systemic immunity.[38]

Certain pharmacologically active protein toxins also do not induce oral tolerance, the best examples being the ADP ribosylating agents cholera toxin (CT) and the related heat labile enterotoxin from *E. coli* (LT).[40,53-55] Both proteins stimulate primary local and systemic immune responses against themselves, and can act as adjuvants for other proteins given orally at the same time. These effects appear to reflect a pharmacological ability of the toxins to abrogate the immunoregulatory mechanisms normally responsible for inducing tolerance and they have been exploited for the development of mucosal vaccines.

Together, these findings may help explain the ability of the intestinal immune system to discriminate between harmless and pathogenic antigens, as most harmful organisms will be invasive, particulate and rich in pharmacologically active toxins, or thymus-independent antigens such as LPS.

Immunological Consequences of Oral Tolerance

CD4 T Cell Dependent Responses

All components of the systemic immune response can be tolerised by appropriate regimes of antigen feeding.[10,12] However, classical cell mediated immune (CMI) responses such as lymphocyte proliferation, delayed type hypersensitivity (DTH) and contact sensitivity are generally easier to tolerise than are humoral immune responses, since they require less antigen and the tolerance persists much longer.[12,17,56,57] A similar pattern has been described in man.[22] When the individual components of T cell dependent immunity are studied, Th1 responses such as IgG2a antibody, IL2 and γIFN production are often easier to inhibit by feeding antigen than Th2-dependent IgG1, IL4, IL5 and IL10 responses.[31,58-62] High doses of antigen suppress the production of all Th1 and Th2 dependent cytokines,[61,63-65] whereas multiple, low doses of antigen may preferentially upregulate production of IL4 and IL10, with concomitant inhibition of Th1 dependent IL2 and γIFN.[61,63] One exception to the general resistance of humoral responses to oral tolerance is IgE antibody production,[10,12] an unusual finding considering that IgE production is highly dependent on IL4. As the effector functions which are most susceptible to oral tolerance in vivo are IgE and DTH, which are the mechanisms most frequently associated with pathological food hypersensitivity, it seems that prevention of food-specific IgE and DTH responses is a critical biological role of oral tolerance.

CD8⁺ T Cells

CD8⁺ T cell dependent responses can also be tolerised by feeding soluble antigens, but this has been a somewhat controversial area, ever since the original suggestions that CD8⁺ "suppressor" cells were one of the most important immunoregulatory mechanisms in oral tolerance.[10] In most cases, the induction of oral tolerance does not require the presence of CD8⁺ T cells;[66-69] we and others have also shown that feeding OVA results in oral tolerance of systemic class I MHC-restricted cytotoxic T cell (CTL) responses.[66,70,71] However, these latter studies examined systemic CTL responses that were dependent on CD4⁺ helper T cells, which are themselves normally highly susceptible to tolerance. The position with CD4-independent CD8⁺ T cell responses is less clear. Although it has been reported that CD4-independent CTL responses to OVA, or to the contact sensitising agent DNCB are fully susceptible to oral tolerance,[68,69] we found that the CD4-independent CD8⁺ T cell responses generated by immunisation with OVA/CFA were unaffected by oral administration of antigen (our unpublished observations). LCMV-specific CD8⁺ CTL responses are also not tolerised by feeding antigen.[62] More contradictions come from the findings that OVA-specific CD8⁺ CTL may actually be primed by feeding tolerogenic doses of antigen to either normal mice[71] or to mice expressing an OVA-specific CD8⁺ transgenic T cell receptor (TcR).[71-74] In the latter cases, this may lead to CD8⁺ T cell dependent immunopathology in tissues expressing OVA as a transgenic antigen. Interestingly, the priming of CD8⁺ CTL responses by feeding antigen to normal mice was found to be dependent on the presence of CD4⁺ T cells and occurred despite the fact that

CD4-dependent CD8[+] CTL responses to subsequent systemic challenge were tolerised.[71] These findings support other, more direct evidence that CD4[+] T cells go through a transient phase of priming before become tolerant to fed antigens (reviewed in ref. 75 and see below).

In our hands, it was impossible to prime CD8[+] T cells simply by feeding OVA to normal mice[66] and understanding the reasons for these discrepant results will be important both for understanding the basis of oral tolerance, and for developing strategies of vaccinating protective CD8[+] T cell responses via the gut. One explanation may be that a state of split tolerance can occur in different functional subsets of CD8[+] T cells depending on the conditions. Thus it has been reported that IL4/IL10 producing CD8[+] regulatory T cells can be primed by feeding antigen, irrespective of whether CD8[+] CTL are tolerised[62,70] or primed[76] by the feeding regime. Split tolerance of mucosal CD8[+] T cell responses has also been described in animals expressing OVA only on intestinal epithelial cells and transferred with OVA-specific TcR transgenic T cells.[74] In this model, CTL activity was preserved, but other functions such as clonal expansion and the production of γIFN and TNFα were tolerant. Similar findings have been made in tolerance of peripheral CD8[+] T cell functions,[77] suggesting that different aspects of CD8[+] T cell function may be regulated differentially by tolerogenic signals. One additional possibility is that CD8[+] T cells in different anatomical locations may behave differently. Thus, it has been shown that a regulatory population of CD8[+] T cells may be required for tolerance of mucosal, but not systemic immunity in protein fed mice.[67] In addition, a recent report has shown that feeding allogeneic spleen cells induces a population of regulatory CD8[+] T cells which accumulate preferentially in subsequent renal allografts.[76] Thus, regulatory CD8[+] T cells may have a predilection to migrate to effector sites, in contrast to regulatory CD4[+] T cells which usually exert their effects in secondary lymphoid organs.

Other Systemic Effects

The locomotor activity of lymphocytes is also inhibited by the induction of oral tolerance, with peripheral lymph node lymphocytes from tolerised mice showing defective migration into three dimensional collagen gels in response to chemokines (Fig. 1). Thus, the induction of tolerance not only affects their effector functions, but may reduce their ability to migrate into appropriate sites in the body.

Effects of Oral Tolerance Regimes on Mucosal Immunity

Initial findings led to the concept that secretory IgA responses and systemic immunity were regulated reciprocally by feeding antigen, with priming of local immunity in the face of systemic tolerance.[78] This would be consistent with more recent evidence that oral tolerance may be associated with upregulated production of TGFβ, a cytokine which acts as a switch factor in the maturation of IgA producing B cells.[79] Nevertheless, IgA antibodies against food antigens are absent in normal individuals, despite the presumed presence of systemic tolerance to these antigens. Experimental studies have also produced conflicting findings on IgA production in oral tolerance, with reports of suppression,[80-84] preservation[80,85] or priming[22,78] of secretory IgA antibody production in man and animals. There is also no consensus on whether different genetic modifications affect local IgA production and oral tolerance in a linked manner. Both are defective in γIFN KO mice and in γδTcR KO mice.[86-88] but only IgA production has been reported as being abnormal in γIFN receptor KO mice[89]and IgA responses are increased in CD8KO mice, in which tolerance is either normal or decreased.[67] One suggested explanation for these discrepant findings is that priming of IgA production only occurs with feeding regimes that selectively induce TGFβ-producing regulatory T cells. Conversely, feeding regimes that induce anergy or deletion of all antigen specific T cells may also suppress IgA production.[11,90] Although compatible with some of the evidence, there are also exceptions to this idea[49,84,87] and more experiments are required to address this issue directly.

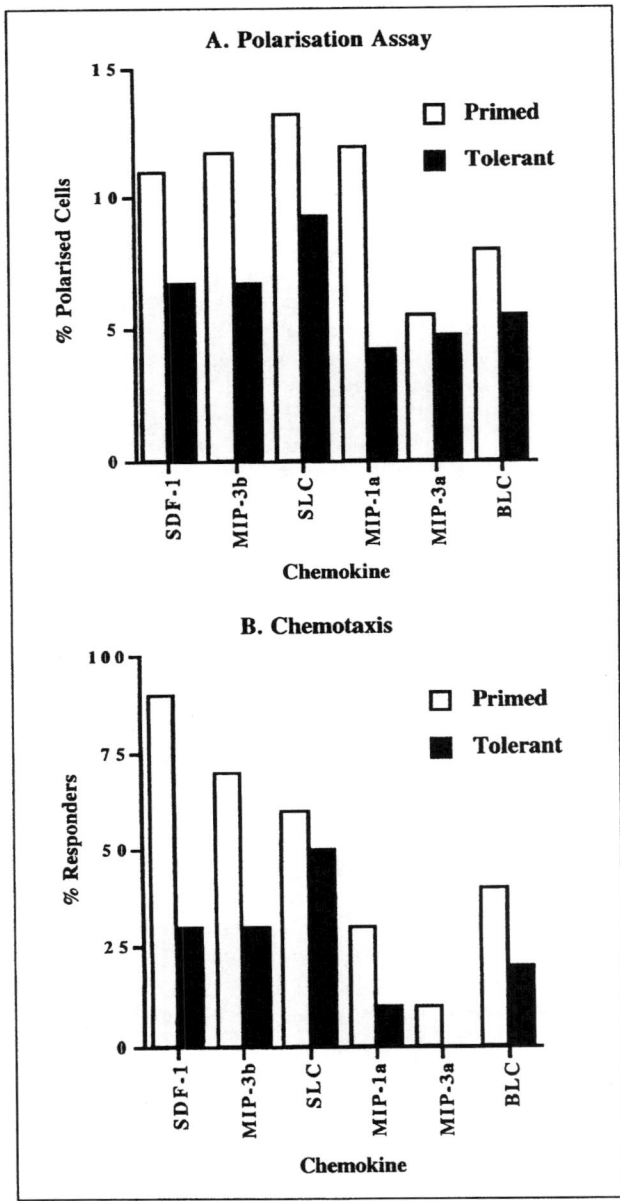

Figure 1. Response of orally primed or tolerised T cells to chemokines in vitro. OVA-specific DO11.10 transgenic T cells were adoptively transferred into normal BALB/c mice, which were then fed 100mg OVA to induce oral tolerance, or with saline as a control. 2 days after feeding, mice were immunised subcutaneously with OVA in Complete Freund's adjuvant and the draining lymph nodes removed 2-4 days later. Primed and tolerised lymphocytes were assayed for shape change (A) or chemotaxis into filters (B) in response to optimal concentrations of chemokines. Results are expressed as the % cells showing polarised morphology (A), or the proportion of individual cultures in which cells migrated through the full thickness of the filter (B).

Using TcR transgenic T cells, it has been reported that expansion of antigen-specific CD4⁺ T cells occurs in the jejunal lamina propria after induction of tolerance in mice[91] (Smith KE et al submitted for publication), perhaps suggesting local T cell responses may be stimulated during the induction of oral tolerance. However, it is important to note that transient expansion of antigen specific T cells occurs in other organs after feeding antigen and appears to be a universal feature of the induction phase of oral tolerance (see below). Therefore it would be important to explore the effector functions of the expanded population of T cells found in the lamina propria of fed mice to determine if they are functionally primed or tolerised. That tolerance of local T cells may occur is suggested by the fact that the experimental colitis caused by activation of mucosal γIFN producing lymphocytes by rectal administration of haptens can be suppressed by feeding haptenated colonic proteins. This is accompanied by reduced local production of γIFN and increased levels of TGFβ.[92] Local immune responses to adenovirus can also be suppressed by feeding viral antigens.[93,94]

Time Course and Duration of Oral Tolerance

Systemic tolerance can be demonstrated within 1-2 days of feeding antigen[78](our unpublished observations) and several components of the resulting tolerance may then persist for many months. Tolerance of DTH responses may then be intact in mice for up to 18 months after a single feed of high dose OVA[95] (our unpublished observations), but other functions such as disease prevention, serum antibodies and cytokine production may return to normal within a few weeks to months [95-97] (our unpublished observations). Proliferative responses may remain significantly inhibited for up to 6-9 months (our unpublished observations).[98] The length of the tolerant period depends markedly on the initial dose of fed antigen and on the nature of the antigen.[12,99]

Effects of Antigen Dose and Frequency on Oral Tolerance

Although a wide range of antigen doses will induce significant oral tolerance, one of the most interesting concepts which has arisen in the last 5-10 years is the idea that the mechanisms responsible for oral tolerance may depend on the dose of fed antigen.[11,58] In mice, a single feed of a few mg of a protein such as OVA is sufficient to induce tolerance and doses of 20 mg and above produce maximal immune suppression.[12,57,100] The exact dose response varies with the antigen used and cell mediated immune responses are more readily tolerised than humoral immune responses or Th2 dependent functions.[12,57,90] Using purified proteins, there has been little evidence of an upper limit to the dose of antigen which can induce tolerance, but there have been isolated reports in which tolerance is not as marked at the highest doses tested[101] and the studies using particulate vectors to administer antigen suggest that systemic priming could result if high enough doses of intact antigen could be given (see above). Extremely low doses of antigen have a paradoxical ability to prime the systemic immune response, with doses in the range of 1-50 µg protein being effective in this respect.[102-104] Again this affects CMI effector responses more than humoral immunity, and it is a phenomenon that has important implications for the therapeutic use of oral tolerance.

The immunological consequences of oral tolerance may be determined by the nature of the feeding regime. Compared with single feeds of antigen, multiple administration of antigen or its inclusion in drinking water or the diet produces more profound tolerance and affects more aspects of the systemic immune response.[61,105,106] Similar findings have been made in previously primed animals,[103,107] and the phenomenon appears to reflect continuous exposure to antigen rather than the total dose administered. As we have noted, the regulatory mechanisms associated with oral tolerance may also depend on the feeding regime, with doses of <5 mg protein stimulating regulatory T cells, while higher amounts (≥20 mg) are considered to cause clonal anergy or deletion of T cells. These are often referred to as "low dose" and "high dose" tolerance[11,58,108] and the distinction between them is of potential practical importance, as it is proposed that only the low dose regime will induce the phenomenon of "bystander suppression", which will be crucial to the use of oral tolerance in treatment of clinical disease (see below). It should be noted that as originally described, the two regimes differ not only in the dose of antigen, but also in the frequency of feeding. "High dose" feeding normally involves a single administration of antigen, whereas "low dose" involves multiple feeds of antigen over the space of 1 week or so. It is therefore unclear whether the different immunological consequences truly reflect the effects of the different amounts of antigen, or if the number of exposures to antigen is also important. Few direct comparisons of this kind have been undertaken. The distinctive effects of differing antigen doses and feeding regimes may reflect differential susceptibility of T cell subsets and B cells to antigen level; alternatively, lower amounts of antigen do not penetrate beyond the gut associated lymphoid tissues (GALT), where the local microenvironment may favour the induction of regulatory T cells of the Th3 or Tr1 subset. In contrast, larger doses of antigen may gain access to systemic immune organs, where they are available to anergise or delete T cells.

Age Dependent Effects of Oral Tolerance

In man, the neonatal and weaning periods are times of high susceptibility to diseases associated with food hypersensitivity. A number of studies have reported that rodents also exhibit defects in oral tolerance induced by oral exposure to antigens until around 3-4 days of age. The adult pattern of susceptibility to tolerance becomes fully established around 7 days old in mice, but there is a further, brief window of defective tolerance around weaning.[109-114] This phenomenon also applies when the antigen is derived from the maternal diet and passed on via breast milk.[111] Calves and piglets can also be sensitised by feeding antigen during the pre-weaning period.[13,14,28,115] The reasons for the defective tolerance in the early neonatal period are not known. Although it may relate to differences in the digestion and uptake of antigen by the neonatal intestine, it does not correlate directly with differences in the amount of protein absorbed and can be corrected by transfer of mature lymphocytes.[109,112] Alternatively, the developing immune system may generate distinct regulatory mechanisms, an idea supported by the finding that equivalent feeding regimes induce mainly clonal anergy in neonatal rats, but active regulation in adults.[106] The altered tolerance at weaning is not related to the age of the animal, but is influenced by the process of weaning itself and is likely to be determined by the alterations in intestinal microenvironment or in systemic hormone levels associated with weaning. It is important to emphasise that full tolerance susceptibility develops rapidly thereafter, both for food proteins[114] and commensal bacteria,[116] indicating how necessary it is to establish this homeostatic process as soon as possible after the introduction of novel antigens into the intestine.

At the other end of the age spectrum, aging mice have been reported to become increasingly resistant to the induction of oral tolerance by feeding OVA.[97,117]

Influence of Intestinal Bacteria on Oral Tolerance

The immunomodulatory effects of LPS and other bacterial products are well known. Germ-free mice have defective systemic immune competence[118-120] and cannot be tolerised by feeding sheep red blood cells (SRBC).[121] Early studies also suggested that it was impossible to induce tolerance by feeding SRBC to C3H/HeJ mice that have a genetically determined inability to respond to LPS[57,81,122,123] However, other works showed that oral tolerance to proteins, haptens and autochthonous gut flora was entirely normal in these mice.[57,124] This discrepancy may reflect the fact that the gene defect in C3H/HeJ mice is an absence of the Toll like receptor 4 (Tlr-4) receptor,[125] which might be expected to have a preferential effect on responses to materials like SRBC. Such responses would require uptake and processing by macrophages whose activity in the gut is dependent on stimulation via factors such as LPS.

Nevertheless, there is increasing evidence that the presence of the intestinal bacterial flora can indeed have an important influence on the induction of oral tolerance to protein antigens. Administration of exogenous LPS at the time of feeding can enhance the induction of tolerance in normal mice fed OVA,[57,126-128] while tolerance to fed OVA is relatively short-lived in germ-free mice.[97,129] In addition, OVA feeding has less effect on Th2 mediated immune responses in germ-free mice than in conventional animals.[120] How the germ free state may influence oral tolerance has not been determined, but in the study by Sudo et al the defective tolerance of Th2 responses was associated with a high basal level of IL4 production in germ-free mice and could be partly restored by neonatal colonisation with a single *Bifidobacterium* species.[120] It seems that the defective tolerance in germ free animals does not reflect altered intestinal handling of antigen, as uptake of tolerogenic OVA into serum is normal in germ free mice.[130] One attractive hypothesis is that LPS or other microbial products present in the microenvironment of the intestine and GALT stimulate the production of immunomodulatory mediators which are required for the generation of tolerogenic mechanisms. In support of this idea, recent studies suggest that exposure to physiological amounts of LPS may be necessary for maintaining the ability of intestinal macrophages to produce immunoregulatory amounts of prostaglandin E2 (PGE_2)[131] (and see below). Together, these findings may also explain the apparent state of tolerance to commensal bacteria which is found in normal animals,[50,51,132] a phenomenon which seems to be induced at the time of first colonisation during weaning.[116] The possible involvement of bacterial products other than LPS has also not been examined.

Oral Tolerance in the Primed Immune System

If oral tolerance is to be an effective therapy for inflammatory conditions, it will need to function once disease has been established for some time. As will be discussed in other chapters in this volume, many groups have observed that tolerance can be induced by feeding antigen to animals with existing experimental autoimmune disease. In addition, a number of studies have shown that oral tolerance can be effective after priming mice parenterally with model antigens.[94,96,98,101,103,107,133-139] However, large doses of fed antigen, or more frequent feeds, are usually required to induce significant tolerance equivalent to that found in naive animals and the tolerant state affects Th1 type responses much more than Th2 responses or antibody production, which may be unaffected or even enhanced.[107,135,136,138] Even if antigen doses or feeding frequency are increased substantially, it can be difficult to induce tolerance of these resistant responses.[138] Of particular note, there is also only a short time after systemic priming when oral tolerance can be induced, a period which is usually 1 week or less.[98,107,136,138] This can occasionally be extended if repeated feeds of antigen are given.[98,103,107] The disappearance of tolerance coincides with the development of the serum antibody response in the primed animals,[136] and circulating antibodies are known to interfere with the induction of oral tolerance.[98,140] However, in our hands it was impossible to extend the period of susceptibility to tolerance using higher doses of antigen, as would be anticipated if the defect was simply due to mopping up of available antigen by antibody.[138] The reasons for the relative resistance of primed mice to oral tolerance remain uncertain, but may reflect an inherent property of antigen-experienced T lymphocytes once they have differentiated fully after systemic priming.[137,138] The mechanisms responsible for tolerance in the primed immune system are also unknown and together with the selectivity of the tolerance induced in primed animals, these factors indicate the difficulties which may need to be overcome if oral tolerance is to be used in clinical practice. However, the encouraging results from experimental models of autoimmune disease show that further mechanistic studies are warranted. Furthermore, the recent demonstration that linking antigen to cholera toxin B subunit may be an efficient way of inducing mucosal tolerance in primed animals, even using very small doses of antigen, supports the view that this may not be an insurmountable difficulty.[139]

Role of Intestinal Absorption and Antigen Uptake

Digestive Functions of the Intestine

As we shall discuss, oral tolerance to protein antigens reflects the manner in which the protein is processed in the intestine (see below). Thus one might predict that any factor that alters either the amount or the chemical nature of the antigen absorbed from the intestine also will influence the immunological consequences of this material. This idea is supported by the high levels of food-specific antibodies that occur in individuals with disorders that cause increased intestinal permeability to macromolecules, for example in Crohn's disease and coeliac disease.[21,141] Although experimental factors which increase the amount of protein entering the circulation frequently are associated with prevention of tolerance induction,[142,143] (Furrie E et al submitted for publication), no direct correlation between intestinal uptake of antigen and the degree of tolerance and/or active immunity has been established.

The role of proteolytic processing in the intestine is also ill-defined, although many workers routinely coadminister agents which inhibit the activity of stomach acid and intestinal proteases. In addition, denatured proteins do not induce tolerance perhaps because they are resistant to the usual digestive processes.[144] However, it has also been reported that administration of the protease inhibitors aprotinin or soya trypsin inhibitor may actually prevent the induction of tolerance by feeding single doses of either MBP or OVA to mice.[103,143] Further conflicting evidence comes from reports that trypsin inhibitors may have no effect on[145] or even enhance tolerance associated with both anergy[146] and bystander suppression.[30] These discrepancies may partly reflect a species difference between rats and mice, as it is suggested that the absence of a gall bladder in rats inhibits effective absorption of proteins, necessitating the use of protease inhibitors to ensure survival of sufficient protein in the lumen.[103] Additionally, individual T cell epitopes which may be required for inducing different mechanisms of tolerance may also vary in their sensitivity to proteolysis.

Tolerance As a Consequence of Defective Antigen Presentation

The ways in which antigen is presented to T cells frequently determine whether tolerance or immunity results. This may reflect the involvement of specific antigen-presenting cells and their cell surface molecules or mediators, or it may be a function of the anatomical site in which these processes occur. The state of oral tolerance appears to involve anergy or functional deviation of CD4$^+$ T cells and this is preceded by partial activation of these T cells (see below). These features are consistent with the view that the initial event in the process is presentation of fed antigen by APC which lack costimulatory molecules, or which possess unusual costimulatory properties.[75] This idea is supported by older evidence that activation of the APC functions of the reticuloendothelial system (RES) by exogenous immunomodulatory agents, or by previous exposure to an unrelated antigen, interferes with the induction of oral tolerance.[147-151]

Routes of Antigen Uptake from the Intestine

A number of sites for the uptake and presentation of antigen have been suggested, including local tissues such as the intestinal epithelium, the lamina propria, the Peyer's patches (PP) or mesenteric lymph nodes, and more distal tissues including the spleen, liver and peripheral lymph nodes. All intestinal antigens must first enter the body by passing across the epithelium of the gut and, as we have noted, many pathogens and particulate materials appear to be taken up preferentially via M cells in the follicle associated epithelium (FAE) of PP. However, there is less evidence for the uptake of soluble antigens by this route and the total surface area of the FAE is small in comparison with conventional, villus mucosa. That a substantial proportion of protein antigen enters either via or between villus enterocytes is

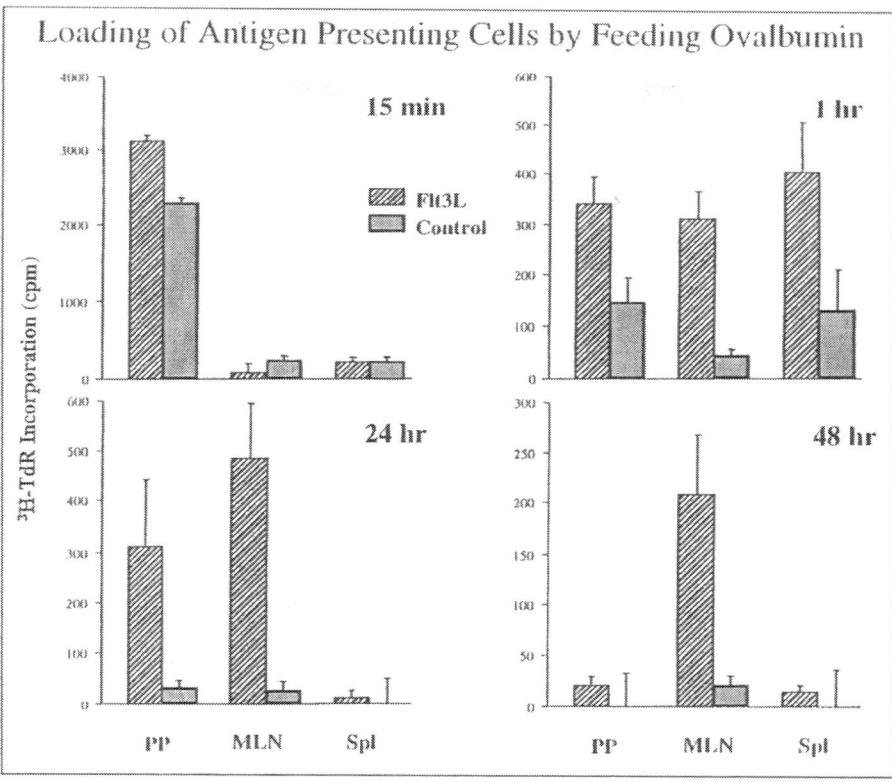

Figure 2. Loading of DC in the GALT and spleen by feeding OVA. APC were isolated at different times after feeding from control mice, or from mice treated for 9 days to expand DC in vivo and incubated with OVA-specific TcR transgenic DO11.10 CD4⁺ T cells in vitro.

suggested by recent morphological studies which have shown orally administered OVA entering endosomal vesicles in enterocytes, before appearing in the intercellular space.[152]

Fed antigen then has to be taken up by APC, and it has proved difficult to determine if these APC are in the PP, villus lamina propria, or both. When mesenteric lymphadenectomised rats are fed OVA, antigen bearing dendritic cells can be isolated readily from the efferent lymph draining the intestine and this phenomenon occurs irrespective of whether PP are present in the drained segment of intestine.[153-155] Antigen-loaded APC have also been isolated from both the PP and villus lamina propria of fed rodents.[156-158] This occurs within a few minutes of feeding and before APC can be found in other tissues (Fig. 2). In the case of the lamina propria, it has been reported that the loaded APC can induce specific tolerance when transferred to naïve mice, suggesting that antigen presentation in this site may play an important role in the induction of oral tolerance.[158] Similar studies have not been carried out with APC from PP, although there is now considerable evidence that PP contain distinctive populations of APC (see below). PP are absent or grossly deficient in B cell-depleted or KO mice, as well as in lymphotoxin β(LTβ) KO mice and in mice treated from birth with a soluble form of the LTβ receptor. However, recent studies have reported that oral tolerance is normal in all these animals, suggesting that the PP and M cells in its FAE are not required to induce compartments through oral tolerance would be important for the prevention of exaggerated or allergic responses to food proteins and allergens. Furthermore, this system could be applied to the treatment and prevention of autoimmune diseases by feeding self antigens.

  Although several possible mechanisms (e.g., B cell tolerance, anti-idiotypic Ab, intestinal antigen-processing events resulting in toleragen formation, and conventional APC processing) have been suggested to be involved in the induction of oral tolerance,[5] most studies now suggest that T cells are the major cell players involved in this immune response.[3, 5-12] In earlier work, it was shown that oral tolerance or systemic unresponsiveness was induced by adoptive transfer of T cells from rats orally fed bovine serum albumin.[13] Subsequently, a large number of studies demonstrated that oral immunization with protein antigen induced CD4+ T helper (Th) cells in mucosa-associated tissues that supported IgA Ab responses, whereas suppressor T cells were induced in systemic compartments such as spleen that downregulated antigen-specific IgM, IgG, and IgE Ab responses.[14-20] Furthermore, the Th cells for IgA responses tended to remain localized in Peyer's patches, whereas the suppressor T cells tended to migrate into the systemic compartment (e.g., the spleen). These observations were considered to be logical explanations for cellular mechanisms of oral tolerance where Peyer's patch-derived CD4+ Th cells supported IgA Ab responses, while splenic T suppressor cells accounted for systemic unresponsiveness. It is now generally agreed that a functional suppressor mechanism exists for the downregulation of systemic immune responses; however, the nature and properties of these suppressor T cells are disputed.

The Role of αβTCR+ T Cells in Oral Tolerance

Th1 versus Th2 Cells and Their Derived Cytokines

  Current dogma suggests that high oral doses of protein induces clonal anergy and perhaps deletion of T cells, while low, spaced oral doses tend to induce active suppression by T cells via secretion of inhibitory cytokines such as TGF-β, IL-10 and perhaps IL-4 (Fig. 1).[3,21-31] Anergy can be defined as T cell tolerance characterized by a lack of IL-2 synthesis with diminished IL-2 receptor (IL-2R) expression.[32] Anergy is readily reversed by culture with exogenous IL-2.[33] Anergic T cells develop following high oral doses of myelin basic protein (MBP)[25] and OVA.[26] With MBP, anergic T cells were of Th1-type, since diminished IL-2 and IFN-γ production was observed.[26] In this regard, it has been suggested that CD4+ Th1-type cells are more sensitive to oral tolerance induction.[28,34] In addition, it is assumed that anergic T cells populate the systemic immune compartment, since it was shown that anergic splenic CD4+ T cells, when transferred to SCID mice, remained unresponsive.[29]

  A second major way that T cells could regulate oral tolerance is by induction of Th1 cells for downregulation of Th2-type or Th2-type cells to suppress Th1-type responses.[35] In this regard, it is thought that Th1-type cells are most affected via cytokines produced by Th2-type cells. Recent studies call into question this type of downregulation of systemic immune responses since high oral doses of OVA inhibited the production of OVA-specific Th1- (IFN-γ and IL-2) and Th2- (IL-4, IL-5 and IL-10) type cytokines.[27] In addition, both IFN-γ-induced IgG2a and IL-4-dependent IgG1 anti-OVA Abs were diminished in mice fed a high dose of OVA.[27] This result would clearly suggest that both Th1 and Th2 cell subsets are sensitive to oral tolerance induction (Fig. 1).

  A third major mechanism for oral tolerance is revealed when prolonged oral administration of lower Ag doses is done (so-called low dose oral tolerance). This often results in Ag-specific CD4+ or CD8+ T cells which secrete TGFβ, IL-4 and IL-10.[3] In this regard, TGF-β effectively downregulates both Th1- and Th2-type T cell responses. Further, both IL-4 and IL-10 effectively downregulate strong CD4+ Th1-type responses.[3] In addition, recent studies have characterized T regulatory 1 (Tr1) cells as those which produce IL-10, and which downregulate this phenomenon.[159,160-162] One study has contested this conclusion, by showing that oral tolerance is defective in mice lacking the type 1 TNF receptor, which also lack normal PP.[163] However, it is important to note that these KO mice have additional alterations in T cell regulation and function, which could account for a defect in oral tolerance.

Sites of Interaction between T Cells and Antigen-Loaded APC

Even if antigen is taken up rapidly by APC in the PP and lamina propria, it is not inevitable that the first interaction between the APC and specific T cell occurs in these sites. The conventional idea that PP are the first place where T cells recognise fed antigen was derived partly from older studies which showed that regulatory T cells could be identified in the PP before appearing in peripheral tissues such as the spleen.[164] Subsequent experiments in which tolerogenic doses of protein antigen have been fed to fully T cell receptor (TcR) transgenic mice have also shown rapid activation and clonal deletion of specific T cells in the PP,[65,165] as well as production of regulatory cytokines by these cells.[166] However, fully TcR transgenic animals are not an appropriate model for assessing immunoregulation under physiological conditions, and studies using the adoptive transfer of identifiable TcR transgenic T cells into normal recipients have produced less definitive findings. Although some workers have found evidence of antigen recognition by CD4+[167,168] (Smith K et al submitted) and CD8+ T cells[168] in the PP soon after feeding antigen to such mice, others have not been able to detect this in either adoptively transferred mice or in mice transgenic only for the TcRβ gene.[169-172] The reasons for these discrepancies are not clear but may reflect a poor ability of the adoptively transferred T cells to enter the PP, meaning that only a low frequency of antigen specific T cells is present to be expanded and identified. The same caveat must be applied to studies using this model to analyse whether the lamina propria is a site for the initial interaction between T cells and APC, as naïve CD4+ T cells do not migrate to this tissue to any extent.[173,174] The paucity of naïve CD4+ T cells in the lamina propria also makes it unlikely that the induction of tolerance could first occur here.

It is important to note that presentation of antigen to T cells in either the PP or lamina propria should prime lymphocytes that recirculate preferentially to mucosal sites[175] and so would be unlikely to account for systemic unresponsiveness. The mesenteric lymph node (MLN) is believed to be a crossover point between the mucosal and systemic immune systems and several pieces of evidence suggest that the first contact of T cells with antigen occurs here. First, rapid activation of CD4+ and CD8+ T cells in the MLN is a constant finding in experiments in which TcR transgenic T cells have been used to study the induction of oral tolerance[167-172] and this may occur within 3-6 hours of feeding antigen (Smith K et al submitted). Secondly, antigen loaded APC can be found in the MLN within 1 hour and persist there for up to 48 hours after feeding, indicating presentation of antigen may occur in this tissue for extended periods after feeding (Fig. 2). This is consistent with the fact that the majority of the dendritic cells emanating from the intestine normally appear to lodge permanently in the MLN.[153-155] Finally, preliminary studies using LTα KO mice, which lack both MLN and PP, suggest that the presence of an MLN is essential for the induction of oral tolerance.[159] Interestingly, work on the respiratory tract indicates that the lymph nodes draining the mucosal tissues may differ from lymph nodes in other anatomical sites and may provide specialised microenvironments for the induction of tolerance. Thus the draining cervical lymph node is necessary for the tolerant state induced by intranasal administration of antigen, and the absence of tolerance that occurs when this node is removed can be restored by transplantation of the appropriate lymph nodes, but not by other, peripheral lymph nodes.[176] The basis of this effect is unknown and whether a similar phenomenon occurs in the MLN has never been studied. Nevertheless, older work has shown that the immunological environment of the MLN may be distinct from that of other lymphoid tissues and that this may relate to local differences in responsiveness to steroid hormones.[177] The unique anatomical and functional properties of mucosally associated lymphoid tissues and their influence on subsequent immune responses is an area worthy of future study.

Despite the clear evidence that fed antigen is rapidly taken up and presented to T cells in local lymphoid tissues of the intestine, it is essential to note that intestinally absorbed proteins also gain access to the systemic circulation within 15-30 minutes (see below). As a result, T cells could also be tolerised directly in peripheral tissues, without the need for APC or T cells themselves to migrate from the gut. In support of this, T cell activation and antigen-loaded APC are found simultaneously in the spleen of mice fed cytochrome c.[172] In addition, it has been shown that the activation of CD4+ T cells in MLN after feeding antigen is paralleled by an equivalent phenomenon in peripheral lymph nodes and spleen, although the extent is considerably less[169-172] (Smith, K. et al., submitted).

The relative contributions of disseminated and local presentation of antigen to systemic tolerance may depend on the dose of antigen. In initial studies using the adoptive transfer of TcR transgenic T cells, it was reported that the T cells that were activated in peripheral lymphoid organs by fed antigen did not progress beyond the expression of activation markers such as CD69, with no entry into cell division. Thus it was believed that any recognition of fed antigen in the periphery was of minimal functional significance. However, more recent studies using higher doses of fed OVA (100 mg) have shown that adoptively transferred transgenic T cells can indeed be induced to divide in the peripheral lymph nodes (Smith K et al, submitted). It is of course difficult to prove definitively that these dividing T cells have not migrated to the periphery after first encountering antigen in mucosal tissues. Nevertheless the speed of the phenomenon makes this seem unlikely and the data suggest that the failure to observe peripheral T cell division in previous studies may relate to the insensitivity of the methods used to detect T cell proliferation in situ. Alternatively, the discrepancies may reflect true dose-dependent effects on the immunoregulatory processes involved in oral tolerance. Thus it may be that low doses of antigen penetrate no further than the intestinal wall and perhaps the MLN, where the local microenvironment and specialised APC determine that activation of regulatory T cells is the result. In contrast, higher doses of antigen may gain direct access to the more conventional APC and T cells in peripheral lymphoid organs, ensuring that generalised T cell anergy predominates over any local regulatory T cell activity that is induced. That distinct regulatory mechanisms could operate in different sites during oral tolerance is suggested by the finding that, although feeding antigen can tolerise both systemic and mucosal immune responses, systemic tolerance is intact in the absence of CD8+ T cells, whereas the local tolerance is not.[67]

Intestinal Processing Generates Tolerogenic Moieties in Serum

Circulating antigen can be found in the serum of both experimental animals and humans after ingestion of protein[178] and, when taken 1 hour after feeding mice, this material induces tolerance when transferred parenterally into naïve animals.[179-184] Serum taken from mice given equivalent doses of protein by parenteral routes does not reproduce the phenomenon,[180] indicating that a unique processing event may occur during intestinal absorption of antigen.

The nature of this tolerogenic material is controversial. Given the speed with which it appears in the circulation, it is unlikely to involve molecules with immunological specificity such as antibody or TcR. The consensus has been that it represents the protein itself, either in the form of ultrafiltered monomers of the whole molecule, or fragments of the protein.[181,183,184] More recently, it has been suggested that at least part of the tolerogenic activity in serum tolerogen may be associated with lipid vesicles ("tolerosomes") that contain antigen bound to class II MHC molecules.[185] Class II MHC positive vesicles of this kind can be identified inside enterocytes and lying free in the lamina propria of normal animals. In addition, vesicles of the appropriate density which induce tolerance in T cells appear in the supernatants of class II

MHC expressing epithelial cells cultured with OVA.[185] Analogous class II MHC expressing vesicles ("exosomes"), which can be recognised directly by T cells, have been found to be released by other APC such as dendritic cells and B cells.[186] It is suggested that fed antigen complexes with class II MHC in enterocytes, with membrane fragments then being released as tolerosomes into the circulation. There they may contribute to the induction of tolerance by interacting outside the intestine with naïve, antigen-specific CD4+ T cells. This hypothesis is consistent with the evidence that although enterocytes normally express class II MHC in most species, they lack the costimulatory molecules for full activation of T cells such as B7.1/B7.2.[187] The tolerosomes would be expected to share these properties. The serum tolerogen is also not generated in immunodeficient scid mice, a defect that can be restored by transferring normal lymphoid cells or by treatment with γIFN, factors which may restore the lack of class II MHC expression on enterocytes in scid mice.[130,185] However, the nature of these novel tolerosomes needs to be confirmed. In particular, their potential role in oral tolerance must be considered in the light of the fact that any antigenic material bound to class II MHC in this way should be in the form of peptide, while the original descriptions of the serum tolerogen showed that it was reactive with antibodies against native protein.[180,181] Of course it is conceivable that both native protein and exosomes contribute to the phenomenon.

A Role for the Liver in Oral Tolerance?

An additional site that has been implicated in the induction of oral tolerance is the liver. Much of the venous blood from the intestine enters the liver via the portal vein and the liver contains large numbers of tolerogenic APC, including a population of distinct dendritic cells that induce IL10 production by T cells.[188] Administration of antigen into the portal vein itself induces a state of systemic unresponsiveness which has many similarities to oral tolerance[189] and some studies in which the liver was bypassed by a porto-caval shunt have suggested that oral tolerance was defective under these conditions.[190] However, earlier work of this kind did not find an effect of liver bypass on oral tolerance[191] and the many side effects of this surgical manoeuvre make interpretation of the results difficult. Thus the exact role of the liver remains to be defined.

Antigen Presenting Cells Involved in Oral Tolerance

The nature of the APC that presents fed antigen such that tolerance of CD4+ T cells occurs is controversial. The class II MHC expressing enterocyte has been a favoured candidate because it is likely to be the first cell that meets intestinal antigen and enterocytes can process and present protein antigens in vitro.[192] In addition, the enterocyte lacks conventional costimulatory molecules. However, as we have noted above, it is difficult to imagine that presentation by intact epithelial cells could initiate the induction of a state of systemic tolerance when there are few recirculating, naive CD4+ T cells available in the lamina propria to be the targets of such effects. Thus it is unsurprising that recent work indicates that the crucial APC involved in oral tolerance is bone marrow derived.[168] However, as discussed above, tolerosomes released from enterocytes could play a role after presentation by more conventional APC. Uptake of fed antigens in association with apoptotic enterocytes by dendritic cells (DC) is an additional way in which epithelial cells could be involved (see below).

Resting B lymphocytes are one bone marrow derived cell type which has received attention as a tolerogenic APC in other models[193-196] and peripheral T cell tolerance cannot be induced by administration of soluble antigen into the anterior chamber of the eye in B cell deficient mice.[197] Although this phenomenon has many parallels to oral tolerance, more than one study has shown recently that the induction of oral tolerance by feeding proteins occurs normally in the absence of B cells.[160-162,198] It therefore seems unlikely that B cells play an essential role in the phenomenon.

Activated macrophages are found in relatively large numbers in the mucosa, especially in the large intestine. However, there is no evidence that these cells can act as APC in oral tolerance. This is not surprising, given that macrophages probably do not present soluble antigens efficiently to T cells. It seems more likely that mucosal macrophages may present phagocytosed particulate antigens in immunogenic form, perhaps accounting for the ability of proteins not to induce oral tolerance when incorporated into particulate vectors.[40-42] However, as discussed below, current evidence indicates that resident macrophages may play an accessory role in maintaining oral tolerance by modulating the function of local DC via the production of PGE_2.

The current consensus is that DC may the the principal population of APC that controls whether orally administered antigen induces tolerance or active immunity. As we have noted, DC are abundant in the intestine and there is continual recirculation of DC from there into the draining lymphoid tissues. They are therefore ideally suited to carry tolerogenic antigen from the intestine to CD4+ T cells in the GALT and periphery. Although initial studies suggested that DC in intestinal lymph that had been loaded by antigen feeding could prime T cells in vivo and in vitro,[153,154,199] more recent studies have shown that selective expansion of DC numbers in vivo using the cytokine flt3 ligand (flt3L) enhances the susceptibility of mice to the induction of oral tolerance by feeding OVA. This is the case even when the doses of antigen that are used have no effect in normal animals, or even prime the systemic immune response.[104,169,200] Flt3L also enhances the ability of antigen feeding to suppress experimental acute encephalomyelitis in mice (Whitacre, C.C . Personal Communication) and to induce tolerance in previously primed mice (our unpublished observations). Interestingly, expansion of DC with flt3L also increases the abortive activation of CD4+ T cells that occurs in mucosal and peripheral lymphoid tissues after feeding antigen.[169] The question therefore arises as to why increased numbers of DC appear to increase susceptibility to oral tolerance when DC have traditionally been associated with immune priming. The explanation may lie in the fact that the DC isolated from the intestine and other tissues of normal and flt3L treated animals are deficient in their expression of costimulatory molecules such as CD40, CD80 or CD86,[104,200] suggesting that these are immature DC with the features of APC that induce tolerance in other models. Other evidence supports the view that DC isolated from the PP also express low levels of costimulatory molecules or pro-inflammatory cytokines (see below). One further intriguing possibility comes from recent work which shows that a subpopulation of DC in intestinal lymph contains fragments of apoptotic enterocytes and that these DC have relatively low stimulatory activity for T cells.[201] In other systems, DC which have ingested apoptotic cells are tolerogenic[202] and it is suggested that intestinal DC may be able to induce tolerance to self antigens, or to luminal antigens that have been taken up by the enterocytes before dying.[201] Although there is no direct evidence for this mechanism, other work has shown that mice are tolerant to OVA when it is expressed only by enterocytes, even when the OVA construct used is not expressed on the cell membrane and cannot be secreted.[74] Apoptosis of effete enterocytes is a constant and normal process and ingestion of these cells by tolerogenic DC could allow systemic tolerance to associated antigens.

A central role for DC in the induction of oral tolerance is consistent with the resting phenotype of intestinal DC noted above and by recent studies on the nature of DC isolated from normal PP. These DC may be relatively immature[203] and may preferentially stimulate the production of IL4 and IL10 by T cells, rather than the IL2 and γIFN induced by DC from other tissues.[204-206] In parallel, freshly isolated PP DC express only low levels of costimulatory molecules such as CD80/CD86 and themselves produce IL10.[205] Together, these results suggest that IL10 producing mucosal DC could be the APC that are responsible for stimulating the IL10 dependent regulatory T cells that have been implicated in oral tolerance.[11,12] When stimulated via CD40, PP DC take on the functions more appropriate to immunostimulatory

APC. An analogous population of DC has been described in the respiratory tract of rats, which are also defective in conventional costimulatory activity and express IL10 mRNA.[207] It is intriguing to speculate how mucosal DC can maintain this non-stimulatory phenotype in an environment which is exposed continually to immunomodulatory factors such as LPS. One possible explanation may come from recent studies which show that macrophages in the lamina propria of normal animals constitutively produce prostaglandin E_2 (PGE_2),[131] a mediator that can modulate the maturation and function of DC, inducing the production of IL10.[208,209] Interestingly, this constitutive production of PGE_2 appears to be dependent on the presence of physiological levels of LPS derived from the gut.[131] In addition to local macrophages, it is possible that intestinal epithelial cells help promote downregulatory pathways in the mucosa, as recent studies show that interactions with commensal bacteria can stimulate the production of inhibitory signals and mediators by enterocytes.[210,211] Thus the intestinal microenvironment may normally be dominated by regulatory mediators such as PGE_2 and IL10 which influence the subsequent differentiation of APC and T cells so that tolerance is maintained under normal circumstances.

Interference with this homeostatic balance may be central to the development of immunopathology[131] (and see below) and modulation of DC activity may be critically important in determining whether intestinal antigens stimulate tolerance, protective immunity or immunopathology. This is suggested by the fact that agents which activate DC, such as IL1, can reverse the tolerance induced by feeding antigen, even when DC numbers have been expanded by flt3L.[200] Flt3L treatment also enhances local protective antibody responses in mice immunised orally with cholera toxin[200] and dramatically increases $CD4^+$ and $CD8^+$ T cell responses to antigen incorporated in immune stimulating complexes (ISCOMS) Beacock-Sharp H et al, in preparation). Both ISCOMS and CT have been shown to target and/or activate DC[212](Beacock-Sharp H et al in preparation). Thus the function of intestinal DC may be to act as the gatekeepers of the mucosal immune response, determining the immunological consequences of oral administration of antigen. Under physiological conditions, the antigen load consists of food antigens and commensal bacteria, which do not induce inflammation or the "danger" signals that are necessary for activating DC. As a result, presentation of these antigens to T cells produces tolerance. Conversely, toxins and invasive pathogens stimulate inflammation, promoting DC activation and allowing protective immunity to develop. This hypothesis is consistent with the current evidence that DC are exquisitely sensitivity to microenvironmental influences that signal danger and which they then transmit to antigen specific T cells via changes in function and APC activity.[208,213]

Induction of Tolerance by Other Mucosal Routes

Other forms of mucosal tolerance have recently been investigated, specifically the administration of antigen via the nasal or aerosol route. These routes appear equally efficient and in some instances may be more effective in suppressing autoimmune diseases in animal models.[214-223] Furthermore, smaller doses of antigen can be administered compared with the oral route, perhaps because there is less degradation of the proteins before they reach the intestinal mucosal surface. The degree of similarity between the mechanisms of oral and nasal tolerance remains to be elucidated. One further route by which an analogous form of tolerance can be induced is by administration of antigen into the anterior chamber of the eye.[9] Although not strictly a mucosal surface, similar effects have been described after application of antigen to the conjunctival surface and the phenomenon of anterior chamber induced immune deviation (ACAID) provides lessons which may be applicable to understanding the basis of oral tolerance. It seems to occur partly because the eye is detached from local secondary lymphoid organs, having no afferent lymphatics. As a result, the only route of antigen absorption is filtration through the local epithelial surface, followed by delivery in the bloodstream to the spleen, where the dominant effect is the induction of tolerance. The aqueous humour that constitutes the fluid content of the anterior chamber is also rich in immunomodulatory mediators such as TGFβ and has been shown to convert APC into a tolerogenic state.[9,224,225] This leads to the activation of regulatory T cells and deviation of the immune response away from Th1 dependent inflammatory responses. Together, these findings emphasise how an immunomodulatory local microenvironment and the rapid uptake of ultrafiltered antigen from an epithelial surface can provoke tolerance as a default mechanism.

Modulation of Oral Tolerance

A number of procedures can enhance the induction of oral tolerance and some of these could offer pointers for better exploitation of the phenomenon for therapeutic purposes. This can be achieved experimentally by administration of anti-IL12, a procedure associated both with increased TGFβ secretion and T cell apoptosis.[165] Exogenous IL2, IL4 or IL10 also enhance tolerance due to active suppressor mechanisms, perhaps reflecting the ability of these cytokines to act as growth and differentiation factors for regulatory T cells.[226,227] These effects may be reproduced using orally administered cytokines.[227]

A further approach, which has received much attention in recent years, is the use of the B subunit of ADP ribosylating toxins as tolerogenic "adjuvants". As we have noted, intact CT or *E. coli* enterotoxin are strongly immunogenic when given orally and can also stimulate primary immune responses to coadministered antigens.[228,229] However, when antigens are coupled to the B subunit of CT (CTB) or LT (LTB), the induction of oral tolerance is greatly enhanced.[230-232] Under these conditions, both naive and primed animals can be tolerised by extremely small amounts of antigen. The scope of the tolerance extends to IgE mediated allergic responses and autoimmune diseases such as type 1 diabetes, arthritis and EAE[139,231,233,234] and the tolerogenic effect of CTB may also be apparent when the nasal[235,236] or parenteral routes are used.[237] It is currently unclear whether this generality also extends to LTB, as some workers have found it to act as an active adjuvant when given nasally.[238] The reasons for the markedly different effects of the holotoxins and their B subunits are still under investigation, but may reflect the ability of CTB/LTB to target antigen to tolerogenic APC such as enterocytes or B cells via their ability to bind to Gm1 ganglioside and without the proinflammatory effects of the CTA subunit. There may also be active interference with antigen presentation, either due to inhibitory signalling by the B subunit-Gm1 complex, to inhibition of costimulatory molecule expression, or to blocking of the trafficking of the vesicular structures involved in class II MHC presentation.[237,239] Irrespective of the molecular mechanisms involved, the overall functional effect in vivo appears to be preferential expansion of CD4$^+$ regulatory T cells producing IL4 and TGFβ[233,234,237] Thus both CTB and LTB could be seen as "adjuvants" which induce a state of immune deviation that appears as tolerance of inflammatory immune responses. Considerable interest is now focussed on clinical trials of this novel approach in autoimmune disease.

Alternative, nonpharmacological approaches to enhancing oral tolerance are suggested by the findings noted above that incorporation of low doses of protein in multiple emulsions[47] or biodegradable microspheres[48] can induce tolerance very readily. It is tempting to believe that combining these particulate vectors with a targeting molecule such as CTB may prove useful in clinical practice.

Breakdown in Oral Tolerance and the Pathogenesis of Disease

We have discussed the concept that oral tolerance is an important physiological phenomenon and that its purpose is to prevent the Th1 dependent reactions to food proteins and commensal bacteria which may underlie coeliac disease and inflammatory bowel disease respectively. In support of this idea, prevention of oral tolerance in experimental animals sensitises the intestine to develop mild enteropathy when the antigen is met subsequently in the diet. This consists of crypt hyperplasia, crypt hypertrophy and increased infiltration of the jejunal epithelium by lymphocytes,[14,102,148,150,240,241] features that are found in naturally occurring enteropathies such as coeliac disease and in the early lesions of Crohn's disease.[242] Although the classical feature of coeliac disease, villus atrophy, was not observed in these studies, this feature has been found more recently when antigen was fed to TcR transgenic mice in combination with inhibition of PGE_2 production.[131] This induction of immunopathology may reflect inhibition of the physiological, macrophage dependent regulatory mechanism discussed above and the results support an important role for this process in actively preventing hypersensitivity to dietary proteins.

Recent work suggests that similar processes may underlie inflammatory bowel disease (IBD). Rodents and humans normally are tolerant to their own gut flora and this state breaks down when IL12/γIFN dependent IBD develops.[50,51] In addition, there are several experimental models of IBD in which a defect in regulatory T cells predisposes to the spontaneous development of IBD.[243] In many cases, the regulatory T cells appear to act via IL10 and/or TGFβ dependent mechanisms[244] and interestingly, in vitro generated, IL10 producing regulatory T cells can prevent experimental IBD in vivo.[244,245] As we have noted, IBD induced by the contact sensitising agent TNBS can also be prevented by feeding soluble TNBS or TNP-conjugated colonic proteins, a phenomenon which appears to be mediated by TGFβ.[80,92,246]

Thus it seems reasonable to conclude that closely related immunoregulatory mechanisms prevent the development of hypersensitivity to food antigens and antigens derived from commensal bacteria. Although defects in such mechanisms have not yet been identified in the clinical conditions, we would predict that these diseases arise when antigens that normally fail to induce costimulatory activity in APC provoke aberrant proinflammatory effects in the mucosal microenvironment. These alterations could occur due to the presence of concomitant inflammation, to inherent defects in cytokine regulation, or to abnormalities in the LPS-induced production of PGE_2 by macrophages. As a result, local APC such as DC are diverted from their normal physiological role of inducing T cell anergy or regulatory activity, becoming able to prime CD4+ T cells productively in the presence of IL12 and so generate unopposed populations of inflammatory Th1 cells.

References

1. Swarbrick ET, Stokes CR, Soothill JF. Absorption of antigens after oral immunization and the simultaneous induction of specific systemic tolerance. Gut 1979; 20(2):121-5.
2. Kilshaw PJ, Cant AJ. The passage of maternal dietary proteins into human breast milk. Int Arch Allergy Appl Immunol 1984; 75:8-15.
3. Husby S, Foged N, Host A et al. Passage of dietary antigens into the blood of children with coeliac disease. Quantification and size distribution of absorbed antigens. Gut 1987; 28:1062-72.
4. Husby S, Jensenius JC, Svehag S-E. Passage of undergraded dietary antigen into the blood of healthy adults. Further characterization of the kinetics of uptake and the size distribution of the antigen. Scand J Immunol 1986; 24:447-52.
5. Harmatz PR, Bloch KJ, Brown M et al. Intestinal adaption during lactation in the mouse. I. Enhanced intestinal uptake of dietary protein antigen. Immunology 1989; 67:92-5.
6. Elson C, Sartor, RB, Tennyson, GS et al. Experimental models of inflammatory bowel disease. Gastroenterology 1995; 109:1344-67.
7. Weiner HL. Oral tolerance: Immune mechanisms and treatment of autoimmune diseases. Immunol Today 1997; 18:335-43.
8. Lowrey JL, Savage ND, Palliser D et al. Induction of tolerance via the respiratory mucosa. Int Arch Allergy Immunol 1998; 116:93-102.
9. Streilein JW. Immunologic privilege of the eye. Springer Semin Immunopathol 1999; 21:95-111.

10. Mowat AM. The regulation of immune responses to dietary protein antigens. Immunol Today 1987; 8:93-8.

11. Faria AMC, Weiner HL. Oral tolerance: Mechanisms and therapeutic applications. Adv Immunol 1999; 73:153-264.

12. Mowat AM, Weiner HL. Oral tolerance: Basic mechanisms and clinical implications. In: Ogra PL, Mestecky J, Lamm ME et al, eds. Mucosal Immunology. 2nd ed. San Diego: Academic Press; 1999:587-617.

13. Miller BG, Newby TJ, Stokes CR et al. Influence of diet on postweaning malabsorption and diarrhoea in the pig. Res Vet Sci 1984; 36:187-93.

14. Stokes CR, Miller BG, Bourne FJ. Animal models of food sensitivity. In: Brostoff J, Challacombe SJ, eds. Food Allergy and Intolerance. Eastbourne: W.B. Saunders 1987:286-300.

15. Cantor HM, Dumont AE. Hepatic suppression of sensitization to antigen absorbed into the portal vein. Nature 1967; 215:744-5.

16. Deplazes P, Penhale WJ, Greene WK et al. Effect on humoral tolerance (IgG and IgE) in dogs by the oral administration of ovalbumin and Der pI. Vet Immunol Immunopathol 1995; 45:361-7.

17. Heppell LM, Kilshaw PJ. Immune reponses in guinea pigs to dietary protein. I. Induction of tolerance by feeding ovalbumin. Int Archs Allergy Appl Immunol 1982; 68:54-61.

18. Bhogal BS, Karkhanis YD, Bell MK et al. Production of auto-anti-idiotypic antibody during the normal immune response. XII. Enhanced auto-anti-idiotypic antibody production as a mechanism for apparent B cell tolerance in rabbits after feeding antigens. Cell Immunol 1986; 101:93-104.

19. Korenblatt PE, Rothberg RM, Minden P et al. Immune responses of adult humans after oral and parenteral exposure to bovine serum albumin. J Allergy 1968; 41:226-35.

20. Lowney ED. Immunologic unresponsiveness to a contact sensitizer in man. J Invest Dermatol 1968; 51(6):411-7.

21. Walker WA. Role of the mucosal barrier in antigen handling by the gut. In: Brostoff J, Challacombe SJ, eds. Food Allergy and Intolerance. Eastbourne: W.B. Saunders 1987:209-22.

22. Husby S, Mestecky J, Moldoveanu Z et al. Oral tolerance in humans: T cell but not B cell tolerance after antigen feeding. J Immunol 1994; 152:4663-70.

23. Matsui M, Hafler DA, Weiner HL. Pilot study of oral tolerance to keyhole limpet hemocyanin in humans. Down regulation of KLH-reactive precursor-cell frequency. Ann NY Acad Sci 1996; 778:398-404.

24. Suko M, Mori A, Ito K et al. Oral immunotherapy may induce T cell anergy. Int Arch Allergy Immunol 1995; 107:278-81.

25. Bagot M, Charue D, Flechet ML et al. Oral desensitization in nickel allergy induces a decrease in nickel-specific T-cells. Eur J Dermatol 1995; 5:614-7.

26. Peri BA, Rothberg RM. Circulating antitoxin in rabbits after ingestion of diphtheria toxin. Infect Immun 1981; 32:1148-54.

27. Silverman GA, Peri BA, Rothberg RM. Systemic antibody responses of different species following ingestion of soluble protein antigens. Dev Comp Immunol 1982; 6(4):737-46.

28. Stokes CR. Induction and control of intestinal immune responses. In: Stokes CR, Newby TJ, eds. Local immune responses of the gut. Boca Raton: CRC Press 1984:97-141.

29. Miller CC, Cook ME. Evidence against the induction of immunological tolerance by feeding antigens to chickens. Poultry Sci 1994; 73:106-12.

30. Miller A, Al-Sabbagh A, Santos LMB et al. Epitopes of myelin basic protein that trigger TGF-β release after oral tolerization are distinct from encephalitogenic epitopes and mediate epitope-driven bystander suppression. J Immunol 1993; 151:7307-15.

31. Gregerson DS, Obritsch WF, Donoso LA. Oral tolerance in experimental autoimmune uveoretinitis: Distinct mechanisms of resistance are induced by low versus high dose feeding protocols. J Immunol 1993; 151:5751-61.

32. Al-Sabbagh A, Miller A, Santos LMB et al. Antigen-driven tissue-specific suppression following oral tolerance: Orally administered myelin basic protein suppresses proteolipid induced experimental autoimmune encephalomyelitis in the SJL mouse. European J Immunol 1994; 24:2104-9.

33. Khare SD, Krco CJ, Griffiths MM et al. Oral administration of an immunodominant human collagen peptide modulates collagen-induced arthritis. J Immunol 1995; 155:3653-9.

34. Javed NH, Gienapp IE, Cox KL et al. Exquisite peptide specificity of oral tolerance in experimental autoimmune encephalomyelitis. J Immunol 1995; 155:1599-605.

35. Wildner G, Hünig T, Thurau SR. Orally induced, peptide-specific g/d TcR+ cells suppress experimental autoimmune uveitis. Eur J Immunol 1996; 26:2140-8.
36. Hoyne GF, Callow MG, Kuo MC et al. Inhibition of T-cell responses by feeding peptides containing major and cryptic eptopes: Studies with the Der p I allergen. Immunology 1994; 83:190-5.
37. Baggi F, Andreeta F, Caspani E et al. Oral administration of an immunodominant T-cell epitope downregulates Th1/Th2 cytokines and prevents experimental myasthenia gravis. J Clin Invest 1999; 104:1287-95.
38. Stokes R, Newby TJ, Huntley JH et al. The immune response of mice to bacterial antigens given by mouth. Immunology 1979; 38:497-502.
39. Rubin D, Weiner HL, Fields BN et al. Immunologic tolerance after oral administration of reovirus: Requirement for two viral gene products for tolerance induction. J Immunol 1981; 127:1697-701.
40. McGhee JR, Mestecky J, Dertzbaugh MT et al. The mucosal immune system: From fundamental concepts to vaccine development. Vaccine 1992; 10:75-88.
41. Maloy KJ, Donachie AM, O'Hagan DT et al. Induction of mucosal and systemic immune responses by immunization with ovalbumin entrapped in poly(lactide-co-glycolide) microparticles. Immunology 1994; 81:661-7.
42. Barone KS, Reilly MR, Flanagan MP et al. Abrogation of oral tolerance by feeding encapsulated antigen. Cell Immunol 2000; 199:65-72.
43. Owen RL. M cells-entryways of opportunity for enteropathogens. J Exp Med 1994; 180:7-9.
44. Ermak T, Dougherty EP, Bhagat HR et al. Uptake and transport of copolymer biodegradable microspheres by rabbit Peyer's patch M cells. Cell Tissue Res 1995; 279:433-6.
45. Jones B, Pascopella L, Falkow S. Entry of microbes into the host: Using M cells to break the mucosal barrier. Curr Opin Immunol 1995; 7:474-8.
46. Michalek SM, Eldridge JH, Curtiss R, III et al. Antigen delivery systems: New approaches to mucosal immunization. In: Ogra PL, Mestecky J, Lamm ME et al, eds. Handbook of Mucosal Immunology. San Diego: Academic Press, Inc. 1994:373-90.
47. Elson CO, Tomasi M, Dertzbaugh MT et al. Oral antigen delivery by way of a multiple emulsion system enhances oral tolerance. Ann NY Acad Sci 1996; 778:156-62.
48. Pecquet S, Leo E, Fritsche R, Pfeifer A et al. Oral tolerance elicited in mice by beta-lactoglobulin entrapped in biodegradable microspheres. Vaccine 2000; 18:1196-202.
49. Garg S, Bal V, Rath S et al. Effect of multiple antigenic exposures in the gut on oral tolerance and induction of antibacterial systemic immunity. Infect Immun 1999; 67:5917-24.
50. Duchmann R, Kaiser I, Hermann E et al. Tolerance exists towards resident intestinal flora but is broken in active inflammatory bowel disease (IBD). Clin Exp Immunol 1995; 102(3):448-55.
51. Duchmann R, Schmitt E, Knolle P et al. Tolerance towards resident intestinal flora in mice is abrogated in experimental colitis and restored by treatment with interleukin-10 or antibodies to interleukin-12. Eur J Immunol 1996; 26:934-8.
52. Titus RG, Chiller JM. Orally-induced tolerance. Definition at the cellular level. Int Arch Allergy Appl Immunol 1981; 65:323-38.
53. Wilson AD, Stokes CR, Bourne FJ. Adjuvant effect of cholera toxin on the mucosal immune response to soluble proteins. Differences between mouse strains and protein antigens. Scand J Immunol 1989; 29:739-45.
54. Van der Heijden PJ, Bianchi ATJ, Dol M et al. Manipulation of intestinal immune responses against ovalbumin by cholera toxin and its B subunit in mice. Immunology 1991; 72:89-93.
55. Gaboriau-Routhiau V, Moreau M. Gut flora allows recovery of oral tolerance to ovalbumin in mice after transient breakdown mediated by cholera toxin or Escherichia coli heat-labile enterotoxin. Pediatr Res 1996; 39(4 I):625-9.
56. Mowat AM, Strobel S, Drummond HE et al. Immunological responses to fed protein antigens in mice. I. Reversal of oral tolerance to ovalbumin by cyclophosphamide. Immunology 1982; 45:104-13.
57. Mowat AM, Thomas MJ, Mackenzie S et al. Divergent effects of bacterial lipopolysaccharide on immunity to orally administered protein and particulate antigens in mice. Immunology 1986; 58:677-84.
58. Weiner HL, Friedman A, Miller A et al. Oral tolerance: Immunologic mechanisms and treatment of animal and human organ-specific autoimmune diseases by oral administration of autoantigens. Ann Rev Immunol 1994; 12:809-38.

59. Melamed D, Friedman A. In vivo tolerization of Th1 lymphocytes following a single feed with ovalbumin: Anergy in the absence of suppression. Eur J Immunol 1994; 24:1974-81.
60. Fishman-Lobell J, Friedman A, Weiner HL. Different kinetic patterns of cytokine gene expression in vivo in orally tolerant mice. Eur J Immunol 1994; 24:2720-4.
61. Melamed D, Fischmann-Lobell J, Uni Z et al. Peripheral tolerance of Th2 lymphocytes induced by continuous feeding of ovalbumin. Int Immunology 1996; 8:717-24.
62. von Herrath MG, Dyrberg T, Oldstone MBA. Oral insulin treatment suppresses virus-induced antigen-specific destruction of b cells and prevents autoimmune diabetes in transgenic mice. J Clin Invest 1996; 98:1324-31.
63. Friedman A, Weiner HL. Induction of anergy or active suppression following oral tolerance is determined by antigen dosage. Proc Natl Acad Sci USA 1994; 91:6688-92.
64. Garside P, Steel M, Worthey EA et al. Th2 cells are subject to high dose oral tolerance and are not essential for its induction. J Immunol 1995; 154:5649-55.
65. Chen Y, Inobe J-I, Marks R et al. Peripheral deletion of antigen-reactive T cells in oral tolerance. Nature 1995; 376:177-80.
66. Garside P, Steel M, Liew FY et al. CD4+ but not CD8+ T cells are required for the induction of oral tolerance. Int Immunol 1995; 7:501-4.
67. Grdic D, Hornquist E, Kjerrulf M et al. Lack of local suppression in orally tolerant CD8-deficient mice reveals a critical regulatory role of CD8+ T cells in the normal gut mucosa. J Immunol 1998; 160:754-62.
68. Desvignes C, Etchart N, Kehren J et al. Oral administration of hapten inhibits in vivo induction of specific cytotoxic CD8+ T cells mediating tissue inflammation: A role for regulatory CD4+ T cells. J Immunol 2000; 164:2515-22.
69. Desvignes C, Bour H, Nicholas JF et al. Lack of oral tolerance but oral priming for contact sensitivity to dinitrofluorobenzene in major histocompatibility antigen deficient mice and in CD4+ T cell-depleted mice. Eur J Immunol 1996; 26:1756-61.
70. Ke Y, Kapp JA. Oral antigen inhibits priming of CD8+ CTL, CD4+ T cells and antibody responses while activating CD8+ suppressor T cells. J Immunol 1996; 156:916-21.
71. Blanas E, Carbone FR, Allison J et al. Induction of autoimmune diabetes by oral administration of autoantigen. Science 1996; 274:1707-9.
72. Kim S-K, Reed DS, Olson S et al. Generation of mucosal cytotoxic T cells against soluble protein by tissue-specific environmental and costimulatory signals. Proc Natl Acad Sci USA 1998; 95:10814-9.
73. Lefrançois L, Olson S, Masopust D. A critical role for CD40-CD40 ligand interactions in amplification of the mucosal CD8 T cell response. J Exp Med 1999; 190:1275-83.
74. Vezys V, Olson S, Lefrancois L. Expression of intestine-specific antigen reveals novel pathways of CD8 T cell tolerance induction. Immunity 2000; 12:505-14.
75. Mowat AM. Oral tolerance: Basic mechanisms and clinical applications. Curr Opin Gastroenterol 1999; 15:546-56.
76. Zhou J, Carr RI, Liwski RS et al. Oral exposure to alloantigen generates intragraft CD8+ regulatory cells. J Immunol 2001; 167:107-13.
77. Tanchot C, Guillaume S, Delon J et al. Modifications of CD8+ T cell function during in vivo memory or tolerance induction. Immunity 1998; 8:581-90.
78. Challacombe SJ, Thomasi TB. Systemic tolerance and secretory immunity after oral immunisation. J Exp Med 1980; 152:1459-72.
79. Kim P-H, Kagnoff MF. Transforming growth factor-b1 is a costimulator for IgA production. J Immunol 1990; 144:3411-6.
80. Elson C, Beagley K, Sharmanov A et al. Hapten-induced model of murine inflammatory bowel disease: Mucosa immune responses and protection by tolerance. J Immunol 1996; 157:2174-85.
81. Kiyono H, McGhee JR, Wannemuehler MJ et al. Lack of oral tolerance in C3H/HeJ mice. J Exp Med 1982; 155:605-10.
82. MacDonald TT. Immunosuprression caused by antigen feeding. II. Suppressor T cells mask Peyer's patch B cell priming to orally administered antigen. Eur J Immunol 1983; 13:138-42.
83. Lycke N, Bromander A, Ekman L et al. The use of knock-out mice in studies of induction and regulation of gut mucosal immunity. Mucosal Immunology Update 1995; 3:1-8.

84. Oliver AR, Silbart LK. Mucosal tolerance to the dinitrophenyl hapten is not broken by cholera toxin. Int Arch Allergy Appl Immunol 1998; 116:318-24.
85. Kelly KA, Whitacre CC. Oral tolerance in EAE: Reversal of tolerance by T helper cell cytokines. J Neuroimmunol 1996; 66:77-84.
86. Fujihashi K, McGhee JR, Kweon M-N et al. γ/δ T cell-deficient mice have impaired mucosal immunoglobulin A responses. J Exp Med 1996; 183:1929-35.
87. Fujihashi K, Dohi T, Kweon M-N et al. gd T cells regulate mucosally induced tolerance in a dose dependent fashion. Int Immunol 1999; 11:1907-16.
88. Kweon M-N, Fujihashi K, VanCott JL et al. Lack of orally induced systemic unresponsiveness in IFN-g knockout mice. J Immunol 1998; 160:1687-93.
89. Kjerrulf M, Grdic D, Lycke N. Impaired mucosal IgA responses but intact oral tolerance in IFN-γ receptor deficient mice. FASEB J 1996; 10(6):A1418.
90. Franco L, Benedetti R, Ferek GA et al. Priming or tolerization of the B and Th2 dependent immune response by the oral administration of OVA-DNP is determined by the antigen dosage. Cell Immunol 1998; 190:1-11.
91. Whitacre CC, Gienapp IE, Meyer A et al. Oral tolerance in experimental autoimmune encephalo-myelitis. Ann NY Acad Sci 1996; 778:217-27.
92. Neurath MF, Fuss I, Kelsall BL et al. Experimental granulomatous colitis in mice is abrogated by induction of TGF-b-mediated oral tolerance. J Exp Med 1996; 183:2605-16.
93. Ilan Y, Prakash R, Davidson A et al. Oral tolerization to adenoviral antigens permits long-term gene expression using recombinant adenoviral vectors. J Clin Invest 1997; 99:1098-106.
94. Ilan Y, Sauter B, Chowdhury NR et al. Oral tolerization to adenoviral proteins permits repeated adenovirus-mediated gene therapy in rats with pre-existing immunity to adenoviruses. Hepatology 1998; 27:1368-76.
95. Strobel S, Ferguson A. Persistence of oral tolerance in mice fed ovalbumin is different for humoral and cell mediated immune responses. Immunology 1987; 60:317-8.
96. Higgins PJ, Weiner H. Suppression of experimental autoimmune encephalomyelitis by oral admin-istration of myelin basic protein and its fragments. J Immunol 1988; 140:440-5.
97. Moreau M, Gaboriau-Routhiau V. The absence of gut flora, the doses of antigen ingested and ageing affect the long-term peripheral tolerance induced by ovalbumin feeding in mice. Res Immunol 1996; 147(1):49-59.
98. Melamed D, Friedman A. Modification of the immune response by oral tolerance: Antigen requirements and interaction with immunogenic stimuli. Cell Immunol 1993; 146:412-20.
99. Kang BI, Kim KM, Kang C-Y. Oral tolerance by a high dose OVA in BALB/c mice is more pronounced and persistent in Th2-mediated immune responses than in Th1 responses. Immunobiology 1999; 200:264-76.
100. Hanson DG, Vaz NM, Maia LCS. Inhibition of specific immune responses by feeding protein Ag's Int Arch Allergy Appl Immunol 1977; 55:526-32.
101. Thompson HS, Staines NA. Could specific oral tolerance be a therapy for autoimmune disease? Immunol Today 1990; 11:396-9.
102. Lamont AG, Mowat AM, Parrott DMV. Priming of systemic and local delayed-type hypersensitiv-ity responses by feeding low doses of ovalbumin to mice. Immunology 1989; 66:595-9.
103. Meyer AL, Benson JM, Gienapp IE et al. Suppression of murine chronic relapsing autoimmune encephalomyelitis by the oral administration of myelin basic protein. J Immunol 1996; 157:4230-8.
104. Viney JL, Mowat AM, O'Malley JM et al. Expanding dendritic cells in vivo enhances the induc-tion of oral tolerance. J Immunol 1998; 160:5815-25.
105. Hirahara K, Hisatune T, Nishijima K-I et al. CD4+ T cells anergized by high dose feeding estab-lish oral tolerance to antibody responses when transferred in SCID and nude mice. J Immunol 1995; 154:6238-45.
106. Lundin BS, Dahlgren UI, Hanson LA et al. Oral tolerization leads to active suppression and bystander tolerance in adult rats, while anergy dominates in young rats. Scand J Immunol 1996; 43:56-63.
107. Peng HJ, Turner MW, Strobel S. The kinetics of oral hyposensitisation to a protein antigen are determined by immune status and the timing, dose and frequency of antigen administration. Immunology 1989; 67:425-30.

108. Liu L, Kuchroo VK, Weiner HL. B7.2 (CD86) but not B7.1 (CD80) costimulation is required for the induction of low dose oral tolerance. J Immunol 1999; 163:2284-90.
109. Hanson DG. Ontogeny of orally induced tolerance in newborns. J Immunol 1981; 127:1518-22.
110. Strobel S, Ferguson A. Immune responses to fed protein antigens in mice. III. Systemic tolerance or priming is related to age at which antigen is first encountered. Pediatr Res 1984; 18(7):588-94.
111. Troncone R, Ferguson A. In mice, gluten in maternal diet primes systemic immune responses to gliadin in offspring. Immunology 1988; 64:533-7.
112. Peng H-J, Turner MW, Strobel S. Failure to induce oral tolerance to protein antigens in neonatal mice can be corrected by transfer of adult spleen cells. Pediatr Res 1989; 26:486-90.
113. Miller A, Lider O, Abramsky O et al. Orally administered myelin basic protein in neonates primes for immune responses and enhances experimental autoimmune encephalomyelitis in adult animals. Eur J Immunol 1994; 24:1026-32.
114. Pecquet S, Pfeifer A, Gauldie S et al. Immunoglobulin E suppression and cytokine modulation in mice orally tolerized to β-lactoglobulin. Immunology 1999; 96:278-85.
115. Barratt MEJ, Powell JR, Allen WD et al. Immunopathology of intestinal disorders in farm animals. In: Marsh MN, ed. Immunopathology of the Small Intestine. Chichester: John Wiley and Sons, 1987:253-8.
116. Karlsson MR, Kahu H, Hanson LA et al. Neonatal colonization of rats induces immunological tolerance to bacterial antigens. Eur J Immunol 1999; 29:109-18.
117. Faria AM, Garcia G, Rios MJ et al. Decrease in susceptibility to oral tolerance induction and occurrence. Immunology 1993; 78(1):147-51.
118. MacDonald TT, Carter PB. Requirement for a bacterial flora before mice generate cells capable of mediating the DTH reaction to sheep red blood cells. J Immunol 1979; 122:2624-9.
119. Collins SR, Campbell JB. Development of delayed hypersensitivity in gnotobiotic mice. Int Archs Allergy Appl Immunol 1980; 61:165-70.
120. Sudo N, Sawamura S, Tanaka K et al. The requirement of intestinal bacterial flora for the development of an IgE production system fully susceptible to oral tolerance induction. J Immunol 1997; 159:1739-45.
121. Wannemuehler MJ, Kiyono H, Babb JL et al. Lipopolysaccharide (LPS) regulation of the immune response: LPS converts germfree mice to sensity to oral tolerance induction. J Immunol 1982; 129(3):959-65.
122. Michalek SM, Kiyono H, Wannemuehler MJ et al. Lipopolysaccharide (LPS) regulation of the immune response: LPS influence on oral tolerance induction. J Immunol 1982; 128:1992-8.
123. Kitamura K, Kiyono H, Fujihashi K et al. Contrasuppressor cells that break oral tolerance are antigen-specific T cells distinct from T helper (L3T4+), T suppressor (Lyt2+) and B cells. J Immunol 1987; 139:3251-9.
124. Saklayen MG, Pesce AJ, Pollak VE et al. Induction of oral tolerance in mice unresponsive to bacterial lipopolysaccharide. Infect Immun 1983; 41(3):1383-5.
125. Poltorak A, He X, Smirnova I et al. Defective LPS signaling in C3H/HeJ and C57BL/10ScCr mice: Mutations in Tlr4 gene. Science 1998; 282:2085-8.
126. Kim JH, Ohsawa M. Oral tolerance to ovalbumin in mice as a model for detecting modulators of the immunologic tolerance to a specific antigen. Biol Pharm Bull 1995; 18:854-8.
127. Khoury SJ, Lider O, Al-Sabbagh A et al. Suppression of experimental autoimmune encephalomyelitis by oral administration of myelin basic protein. III. Synergistic effect of lipopolysaccharide. Cell Immunol 1990; 131:302-10.
128. Khoury SJ, Hancock WW, Weiner HL. Oral tolerance to myelin basic protein and natural recovery from experimental autoimmune encephalomyelitis are associated with downregulation of inflammatory cytokines and differential upregulation of transforming growth factor b, interleukin 4, and prostaglandin E expression in the brain. J Exp Med 1992; 176:1355-64.
129. Moreau MC, Corthier G. Effect of the gastrointestinal microflora on induction and maintenance of oral tolerance to ovalbumin in C3H/HeJ mice. Infect Immunol 1988; 56:2766-8.
130. Furrie E, Turner MW, Strobel S. Failure of scid mice to generate an oral tolerogen after a feed of ovalbumin: A role for a functioning gut-associated lymphoid system. Immunology 1994; 83:562-7.
131. Newberry RD, Stenson WP, Lorenz RG. Cyclooxygenase-2-dependent arachidonic acid metabolites are essential modulators of the intestinal immune response to dietary antigen. Nat Med 1999; 5:900-6.

132. Macpherson AJ, Maloy KJ, Bjarnason I. Intolerance of the dirty intestine. Gut 1999; 44:774-5.
133. Lafont S, Andre C, Andre F et al. Abrogation by subsequent feeding of antibody response, including IgE in parenterally immunised mice. J Exp Med 1982; 155:1573-8.
134. Lider O, Santos LMB, Lee CSY et al. Suppression of experimental autoimmune encephalomyelitis by oral administration of myelin basic protein. II. Suppression of disease and in vitro immune responses is mediated by antigen-specific CD8+ T lymphocytes. J Immunol 1989; 142:748-52.
135. Lamont AG, Bruce MG, Watret KC et al. Suppression of an established DTH response to ovalbumin in mice by feeding antigen after immunization. Immunology 1988; 64:135-40.
136. Leishman AJ, Garside P, Mowat AM. Intervention in established immune responses by induction of oral tolerance. Cell Immunol 1998; 183:137-48.
137. Chung Y, Chang S-Y, Kang C-Y. Kinetic analysis of oral tolerance: Memory lymphocytes are refractory to oral tolerance. J Immunol 1999; 163:3692-8.
138. Leishman AJ, Garside P, Mowat AM. Induction of oral tolerance in the primed immune system: Influence of antigen persistence and adjuvant form. Cell Immunol 2000; 202:71-8.
139. Rask C, Holmgren J, Fredriksson M et al. Prolonged oral treatment with low doses of allergen conjugated to cholera toxin B subunit suppresses immunoglobulin E antibody responses in sensitized mice. Clin Exp Allergy 2000; 30:1024-32.
140. Hanson DG, Vaz NM, Rawlings LA et al. Inhibition of specific immune responses by feeding protein Ag's II. Effects of prior passive and active immunisation. J Immunol 1979; 122:2261-6.
141. Cunningham-Rundles C. Failure of antigen exclusion. In: Brostoff J, Challacombe SJ, eds. Food Allergy and Intolerance. Eastbourne: WB Saunders 1987:223-36.
142. Louis E, Franchimont D, Deprez M et al. Decrease in systemic tolerance to fed ovalbumin in indomethacin-treated mice. Int Arch Allergy Appl Immunol 1996; 109:21-6.
143. Hanson DG, Roy MJ, Green GM et al. Inhibition of orally-induced immune tolerance in mice by prefeeding an endopeptidase inhibitor. Reg Immunol1993; 5:76-84.
144. Peng HJ, Chang Z-N, Han S-H et al. Chemical denaturation of ovalbumin abrogates the induction of oral tolerance of specific IgG antibody and DTH responses in mice. Scand J Immunol 1995; 42:297-304.
145. Saklayen MG, Pesce AJ, Pollak VE et al. Kinetics of oral tolerance: Study of variables affecting tolerance induced by oral administration of antigen. Int Arch Allergy Appl Immunol 1984; 73:75-9.
146. Migita K, Ochi A. Induction of clonal anergy by oral administration of staphylococcal enterotoxin B. Eur J Immunol 1994; 24(9):2081-6.
147. Stokes CR, Newby TJ, Bourne FJ. The influence of oral immunization on local and systemic immune responses to heterologous antigens. Clin Exp Immunol 1983; 52:399-406.
148. Mowat AMI, Parrott DMV. Immunological responses to fed protein antigens in mice. IV. Effects of stimulating the reticuloendothelial system on oral tolerance and intestinal immunity to ovalbumin. Immunology 1983; 50:547-54.
149. Strobel C, Mowat AM, Ferguson A. Prevention of oral tolerance induction to ovalbumin and enhanced antigen presentation during a graft-versus-host reaction in mice. Immunology 1985; 56:57-64.
150. Strobel S, Ferguson A. Modulation of intestinal and systemic immune responses to a fed protein. Gut 1986; 27:829-37.
151. Zhang Z, Michael JG. Orally inducible immune unresponsiveness is abrogated by IFNγ treatment. J Immunol 1990; 144(11):4163-5.
152. Zimmer KP, Buning J, Weber P et al. Modulation of antigen trafficking to MHC class II-positive late endosomes of enterocytes. Gastroenterology 2000; 118:128-37.
153. Liu L, MacPherson G. Antigen acquisition by dendritic cells: Intestinal dendritic cells acquire antigen administered orally and can prime naive T cells in vivo. J Exp Med 1993; 177:1299-307.
154. Liu L, MacPherson GG. Rat intestinal dendritic cells: Immunostimulatory potency and phenotypic characterization. Immunology 1995; 85:88-93.
155. MacPherson GG, Jenkins CD, Stein MJ et al. Endotoxin-mediated dendritic cell release from the intestine. Characterization of released dendritic cells and TNF dependence. J Immunol 1995; 154:1317-22.
156. Galliaerde V, Desvignes C, Peyron E et al. Oral tolerance to haptens: Intestinal epithelial cells from 2,4-dinitrochlorobenzene-fed mice inhibit hapten-specific T cell activation in vitro. Eur J Immunol 1995; 25:1385-90.

157. Richman L, Graeff, AS, Strober W. Antigen presentation by macrophage-enriched cells from the mouse Peyer's patch. Cell Immunol 1981; 62:110-8.
158. Harper H, Cochrane L, Williams NA. The role of small intestinal antigen-presenting cells in the induction of T-cell reactivity to soluble protein antigens: Association between aberrant presentation in the lamina propria and oral tolerance. Immunology 1996; 89:449-56.
159. Spahn TW, Koni PA, Marino MW et al. A critical role for the gut-associated lymphatic tissue in the induction of oral tolerance. Immunol Letters 1999; 69:86A.
160. Hashimoto A, Yamada H, Matsuzaki G et al. Successful priming and tolerization of T cells to orally administered antigens in B-cell-deficient mice. Cell Immunol 2001; 207:36-40.
161. Alpan O, Rudomen G, Matzinger P. The role of dendritic cells, B cells and M cells in gut-oriented immune responses. J Immunol 2001; 166:4843-52.
162. Peng H-J, Chang Z-N, Lee C-C et al. B-cell depletion fails to abrogate the induction of oral tolerance of specific Th1 immune responses in mice. Scand J Immunol 2000; 51:454-60.
163. Gardine CA, Kouki T, DeGroot L. Characterization of the T lymphocyte subsets and lymphoid populations involved in the induction of low dose oral tolerance to human thyroglobulin. Cell Immunol 2001; 212:1-15.
164. Mattingly JA, Waksman BH. Immunologic suppression after oral administration of antigen. I. Specific suppressor cells formed in rat Peyer's patches after oral administration of sheep erythrocytes and their systemic migration. J Immunol 1978; 121:1878-83.
165. Marth T, Strober W, Kelsall BL. High dose oral tolerance in ovalbumin TcR-transgenic mice: Systemic neutralisation of interleukin 12 augments TGFβ secretion and T cell apoptosis. J Immunol 1996; 157:2348-57.
166. Gonnella PA, Chen Y, Inobe J-I et al. In situ immune response in gut-associated lymphoid tissue (GALT) following oral antigen in TCR-transgenic mice. J Immunol 1998; 160:4708-18.
167. Chen Y, Inobe J-I, Weiner HL. Inductive events in oral tolerance in the TcR transgenic adoptive transfer model. Cell Immunol 1997; 178:62-8.
168. Blanas E, Carbone FR, Heath WR. A bone marrow-derived APC in the gut-associated lymphoid tissue captures oral antigens and presents them to both CD4+ and CD8+ T cells. J Immunol 2000; 164:2890-6.
169. Williamson E, O'Malley JM, Viney JL. Defining the role of dendritic cells in oral tolerance induction by visualizing the T cell response elicited by oral administration of soluble protein antigen. Immunology 1999; 97:565-72.
170. Van Houten N, Blake SF. Direct measurement of anergy of antigen-specific T cells following oral tolerance induction. J Immunol 1996; 157:1337-41.
171. Sun J, Dirden-Kramer B, Ito K et al. Antigen-specific T cell activation and proliferation during oral tolerance induction. J Immunol 1999; 162:5865-75.
172. Gütgemann I, Fahrer AM, Davis MM et al. Induction of rapid T cell activation and tolerance by systemic presentation of an orally administered antigen. Immunity 1998; 8:667-73.
173. Saparov A, Elson CO, Devore-Carter D et al. Single-cell analysis of CD4+ T cells from ab T cell receptor transgenic mice: A distinct mucosal cytokine phenotype in the absence of transgene-specific antigen. Eur J Immunol 1997; 27:1774-81.
174. Hurst SD, Cooper CJ, Sitterding SM et al. The differentiated state of intestinal lamina propria CD4+ T cells results in altered cytokine production, activation threshold, and costimulatory requirements. J Immunol 1999; 163:5937-45.
175. Mowat AM, Viney JL. The anatomical basis of mucosal immune responses. Immunol Rev 1997; 156:145-66.
176. Wolvers DAW, Coenen-De Roo CJJ, Mebius RE et al. Intranasally induced immunological tolerance is determined by characteristics of the draining lymph nodes: Studies with OVA and human cartilage gp39. J Immunol 1999; 162:1994-8.
177. Daynes RA, Araneo BA, Dowell TA et al. Regulation of murine lymphokine production in vivo. III. The lymphoid tissue microenvironment exerts regulatory influences over T helper cell function. J Exp Med 1990; 171:979-96.
178. Strobel S, Mowat AM. Immune responses to dietary antigens: Oral tolerance. Immunol Today 1998; 19:173-81.

179. Strobel S, Mowat AM, Drummond HE et al. Immunological responses to fed protein antigens in mice. 2. Oral tolerance for CMI is due to activation of cyclophosphamide sensitive cells by gut processed antigen. Immunology 1983; 49:451-6.

180. Bruce MG, Ferguson A. Oral tolerance to ovalbumin in mice: Studies of chemically modified and of "biologically filtered" antigen. Immunology 1986; 57:627-30.

181. Bruce MG, Ferguson A. The influence of intestinal processing on the immunogenicity and molecular size of absorbed, circulating ovalbumin in mice. Immunology 1986; 59:295-300.

182. Kay RAF. The immunological consequences of feeding cholera toxin. II. Mechanisms responsible for the induction of oral tolerance for DTH. Immunology 1989; 66:416-21.

183. Peng H-J, Turner MW, Strobel S. The generation of a 'tolerogen' after the ingestion of ovalbumin is time-dependent and unrelated to serum levels of immunoreactive antigen. Clin Exp Immunol 1990; 81:510-15.

184. Furrie E, Turner MW, Strobel S. Partial characterization of a circulating tolerogenic moiety which, after a feed of ovalbumin, suppresses delayed-type hypersensitivity in recipient mice. Immunology 1995; 86:480-6.

185. Karlsson M, Kahu K, Hanson LA et al. 70,000g pellet from serum transfer tolerance: Role of major histocompatibility complex class II. Immunol Letters 1999; 69:87(A).

186. Zitvogel L, Regnault A, Lozier A et al. Eradication of established murine tumors using a novel cell-free vaccine: Dendritic cell-derived exosomes. Nat Med 1998; 4:594-600.

187. Sanderson I, Ouellette AJ, Carter EA et al. Differential regulation of B7 mRNA in enterocytes and lymphoid cells. Immunology 1993; 79:434-8.

188. Thomson AW, Drakes ML, Zahorchak AF et al. Hepatic dendritic cells: Immunobiology and role in liver transplantation. J Leukoc Biol 1999; 66:322-30.

189. Mowat AM. Induction of peripheral tolerance by portal vein administration of antigen. In: Crispe IN, ed. The Immunology of the Liver. New York: John Wiley & Sons Inc., 1999:101-15.

190. Yang R, Liu Q, Grosfeld JL et al. Intestinal drainage through liver is a pre-requisite for oral tolerance induction. J Paediatr Surg 1994; 29:1145-8.

191. Thomas HC, Ryan CJ, Benjamin IS et al. The immune system response in cirrhotic rats. The induction of tolerance to orally administered protein antigens. Gastroenterology 1976; 71(1):114-7.

192. Hershberg RM, Mayer LM. Antigen processing and presentation by intestinal epithelial cells—polarity and complexity. Immunol Today 2000; 21:123-8.

193. Fuchs EJ, Matzinger P. B cells turn off virgin but not memory T cells. Science 1992; 258:1156.

194. Buhlmann JE, Foy TM, Aruffo A et al. In the absence of a CD40 signal, B cells are tolerogenic. Immunity 1995; 2:645-53.

195. Gilbert KM, Weigle WO. B cell presentation of a tolerogenic signal to Th clones. Cell Immunol 1992; 139:58.

196. Jenkins MK, Burrell E, Ashwell JD. Antigen presentation by resting B cells. Effectiveness at inducing T cell proliferation is determined by costimulatory signals, not T cell receptor occupancy. J Immunol 1990; 144:1585.

197. D'Orazio TJ, Niederkorn JY. Splenic B cells are required for tolerogenic antigen presentation in the induction of anterior chamber-associated immune deviation (ACAID). Immunology 1998; 95:47-55.

198. Yoshida H, Hachimura S, Hirahara K et al. Induction of oral tolerance in splenocyte-reconstituted SCID mice. Clin Immunol Immunopathol 1998; 87:282-91.

199. Liu LM, MacPherson GG. Lymph-borne (veiled) dendritic cells can acquire and present intestinally administered antigens. Immunology 1991; 73:281.

200. Williamson E, Westrich GM, Viney JL. Modulating dendritic cells to optimize mucosal immunization protocols. J Immunol 1999; 163:3668-75.

201. Huang FP, Platt N, Wykes M et al. A discrete subpopulation of dendritic cells transports apoptotic intestinal epithelial cells to T cell areas of mesenteric lymph nodes. J Exp Med 2000; 191:435-44.

202. Steinman RM, Turley S, Mellman I et al. The induction of tolerance by dendritic cells that have captured apoptotic cells. J Exp Med 2000; 191:411-6.

203. Ruedl C, Hubele S. Maturation of Peyer's patch dendritic cells in vitro upon stimulation via cytokines or CD40 triggering. Eur J Immunol 1997; 27:1325-30.

204. Kelsall B, Strober W. Distinct populations of dendritic cells are present in the subepithelial dome and T cell regions of the murine Peyer's patch. J Exp Med 1996; 183:237-47.

205. Iwasaki A, Kelsall BL. Mucosal immunity and inflammation. I. Mucosal dendritic cells: Their specialized role in initiating T cell responses. Am J Physiol 1999; 276:G1074-8.

206. Iwasaki A, Kelsall BL. Freshly isolated Peyer's patch, but not spleen, dendritic cells produce interleukin 10 and induce the differentiation of T helper type 2 cells. J Exp Med 1999; 190:229-39.

207. Stumbles PA, Thomas JA, Pimm CL et al. Resting respiratory tract dendritic cells preferentially stimulate helper cell type 2 (Th2) responses and require obligatory cytokine signals for induction of Th1 immunity. J Exp Med 1998; 188:2019-31.

208. Kalinski P, Hilkens CMU, Wierenga EA et al. T-cell priming by type-1 and type-2 polarized dendritic cells: The concept of a third signal. Immunol Today 1999; 20(561-7.).

209. Huang M, Stolina M, Sharma S et al. Non-small cell lung cancer cyclooxygenase-2-dependent regulation of cytokine balance in lymphocytes and macrophages: Up-regulation of interleukin 10 and down-regulation of interleukin 12 production. Cancer Res 1998; 58:1208-16.

210. Khoo UY, Proctor IE, Macpherson AJ. CD4+ T cell down-regulation in human intestinal mucosa: Evidence for intestinal tolerance to luminal bacterialantigens. J Immunol 1997; 158:3626-34.

211. Neish AS, Gewirtz AT, Zeng H et al. Prokaryotic regulation of epithelial responses by inhibition of IkappaB-alpha ubiquitination. Science 2000; 289:1560-3.

212. Gagliardi MC, Sallusto F, Marinaro M et al. Cholera toxin induces maturation of human dendritic cells and licences them for Th2 priming. Eur J Immunol 2000; 30:2394-403.

213. Banchereau J, Briere F, Caux C et al. Immunology of dendritic cells. Ann Rev Immunol 2000; 18:767-811.

214. Harrison LC, Dempsey-Collier M, Kramer DR et al. Aerosol insulin induces regulatory CD8 gd T cells that prevent murine insulin-dependent diabetes. J Exp Med 1996; 184:2167-74.

215. Ma C-G, Zhang G-X, Xiao B-G et al. Suppression of experimental autoimmune myasthenia gravis by nasal administration of acetylcholine receptor. J Neuroimmunol 1995; 58:51-60.

216. Metzler B, Wraith DC. Inhibition of experimental autimmune encephalomyelitis by inhalation but not oral administration of the encephalitogenic peptide: Influence of MHC binding affinity. Int Immunol 1993; 5(9):1159-65.

217. Daniel D, Wegmann DR. Protection of nonobese diabetic mice from diabetics by intranasal or subcutaneous administration of insulin peptide B-(9-23). Proc Natl Acad Sci USA 1996; 93:956-60.

218. Dick AD, Cheng YF, McKinnon A et al. Nasal administration of retinal antigens suppresses the inflammatory response in experimental allergic uveoretinitis. A preliminary report of intranasal induction of tolerance with retinal antigens. Br J Ophthalmol 1993; 77:171-5.

219. Dick AD, Cheng YF, Liversidge J et al. Intranasal administration of retinal antigens suppresses retinal antigen-induced experimental autoimmune uveoretinitis. Immunology 1994; 82:625-31.

220. Staines NA, Harper N, Ward FJ et al. Mucosal tolerance and suppression of collagen-induced arthritis (CIA) induced by nasal inhalation of synthetic peptide 184-198 of bovine type II collagen (CII) expressing a dominant T cell epitope. Clin Exp Immunol 1996; 103:368-75.

221. Al-Sabbagh A, Nelson P, Sobel RA et al. Antigen-driven peripheral immune tolerance: Suppression of experimental autoimmune encephalomyelitis and collagen induced arthritis by aerosol administration of myelin basic protein or type II collagen. Cell Immunol 1996; 171:111-9.

222. Tian J, Atkinson MA, Clare-Salzler M et al. Nasal administration of glutamate decarboxylase (GAD65) peptides induces Th2 repsonses and prevents murine insulin-dependent diabetes. J Exp Med 1996; 183:1561-7.

223. Hoyne GF, O'Hehir RE, Wraith DC et al. Inhibition of T cell and antibody responses to house dust mite allergen by inhalation of the dominant T cell epitope in naive and sensitized mice. J Exp Med 1993; 178:1783-8.

224. D'Orazio TJ, Niederkorn JY. A novel role for TGF-β and IL-10 in the induction of immune privilege. J Immunol 1998; 160:2089-98.

225. Takeuchi M, Alard P, Streilein JW. TGF-β promotes immune deviation by altering accessory signals of antigen-presenting cells. J Immunol 1998; 160:1589-97.

226. Rizzo LV, Miller-Rivero NE, Chan C-C et al. Interleukin-2 treatment potentiates induction of oral tolerance in a murine model of autoimmunity. J Clin Invest 1994; 94:1668-72.

227. Inobe J-I, Slavin AJ, Komagata Y et al. IL-4 is a differentiation factor for transforming growth factor-β secreting Th3 cells and oral administration of IL-4 enhances oral tolerance in experimental allergic encephalomyelitis. Eur J Immunol 1998; 28:2780-90.

228. Elson CO, Dertzbaugh MT. Mucosal Adjuvants. In: Ogra PL, Mestecky J, Lamm ME et al, eds. Mucosal Immunology, 2nd Edition. San Diego: Academic Press 1999:818-38.
229. McGhee JR, Czerkinsky C, Mestecky J. Mucosal vaccines: An overview. In: Ogra PL, Mestecky J, Lamm ME et al, eds. Mucosal Immunology, 2nd ed. San Diego: Academic Press 1999:741-57.
230. Sun JB, Holmgren J, Czerkinsky C. Cholera toxin B subunit: An efficient transmucosal carrier-delivery system for induction of peripheral immunological tolerance. Proc Natl Acad Sci USA 1994; 91:10795-9.
231. Sun JB, Rask C, Olsson T et al. Treatment of experimental autoimmune encephalomyelitis by feeding myelin basic protein conjugated to cholera toxin B subunit. Proc Natl Acad Sci USA 1996; 93:7196-201.
232. Bergerot I, Fioix C, Peterson J et al. A cholera toxoid-insulin conjugate as an oral vaccine against spontaneous autoimmune diabetes. Proc Natl Acad Sci USA 1997; 94:4610-4.
233. Ploix C, Bergerot I, Durand A et al. Oral administration of cholera toxin B-insulin conjugates protects NOD mice from autoimmune diabetes by inducing CD4+ regulatory T-cells. Diabetes 1999; 48:2150-6.
234. Sun J-B, Xiao B-G, Lindblad M et al. Oral administration of cholera toxin B subunit conjugated to myelin basic protein protects against experimental autoimmune encephalomyelitis by inducing TGF-β secreting cells and suppressing chemokine expression. Int Immunol 2000; 12:1449-57.
235. McSorley SJ, Rask C, Pichot R et al. Selective tolerization of Th1-like cells after nasal administration of a cholera toxoid-LACK conjugate. Eur J Immunol 1998; 28:424-32.
236. Czerkinsky C, Anjuere F, McGhee JR et al. Mucosal immunity and tolerance: Relevance to vaccine development. Immunol Rev 1999; 170:197-222.
237. Williams NA, Hirst TR, Nashar TO. Immune modulation by the cholera-like enterotoxins: From adjuvant to therapeutic. Immunol Today 1999; 20:95-101.
238. O'Dowd AM, Botting CH, Precious B et al. Novel modifications to the C-terminus of LTB that facilitate site-directed chemical coupling of antigens and the development of LTB as a carrier for mucosal vaccines. Vaccine 1999; 17:1442-53.
239. Lencer WI, Hirst TR, Holmes RK. Membrane traffic and the cellular uptake of cholera toxin. Biochim Biophys Acta 1999; 1450:177-90.
240. Mowat AM, Ferguson,A. Hypersensitivity in the small intestinal mucosa. V. Induction of cell mediated immunity to a dietary antigen. Clin Exp Immunol 1981; 43:574-82.
241. Mowat AM. Depletion of suppressor T cells by 2'-deoxyguanosine abrogates tolerance in mice fed ovalbumin and permits the induction of intestinal delayed-type-hypersensitivity. Immunology 1986; 58:179-84.
242. Mowat AM. The immunopathogenesis of food sensitive enteropathies. In: Newby TJ, Stokes CR, eds. Local Immune Responses of the Gut. Boca Raton: CRC Press 1984:199-225.
243. Bhan AK, Mizoguchi E, Smith RN et al. Colitis in transgenic and knockout animals as models of human inflammatory bowel disease. Immunol Rev 1999; 169:195-207.
244. Groux H, Powrie F. Regulatory T cells in inflammatory bowel disease. Immunol Today 1999; 20:442-6.
245. Groux H, O'Garra A, Bigler M et al. A CD4+ T-cell subset inhibits antigen-specific T-cell responses and prevents colitis. Nature 1997; 389:737-42.
246. Neurath MF, Fuss I, Kelsall BL et al. Antibodies to IL-12 abrogate established experimental colitis in mice. J Exp Med 1995; 182:1281-90.

CHAPTER 3

A Revisit of Current Dogma for the Cellular and Molecular Basis of Oral Tolerance

Kohtaro Fujihashi, Hirotomo Kato and Jerry R. McGhee

Abstract

Studies of the cellular and molecular mechanisms for oral tolerance have focused on the central importance of CD4[+] T cells and their surface co-stimulatory molecules as well as derived cytokines. In addition γδ T cells play critical roles in the induction of mucosally (orally and nasally) induced systemic unresponsiveness. In order to understand the precise mechanisms of regulation of induction of oral tolerance, the investigation of the cell intranet among immune competent cells in mucosal sites will be necessary in order to provide further information for our understanding of this fertile field of investigation.

We have revisited the established notion that oral tolerance should be defined as suppression of Ag-specific systemic immune responses in the presence of mucosal S-IgA Ab responses by using oral immunization regimen (antigen plus CT as mucosal adjuvant) which can induce both systemic and mucosal immune responses. Our results clearly support the new concept that oral tolerance which results from oral delivery of protein Ag simultaneously elicits a state of systemic and mucosal immune unresponsiveness to subsequent encounters with the same Ag. A new model system has been developed to assess the cellular and molecular mechanisms of orally induced unresponsiveness in both the systemic and mucosal immune compartments.

A novel requirement for Peyer's patches in the induction of oral tolerance was also revealed in recent studies. Studies in Peyer's patch-null mice showed a lack of OVA-specific oral tolerance and clearly indicated that GALT provides the necessary environment for downregulatory responses to ingested protein antigens. Since in utero treatment only affected Peyer's patches but not other mucosa-associated lymph nodes, use of this LTβR-Ig-treated mouse model will provide essential information for understanding the cellular and molecular mechanisms of Peyer's patches in the induction of oral tolerance.

Introduction

Oral tolerance is a unique immune reaction characterized by the fact that experimental animals fed large quantities of protein antigen (Ag) become refractory or have a diminished capacity to develop an immune response when re-exposed to that same Ag introduced by the systemic route (e.g., by injection).[1-5] This unique response appears to be an important natural physiological mechanism whereby the host avoids development of cell mediated immunity (CMI) or delayed type hypersensitivity (DTH) and formation of potentially harmful antibodies (Abs), i.e., IgE to many ingested food proteins and similar antigens.[2] For example, inhibition of antigen-specific immune responses in both the systemic and/or mucosal immune

Oral Tolerance: The Response of the Intestinal Mucosa to Dietary Antigens,
edited by Olivier Morteau. ©2004 Eurekah.com and Kluwer Academic / Plenum Publishers.

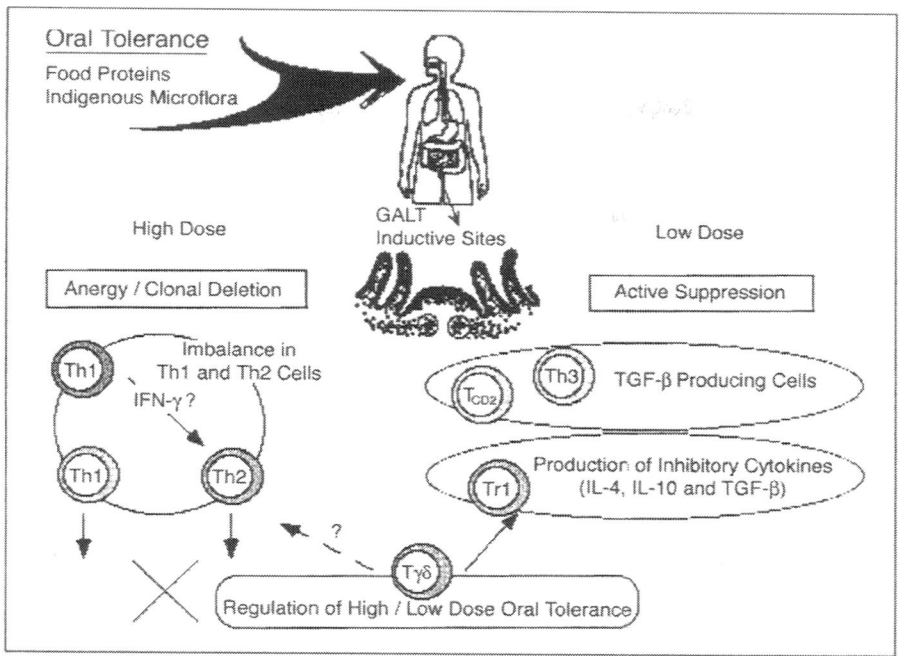

Figure 1. It is now generally agreed that mucosally induced tolerance is established and maintained at the level of T cells. Oral tolerance is possibly associated with selective downregulation of Th1 cells. These T cells may be more sensitive to tolerance induction by Th2 cells via their respective cytokines in systemic sites. However, our recent studies have suggested that both Th1 and Th2 cell subsets are involved in the induction of oral tolerance. In addition, it has been shown that TGF-β-producing CD4[+] or CD8[+] T cells (or Th3 cells) play important roles for inducing unresponsiveness and inhibiting experimental autoimmune diseases. It was recently proposed that Tr1 cells downregulate systemic immune responses through production of cytokines such as IL-10. Finally, γδ T cells also play important roles in oral tolerance induction as well as mucosal IgA regulation, in addition to CD4[+] αβ T cells.

T cell proliferative responses in an Ag-specific manner (Fig. 1).[36] Of relevance, Tr1 cells were shown to prevent the development of T cell-dependent inflammatory bowel disease in a murine model of colitis.[36] These results suggest that Tr1 cells produce IL-10 whose net effect appears to be downregulation of CMI or DTH responses mediated by Th1-type cells. In addition to IL-10, a recent study showed that monocyte chemotactic protein (MCP)-1, a CC chemokine, enhanced Th2-type cytokine responses when transgenic T cells were stimulated via the TCR-CD3 complex.[37] In this regard, it appeared that MCP-1, like IL-10 in other studies, played an immunoregulatory role in oral tolerance by inhibition of Th1-type responses.[38] From this brief summary, it now appears that Th2-type cytokines and related chemokines possess potential regulatory functions for the induction of low dose oral tolerance.

Some confusion currently exists on the potential role of Th1 cell-derived IFN-γ in oral tolerance. Our previous studies showed that CD4[+] T cells isolated shortly after delivery of a high oral dose of OVA resulted in OVA-specific CD4[+] Th1 cells producing IFN-γ. This subset may contribute to downregulation of Th2 cells and cytokines for B cell and Ab responses and may explain why serum IgG Abs are usually reduced in oral tolerance. Of interest was the finding that IFN-γ knockout (IFN-γ[-/-]) mice, when given a large oral dose of OVA, manifested normal serum IgG anti-OVA Ab responses.[39] Others have also shown that splenic T cells from mice orally tolerized with OVA also produce OVA-specific IFN-γ.[40] Interestingly, this T cell subset may arise in the Peyer's patches themselves since repeated high oral doses of OVA given to OVA TCR-transgenic mice resulted in a dominant CD4$^+$ Th1 cell subset producing IFN-γ in this site.[41]

The precise mechanisms whereby IFN-γ regulates mucosally induced tolerance is not yet known; however, it is well established that IFN-γ contributes to inhibition of IL-4-producing, Th2-type cells which themselves tend to favor production of IgG B cell and Ab responses. In addition, a recent study pointed to the importance of IFN-γ induced by oral OVA with a reduction in DTH responses in normal BALB/c mice adoptively transferred with T cells derived from DO11.10 x RAG-1$^{-/-}$ transgenic mice. Thus, IFN-γ clearly played an important role in reducing the migration of T cells into skin areas where DTH responses occur.[42] In contrast to the above studies, others have used mice depleted of IFN-γ by mAb treatment, or IFN-γ receptor$^{-/-}$ or p40 IL-12$^{-/-}$ mice to show that oral tolerance develops normally.[43,44] These seemingly contradictory results may be reconciled by suggesting that an early event in oral tolerance induction involves CD4$^+$ Th1 cell production of IFN-γ, which influences later events such as Th2-type T cell development. In the absence of IFN-γ or IFN-γ R pathways, the mouse would undergo CD4$^+$ Th2-type tolerance through direct effects on this cell type. Thus, Th1-type cells may not be more sensitive to oral tolerance after all and may initially downregulate Th2-type responses (Fig. 1).

Involvement of Co-Stimulatory Molecules in Oral Tolerance

Signalling via the TCR alone in the absence of co-stimulation is thought to be of central importance in tolerance induction. In this regard, a recent study reported that selective blockade of B7-CTLA-4 interactions completely inhibited systemic tolerance induced by a high dose of Ag.[45] In addition, monoclonal anti-CD86 Ab but not anti-CD80 mAb treatment failed to induce low dose oral tolerance.[46] Further, blockade of CD40L-CD40 interactions by anti-CD40 ligand (L) mAb resulted in T cell tolerance to the hapten 2, 4, 6 dinitrofluorobenzene sulfonic acid (TNBS) as manifested by reduced TNBS contact hypersensitivity.[47] In support of this, it has been shown that anergic Th1-type cells express reduced levels of CD40L.[48] To explore a possible role for co-stimulatory signals transduced by the CD40L-CD40 interactions for induction of oral tolerance, CD40L$^{-/-}$ and CD40L$^{+/+}$ mice were given a high dose of OVA by the oral route. As one might expect, oral administration of 25 mg of OVA to CD40L$^{+/+}$ mice resulted in the induction of systemic T cell unresponsiveness where OVA-specific DTH and proliferative responses as well as Th1- and Th2-type cytokine synthesis were reduced in splenic CD4$^+$ T cells, when compared to those of mice given oral PBS only. In contrast, when the same experimental protocol was performed in CD40L$^{-/-}$ mice, OVA-specific systemic T cells developed and were fully responsive to OVA.[49] These findings indicate that the co-stimulatory signals transduced via the CD40L-CD40 interaction serve an important role in the induction of systemic T cell unresponsiveness following oral administration of a high dose of protein Ag. One possible mechanism for loss of oral tolerance is that interruption of CD40L-CD40 signalling leads to a subsequent loss of negative signals generated by interactions between CD86 and CTLA-4 in CD40L$^{-/-}$ mice. In support of this notion, previous studies have demonstrated that CD40L and CD40 interactions are involved in the regulation of CD80/CD86 expression by APCs.[50] In addition, the interaction of CD80/CD86 and CTLA-4 provide negative signals for the inhibition of activated T cells.[51,52] A lack of oral tolerance in CD40L$^{-/-}$ mice suggests that the interactions between CD40L and CD40 are necessary for the expression of CD80/CD86 molecules which affect T cell activation or unresponsiveness; however, the relationship between T cell activation and unresponsiveness as determined by CD28 or CTLA-4 engagement of CD80/CD86 molecules remains to be defined.

TGF-β Producing T Cells in Oral Tolerance

It is well established that TGF-β is a key cytokine for the induction of low-dose oral tolerance.[23] For example, the Peyer's patches of OVA-Tg mice given a high oral dose of OVA manifested increased production of TGF-β.[41,53] Interestingly, it was also shown that TGF-β plays a key role in the induction of mucosal unresponsiveness when STAT4 or STAT6 signaling cascades were absent.[54] Oral administration of MBP induced TGF-β-producing, CD8[+] T cells (Fig. 1),[22,23,31,55] which inhibited MBP-specific immune responses. These TGF-β-producing, CD8[+] T cells were found in Peyer's patches 24-48 hrs following oral administration of MBP, indicating that they were initially induced in the GALT itself.[3] It could be suggested that these GALT-derived T cells migrate to systemic sites and mediate active bystander suppression. Thus, T cells from MBP-fed mice suppressed OVA-specific responses when restimulated with MBP in vitro, whereas T cells from OVA-fed mice inhibited MBP responses after restimulation with the fed antigen.[56] Induction of active suppression was dependent upon antigen dosage and frequency of feeding (e.g., low dose oral tolerance).[24] MBP-specific T cell lines derived from patients with multiple sclerosis who had been orally treated with MBP daily for two years also provided evidence for the presence of MBP-specific, TGF-β-producing T cells.[55] When co-production of Th1 (IFN-γ) or Th2 (IL-4) cytokines was examined, the majority of antigen-specific TGF-β-producing T cells did not produce either IFN-γ or IL-4.[57] Thus, it was suggested that these unique subsets of T cells should be termed Th3 cells since oral administration of MBP induced a TGF-β-secreting subset of T cells which appeared to be responsible for the generation of oral tolerance. However, a recent study in TGF-β1[-/-] mice demonstrated that this cytokine was not essential for the induction of low- or high-dose oral tolerance.[55] To further address the potential role of TGF-β in oral tolerance, it will be essential to assess the levels of TGF-β at various time points, as well as the major T cell subsets which produce this cytokine and their tissue locale in mice fed low or high doses of Ag.

A Distinct Role for γδ T Cells in Low Dose Oral Tolerance

Most investigators agree that a subset of regulatory T cells in mucosa-associated tissues plays an important role in maintaining Ag-specific mucosal IgA Ab responses in the presence of systemic unresponsiveness (Fig. 1). It is well established that mucosal immune compartments such as the intestinal epithelium contain large numbers of γδ T cells in addition to αβ T cells,[58] as does the lamina propria region of the small intestine.[59] Since γδ T cells are localized in the mucosa-associated tissues, one could hypothesize that mucosal γδ T cells may be involved in maintenance of antigen-specific IgA Ab responses in the presence of systemic unresponsiveness following oral administration of Ags. To test this possibility, intraepithelial lymphocyte (IEL) T cells from mice immunized orally with sheep erythrocytes (SRBC) were separated into γδ and αβ T cell fractions. When purified γδ and αβ T cells were adoptively transferred to mice orally tolerized with SRBC, a conversion of systemic unresponsiveness to systemic IgM, IgG and IgA anti-SRBC Ab responses was achieved in mice that received γδ but not αβ T cells.[60] Recent studies have also implied that γδ T cells isolated from mucosa-associated tissues of mice immunized orally with the Escherichia coli labile toxin B subunit (LT-B) exhibit the ability to abrogate oral tolerance. Thus, IEL γδ T cells from LT-B-fed mice (which were tolerized) abrogated systemic unresponsiveness following adoptive transfer to syngeneic mice orally tolerized with LT-B.[61] Thus, γδ T cells appear to be important in the maintenance of appropriate immunological homeostasis in the GI tract.

To directly address the role of γδ T cells in mucosal immunity and tolerance, genetically-induced, mutant mice, which do not possess γδ T cells have been used to evaluate mucosal IgA immunity and oral tolerance. In addition, studies by others have shown that γδ T cells are essential for the induction of oral tolerance using mAb anti- γδ TCR treated and TCRδ[-/-] mice.[62] In marked contrast, it has been shown that γδ T cells are not essential for the induction of aerosol-induced IgE unresponsiveness to OVA.[63] In addition, the results of our separate study indicate that $\gamma\delta$ T cell involvement in oral tolerance depends upon the dose of oral Ag used. For example, $\gamma\delta$ T cells were not required for systemic B or T cell unresponsiveness to high doses of orally administered Ag.[64] In contrast, low oral doses of protein induce $\gamma\delta$ T cells which regulated the production of IL-10 by CD4$^+$ T cells in normal mice (Fig. 1). Interestingly, this pathway was absent in TCR$\delta^{-/-}$ mice, and low dose oral tolerance was absent.[64] This Ag dose-dependent regulatory $\gamma\delta$ T cell dichotomy provides an interesting paradox with regard to the functions of IEL $\gamma\delta$ T cells in response to oral Ag. The sentinel location and increased numbers of $\gamma\delta$ T cells in the intestinal epithelium intuitively suggests a significant role in immune responses to orally administered Ags. Their absence has been associated with a loss of certain epithelial cell functions[65] and to diminishing mucosal IgA responses to oral Ags.[66] The absence of the $\gamma\delta$ T cell subset would therefore be expected to influence the immunologic homeostasis involved in mucosally induced hyporesponsiveness, and our findings indeed indicate compromised oral tolerance in TCR$\delta^{-/-}$ mice given relatively low doses of OVA. This study further demonstrated that $\gamma\delta$ T cells are able to upregulate IL-10 synthesis in TCR$\delta^{+/+}$ mice tolerized with low oral Ag doses. This finding provides direct evidence that $\gamma\delta$ T cells regulate IL-10 synthesis by CD4$^+$ T cells for the induction of low-dose oral tolerance. These results also confirm studies in which $\gamma\delta$ T cells were shown to regulate the induction and maintenance of systemic tolerance to Ags administered via oral,[62,67] respiratory mucosa[68] or portal venous routes.[69,70]

A Revisit of the Notion of Concomitant Systemic Unresponsiveness and Mucosal IgA Immunity

Mucosal Immune Responses in the Presence of Oral Tolerance

Approximately 20 years ago it was shown that oral administration of a streptococcal Ag or ovalbumin (OVA) to mice simultaneously resulted in suppression of Ag-specific systemic immune responses in the presence of salivary secretory IgA (S-IgA) Ab responses.[4] This dual state of systemic unresponsiveness and mucosal S-IgA immunity was dubbed oral tolerance.[1,4] Most studies in this area have tended to focus on systemic unresponsiveness after oral delivery and assume that mucosal S-IgA Abs are concurrently induced. Oral tolerance experiments have essentially been performed by initially feeding a protein Ag followed by systemic immunization with the same Ag given in complete Freund's adjuvant (CFA). In these experiments, a decline in serum IgG and IgE Ab responses together with diminished T cell responses are considered to be the hallmarks of oral tolerance.[5,71] This mode of systemic immunization with Ag with the potent adjuvant CFA does not allow one to determine if tolerance extends to the mucosal compartment as well. It is now well established that parenteral immunization elicits systemic immunity in the absence of mucosal immune responses, and thus one cannot evaluate oral tolerance at the level of the GI tract mucosa.[72] It has been shown that oral tolerance cannot be established and Ag-specific mucosal IgA Ab responses are normally induced when oral proteins are given with cholera toxin (CT) as a mucosal adjuvant.[73,74] Based on these studies, mucosal immunization strategies using adjuvants such as CT and the related *Escherichia coli* labile toxin (LT) have been developed.[72] One of the advantages of mucosal immunization is that this mode can elicit both systemic and mucosal immune responses.[72] In addition, this strategy also provides a unique way to address the mechanisms of induction and regulation of mucosal immune responses as manifested by S-IgA Ab production.

Oral tolerance has continued to be defined as systemic unresponsiveness with the maintenance of mucosal Ab responses. This finding preceded our knowledge that mucosal adjuvants such as CT or LT can prevent oral tolerance induction and induce potent mucosal IgA and systemic immune responses. Therefore, it was important to revisit this notion and to determine if oral tolerance also influences mucosal immune responses, since oral tolerance has been mainly assessed by parenteral boosting with Ag in CFA. Further, studies should address whether potent mucosal adjuvants such as CT can reverse existing oral tolerance and induce both systemic and mucosal Ab responses. To this end, our most recent study addressed these two important issues by gastric administration of OVA followed by an oral immunization protocol with OVA and CT as mucosal adjuvant. We have shown that a single high oral dose of OVA downregulates both systemic and mucosal immune responses as assessed by a novel oral immunization strategy using OVA and CT as mucosal adjuvant.[75] OVA-specific serum IgG, especially IgG1 subclass and IgA Ab responses were diminished in OVA-fed mice when compared with mice given oral PBS. Further, the numbers of OVA-specific IgG and IgA antibody forming cells (AFC) in spleen were also dramatically reduced by OVA feeding prior to oral immunization. Of equal importance, mucosal IgA anti-OVA Abs were also reduced in OVA-fed mice subsequently challenged with OVA plus CT as mucosal adjuvant.[75] The most direct test of the hypothesis that oral OVA would diminish mucosal IgA immunity came from studies which assessed IgA AFC in the gastrointestinal (GI) tract. Dramatically reduced OVA- but normal CT-B-specific AFC were seen in the intestinal lamina propria of mice fed OVA when compared with PBS-fed mice. Significant reductions in CD4[+] T cell proliferative responses and Th2-type cytokine production were also observed in mice fed OVA prior to oral immunization with OVA and CT as mucosal adjuvant. Further, CD4[+] T cells from Peyer's patches of OVA-fed mice subsequently orally immunized with OVA plus CT exhibited unresponsiveness to OVA, while Peyer's patch CD4[+] T cell from PBS-fed mice showed significant OVA-specific proliferative and Th2-type cytokine responses.[75] These results indicate that oral administration of a soluble protein Ag blocks the induction of mucosal immune responses, including CD4[+] T cell responses as well as IgA Ab production in the gastrointestinal tract. Further, a single high dose feeding of protein Ag induces a state of Ag-specific immune unresponsiveness in mucosal compartments, indicating that CT does not break already established oral tolerance either in mucosal or systemic immune compartments.

The Role of Peyer's Patches in Oral Tolerance Induction

The Peyer's patches or GALT have been mainly viewed as major mucosal inductive sites for the generation of Ag-specific, mucosal IgA responses. Nevertheless, the GALT may also be an important site for dispatching immune suppressive signals to continuously ingested antigens. Oral tolerance (or systemic unresponsiveness) represents the most common and important response of the host to environmental antigens, including food and commensal bacterial components, for the maintenance of an appropriate immunological homeostasis. It is also important to consider that induction of mucosal and systemic immunity by oral immunization with protein antigen alone is rather difficult and requires use of potent mucosal adjuvants, vectors or other special delivery systems. Thus, it is logical to consider that Peyer's patches would play a more important role in the maintenance of oral tolerance in normal situations, instead of induction of Ag-specific IgA Ab responses (Fig. 2).

The importance of lymphotoxin (LT) signaling pathways in lymphoid tissue development has been studied by using both LT-α and LT-β gene disrupted mice. LT-α knockout mice do not possess Peyer's patches or associated lymph nodes.[76,77] Mice without LT-β gene expression lack Peyer's patches and peripheral lymph nodes, but possess mesenteric, sacral and cervical lymph nodes.[78-80] Recent studies have used LTβ receptor (LTβR) gene knockout mice to block the LTβR signaling pathway,[81] soluble LTβR-immunoglobulin (Ig) fusion protein as a treatment,[82] and an agonist antibody to the LTβR.[83] All these studies resulted in the aberrant development of peripheral lymphoid tissues. Administration of LTβR-Ig during gestation also

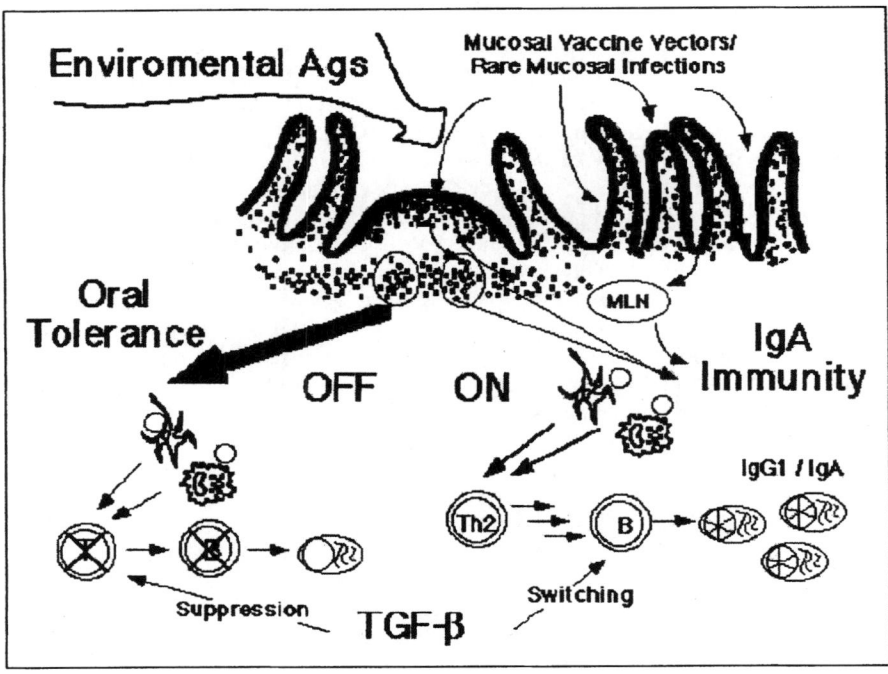

Figure 2. The importance of gut-associated lymphoreticular tissues (GALT) as inductive sites for mucosally induced tolerance or mucosal IgA immunity is illustrated here. The host responds to the constant bombardment by food proteins or indigenous flora proteins by development of systemic unresponsiveness. High oral doses lead to anergy or clonal deletion, while lower doses elicit active suppression. In deliberate oral vaccination, use of mucosal adjuvants such as cholera toxin may induce CD4+ Th2-type cells for mucosal S-IgA and systemic IgG1 Ab responses. Live, recombinant viruses or bacteria such as Salmonella may induce CD4+ Th1-type responses for systemic IgG2a Abs and CD4+ Th cells producing IL-5, IL-6 and IL-10 for mucosal S-IgA Ab responses.

disrupted the development of peripheral lymph nodes and Peyer's patches; however, mesenteric, sacral and cervical lymph nodes remained intact.[82,84] Thus, the LTβR-Ig fusion protein system provides a unique and useful model to elucidate the role of Peyer's patches in the induction of oral tolerance.

In order to precisely address the role of Peyer's patches in the induction of oral tolerance, mice which lack Peyer's patches, but which possess brachial, cervical, mesenteric and sacral lymph nodes have been generated by administration of LTβR-Ig fusion protein to pregnant mice in utero. The immune responses in offspring of LTβR-Ig fusion protein-treated (Peyer's patch-null) and control mice given high oral doses of OVA prior to systemic challenge were examined. In marked contrast to low OVA-specific IgG Ab responses in serum and spleen of normal mice fed OVA, significant Ab responses were seen in Peyer's patch-null mice given oral OVA.[85] Further, high T cell proliferative and DTH responses were seen in Peyer's patch-null mice given oral OVA before systemic challenge.[82] Higher levels of CD4+ T cell-derived IFN-γ, IL-4, IL-5 and IL-10 synthesis were noted in Peyer's patch-null mice fed OVA, while OVA fed, normal mice had suppressed cytokine levels.[85]

These findings show that organized Peyer's patches are required for oral tolerance to proteins. To support this view, it has been shown that germ-free mice possessed a profound hypotropy of Peyer's patches,[86] and these mice do not elicit systemic unresponsiveness when fed sheep red blood cells for prolonged periods.[87] Furthermore, it was shown that the absence of IgA Abs in mother's milk, in addition to a lack of passive immunity for protection, accelerated the development of Peyer's patches in the neonate,[88] perhaps due to the induction of tolerance to environmental antigens which can easily invade the intestinal epithelium. Nevertheless, it seems that Peyer's patches possess important dual functions for the induction of IgA Ab responses and tolerance. Indeed, TGF-β in Peyer's patches has been shown to play a central role in isotype switching of surface IgM to IgA B cells,[89,90] and this same cytokine has been detected in Peyer's patches as a key factor in the induction of oral tolerance (Fig. 2).[44,53] Although Peyer's patches possess dual functions in the induction of mucosal immunity and oral tolerance, it seems that establishment of oral tolerance by protein antigens is more dependent on the presence of organized GALT. Thus, it has been shown that intact mucosal IgA responses were induced in Peyer's patch-null mice orally immunized with OVA and CT as mucosal adjuvant.[91] Further support for a requirement of GALT in oral tolerance induction was provided by in vivo treatment with flt3 ligand. This treatment resulted in an expansion of dendritic cells in Peyer's patches with enhanced oral tolerance induction.[92] Taken together, these findings indicate that GALT provides necessary downregulatory signals in order to induce systemic unresponsiveness.

Acknowledgments

We thank Ms. Sheila D. Turner for the final preparation of this manuscript. This work is supported by U.S. Public Health Service Grants AI 35932, DE 09837, AI 18958, DK 44240, AI 43197, DE 12242, P30 DK 54781 and contracts AI 65298 and AI 65299.

References

1. Tomasi TB, Jr. Oral tolerance. Transplantation 1980; 29:353-356.
2. Mowat AM. The regulation of immune responses to dietary protein antigens. Immunol Today 1987; 8:93-98.
3. Weiner HL, Friedman A, Miller A et al. Oral tolerance: Immunologic mechanisms and treatment of animal and human organ-specific autoimmune diseases by oral administration of autoantigens. Annu Rev Immunol 1994; 12:809-837.
4. Challacombe SJ, Tomasi TB Jr. Systemic tolerance and secretory immunity after oral immunization. J Exp Med 1980; 152:1459-1472.
5. Mowat AM, Weiner HL. Oral tolerance: Physiological basis and clinical applications. In: Ogra PL, et al, eds. Mucosal Immunology. San Diego: Academic Press 1998:587-618.
6. Mayer L. Oral tolerance: New approaches, new problems. Clin Immunol 2000; 94:1-8.
7. Wardrop RM 3rd, Whitacre CC. Oral tolerance in the treatment of inflammatory autoimmune diseases. Inflamm Res 1999; 48:106-119.
8. MacDonald TT. T cell immunity to oral allergens. Curr Opin Immunol 1998; 10:620-627.
9. Holt PG. Mucosal immunity in relation to the development of oral tolerance/sensitization. Allergy 1998; 53:16-19.
10. Strobel S, Mowat AM. Immune responses to dietary antigens: oral tolerance. Immunol Today 1998; 19:173-181.
11. Strober W, Kelsall B, Marth B. Oral tolerance. J Clin Immunol 1998; 18:1-30.
12. Fujihashi K, McGhee JR, Yamamoto M et al. Role of γδ T cells in the regulation of mucosal IgA response and oral tolerance. Ann New York Acad Sci 1996; 778:55-63.
13. Thomas HC, Parrott MV. The induction of tolerance to a soluble protein antigen by oral administration. Immunology 1974; 27:631-639.

14. Kagnoff MF. Effects of antigen-feeding on intestinal and systemic immune responses. IV. Similarity between the suppressor factor in mice after erythrocyte-lysate injection and erythrocyte feeding. Gastroenterology 1980; 79:4-61.

15. Kiyono H, Babb JL, Michalek SM et al. Cellular basis for elevated IgA responses in C3H/HeJ mice. J Immunol 1980; 125:732-737.

16. Kiyono H, McGhee JR, Wannemuehler MJ et al. Lack of oral tolerance in C3H/HeJ mice. J Exp Med 1982; 155:605-610.

17. Mattingly JA, Waksman BH. Immunologic suppression after oral administration of antigen. I. Specific suppressor cells formed in rat Peyer's patches after oral administration of sheep erythrocytes and their systemic migration. J Immunol 1978; 121:1878-1883.

18. Mowat AM, Lamont AG, Parrott DM. Suppressor T cells, antigen-presenting cells and the role of I-J restriction in oral tolerance to ovalbumin. Immunology 1988; 64:141-145.

19. Richman LK, Graeff AS, Yarchoan R et al. Simultaneous induction of antigen-specific IgA helper T cells and IgG suppressor T cells in the murine Peyer's patch after protein feeding. J Immunol 1981; 126:2079-2083.

20. Ngan J, Kind LS. Suppressor T cells for IgE and IgG in Peyer's patches of mice made tolerant by the oral administration of ovalbumin. J Immunol 1978; 120:861-865.

21. Chen Y, Inobe J, Marks R et al. Peripheral deletion of antigen-reactive T cells in oral tolerance. Nature 1995; 376:177-180.

22. Chen Y, Inobe J, Weiner HL. Induction of oral tolerance to myelin basic protein in CD8-depletion mice: both CD4$^+$ and CD8$^+$ cells mediate active suppression. J Immunol 1995; 155:910-916.

23. Khoury SJ, Hancock WW, Weiner HL. Oral tolerance to myelin basic protein and natural recovery from experimental autoimmune encephalomyelitis are associated with downregulation of inflammatory cytokines and differential upregulation of transforming growth factor β, interleukin 4, and prostaglandin E expression in the brain. J Exp Med 1992; 176:1355-1364.

24. Friedman A, Weiner HL. Induction of anergy or active suppression following oral tolerance is determined by antigen dosage. Proc Natl Acad Sci USA 1994; 91:6688-6692.

25. Whitacre CC, Gienapp IE, Orosz CG et al. Oral tolerance in experimental autoimmune encephalomyelitis III. Evidence for clonal anergy. J Immunol 1991; 147:2155-2163.

26. Melamed D, Friedman A. Direct evidence for anergy in T lymphocytes tolerized by oral administration of ovalbumin. Eur J Immunol 1993; 23:935-942.

27. Garside P, Steel M, Worthey EA et al. T helper 2 cells are subject to high dose oral tolerance and are not essential for its induction. J Immunol 1995; 154:5649-5655.

28. Gregerson DS, Obritsch WF, Donoso LA. Oral tolerance in experimental autoimmune uveoretinitis. Distinct mechanisms of resistance are induced by low dose vs. high dose feeding protocols. J Immunol 1993; 151:5751-5761.

29. Hirahara K, Hisatsune T, Nishijima K et al. CD4$^+$ T cells anergized by high dose feeding establish oral tolerance to antibody responses when transferred in SCID and nude mice. J Immunol 1995; 154:6238-6245.

30. Melamed D, Friedman A. In vivo tolerization of Th1 lymphocyte following a single feeding with ovalbumin: anergy in the absence of suppression. Eur J Immunol 1994; 24:1974-1981.

31. Miller A, Lider O, Roberts AB et al. Suppressor T cells generated by oral tolerization to myelin basic protein suppress both in vitro and in vivo immune responses by the release of transforming growth factor β after antigen-specific triggering. Proc Natl Acad Sci USA 1992; 89:421-425.

32. Schwartz RH. A cell culture model for T lymphocyte clonal anergy. Science 1990; 248:1349-1356.

33. DeSilva DR, Urdahl KB, Jenkins MK. Clonal anergy is induced in vitro by T cell receptor occupancy in the absence of proliferation. J Immunol 1991; 147:3261-3267.

34. Williams ME, Lichtman AH, Abbas AK. Anti-CD3 antibody induces unresponsiveness to IL-2 in Th1 clones but not in Th2 clones. J Immunol 1990; 144:1208-1214.

35. Burstein HJ, Abbas AK. In vivo role of interleukin 4 in T cell tolerance induced by aqueous protein antigen. J Exp Med 1990; 177:457-463.

36. Groux H, O'Garra A, Bigler M et al. A CD4$^+$ T-cell subset inhibits antigen-specific T-cell responses and prevents colitis. Nature 1997; 389:737-742.

37. Karpus WJ, Lukacs NW, Kennedy KJ et al. Differential CC chemokine-inducedenhancement of T helper cell cytokine production. J Immunol 1997; 158:4129-4136.

38. Karpus WJ, Kennedy KJ, Kunkel SL et al. Monocyte chemotactic protein 1 regulates oral tolerance induction by inhibition of T helper cell 1-related cytokines. J Exp Med 1998; 187:733-741.

39. Kweon MN, Fujihashi K, VanCott JL et al. The role of Th1 cells in tolerance: Lack of mucosally-induced unresponsiveness in interferon-gamma knockout mice. J Immunol 1998; 160:1687-1693.

40. Mowat AM, Steel M, Worthey EA et al. Inactivation of Th1 and Th2 cells by feeding ovalbumin. In: Weiner HL and Mayer LF, eds. Oral tolerance: Mechanisms and applications. Ann N Y Acad Sci 1996; 778:122-132.

41. Marth T, Strober W, Kelsall BL. High dose oral tolerance in ovalbumin TCR-transgenic mice: Systemic neutralization of IL-12 augments TGF-β secretion and T cell apoptosis. J Immunol 1996; 157:2348-2357.

42. Lee HO, Miller SD, Hurst SD et al. Interferon gamma induction during oral tolerance reduces T-cell migration to sites of inflammation. Gastroenterology 2000; 119:129-138.

43. Kjerrulf M, Grdic D, Ekman L et al. Interferon-γ receptor-deficient mice exhibit impaired gut mucosal immune responses but intact oral tolerance. Immunology 1997; 92:60-68.

44. Mowat AM, Steel M, Leishman AJ et al. Normal induction of oral tolerance in the absence of a functional IL-12-dependent IFN-γ signaling pathway. J Immunol 1999; 163:4728-4736.

45. Samoilova EB, Horton JL, Zhang H et al. CTLA-4 is required for the induction of high dose oral tolerance. Intern Immunol 1998; 10:491-498.

46. Liu L, Kuchroo VK, Weiner HL. B7.2 (CD86) but B7.1 (CD80) costimulation is required for the induction of low dose oral tolerance. J Immunol 1999; 163:2284-2290.

47. Tang A, Judge TA, Turka LA. Blockade of CD40-CD40 ligand pathway induces tolerance in murine contact hypersensitivity. Eur J Immunol 1997; 27:3143-3150.

48. Bowen F, Haluskey J, Quill H. Altered CD40 ligand induction in tolerant T lymphocytes. Eur J Immunol 1995; 25:2830-2834.

49. Kweon MN, Fujihashi K, Wakatsuki Y et al. Mucosally induced systemic T cell unresponsiveness to ovalbumin requires CD40 ligand-CD40 interactions. J Immunol 1999; 162:1904-1909.

50. Ranheim EA, Kipps TJ. Activated T cells induce expression of B7/BB1 on normal or leukemic B cells through a CD40-dependent signal. J Exp Med 1993; 177:925-935.

51. Krummel MF, Allison JP. CD28 and CTLA-4 have opposing effects on the response of T cells to stimulation. J Exp Med 1995; 182:459-465.

52. Perez VL, Van Parijs L, Biuckians A et al. Induction of peripheral T cell tolerance in vivo requires CTLA-4 engagement. Immunity 1997; 6:411-417.

53. Gonnella PA, Chen Y, Inobe J et al. In situ immune response in gut-associated lymphoid tissue (GALT) following oral antigen in TCR-transgenic mice. J Immunol 1998; 160:4708-4718.

54. Shi HN, Grusby MJ, Nagler-Anderson C. Orally induced preipheral nonresponsiveness is maintained in the absence of functional Th1 and Th2 cells. J Immunol 1999; 162:5143-5148.

55. Lider O, Santos LM, Lee CS et al. Suppression of experimental autoimmune encephalomyelitis by oral administration of myelin basic protein II. Suppression of disease and in vitro immune responses is mediated by antigen-specific CD8⁺ T lymphocytes. J Immunol 1989; 142:748-752.

56. Miller A, Lider O, Weiner HL. Antigen-driven bystander suppression after oral administration of antigens. J Exp Med 1991; 174:791-798.

57. Fukaura H, Kent SC, Pietrusewicz MJ et al. Induction of circulating myelin basic protein and proteolipid protein-specific transforming growth factor-β1-secreting Th3 T cells by oral administration of myelin in multiple sclerosis patients. J Clin Invest 1996; 98:70-77.

58. Kiyono H, McGhee JR. Mucosal Immunology: Intraepithelial lymphocytes. Adv Host Defense Mechanisms 1994; 9:1-204.

59. Aicher WK, Fujihashi K, Yamamoto M et al. Effects of the lpr/lpr mutation on T and B cell populations in the lamina propria of the small intestine, a mucosal effector site. Intern Immunol 1992; 4:959-968.

60. Fujihashi K, Taguchi T, Aicher WK et al. Immunoregulatory functions for murine intraepithelial lymphocytes: γ/δ T cell receptor-positive (TCR⁺) T cells abrogate oral tolerance, while α/β TCR⁺ T cells provide B cell help. J Exp Med 1992; 175:695-707.

61. Takahashi I, Nakagawa I, Kiyono H et al. Mucosal T cells induce systemic anergy for oral tolerance. Biochem Biophys Res Commun 1995; 206:414-420.

62. Ke Y, Pearce K, Lake JP et al. γδ T lymphocytes regulate the induction and maintenance of oral tolerance. J Immunol 1997; 158:3610-3818.

63. Seymor BWP, Gershwin LJ, Coffman RL. Aerosol-induced immunoglobulin (Ig)-E unresponsiveness to ovalbumin does not require CD8⁺ or T cell receptor (TCR)- γ/δ T cells or interferon (IFN)-γ in a murine model of allergen sensitization. J Exp Med 1998; 187:721-731.

64. Fujihashi K, Dohi T, Kweon MN et al. γδ T cells regulate mucosally induced tolerance in a dose dependent fashion. Intern Immunol 1999; 11:1907-1916.

65. Komano H, Fujiura Y, Kawaguchi M et al. Homeostatic regulation of intestinal epithelia by intraepithelial γδ T cells. Proc Natl Acad Sci USA. 1995; 92:6147-6151.

66. Fujihashi K, McGhee JR, Kweon MN et al. γδ T cell deficient mice have impaired mucosal IgA responses. J Exp Med 1996; 183:1929-1935.

67. Mengel J, Cardillo F, Aroeira LS et al. Anti- γδ T cell antibody blocks the induction and maintenance of oral tolerance to ovalbumin in mice. Immunol. Letters 1995; 48:97-102.

68. McMenamin C, Pimm C, McKersey M et al. Regulation of IgE responses to inhaled antigen in mice by antigen-specific γδ T cells. Science 1994; 265:1869-1871.

69. Gorczynski RM, Cohen Z, Leung Y et al. γδ TCR⁺ hybridomas derived from mice preimmunized via the portal vein adoptively transfer increased skin allograft survival in vivo. J Immunol 1996; 157:574-581.

70. Gorczynski RM, Chen Z, Zeng H et al. Specificity for in vivo graft prolonation in γδ T cell receptor hybridomas derived from mice given portal vein donor-specific preimmunization and skin allografts. J Immunol 1997; 159:3698-3706.

71. Czerkinsky C, Anjuere F, McGhee JR et al. Mucosal immunity and tolerance: relevance to vaccine development. Immunol Rev 1999; 170:197-222.

72. McGhee JR, Kiyono H. The Mucosal Immune System. Fundamental Immunology, Fourth Edition. edited by William E. Paul, Academic Press, San Diego 1999:909-945.

73. Elson CO, Ealding W. Cholera toxin feeding did not induce oral tolerance in mice and abrogated oral tolerance to an unrelated protein antigen. J Immunol 1984; 133:2892-2897.

74. Elson CO, Ealding W. Generalized systemic and mucosal immunity in mice after mucosal stimulation with cholera toxin. J Immunol 1984; 132:2736-2741.

75. Kato, H, Fujihashi K, Kato R et al. Oral tolerance revisited: prior oral tolerization abrogates cholera toxin-induced mucosal IgA responses. J Immunol 2001; 166:3114-21.

76. De Togni P, Goellner J, Ruddle NH et al. Abnormal development of peripheral lymphoid organs in mice deficient in lymphotoxin. Science 1994; 264:703-707.

77. Banks TA, Rouse BT, Kerley MK et al. Lymphotoxin-α-deficient mice. Effects on secondary lymphoid organ development and humoral immune responsiveness. J Immunol 1995; 155:1685-1693.

78. Alimzhanov MB, Kuprash DV, Kosco VM et al. Abnormal development of secondary lymphoid tissues in lymphotoxin β-deficient mice. Proc Natl Aca Sci USA 1997; 94:9302-9307.

79. Koni PA, Sacca R, Lawton P et al. Distinct roles in lymphoid organogenesis for lymphotoxins α and β revealed in lymphotoxin β-deficient mice. Immunity 1997; 6:491-500.

80. Koni PA, Flavell RA. A role for tumor necrosis factor receptor type 1 in gut-associated lymphoid tissue development: genetic evidence of synergism with lymphotoxin β. J Exp Med 1998; 187:1977-1983.

81. Futterer A, Mink K, Luz A et al. The lymphotoxin β receptor controls organogenesis and affinity maturation in peripheral lymphoid tissues. Immunity 1998; 9:59-70.

82. Rennert PD, Browning JL, Mebius R et al. Surface lymphotoxin α/β complex is required for the development of peripheral lymphoid organs. J Exp Med 1996; 184:1999-2006.

83. Rennert PD, James D, Mackay F et al. Lymph node genesis is induced by signaling through the lymphotoxin β receptor. Immunity 1998; 9:71-79.

84. Rennert PD, Browning JL, Hochman PS. Selective disruption of lymphotoxin ligands reveals a novel set of mucosal lymph nodes and unique effects on lymph node cellular organization. Intern Immunol 1997; 9:1627-1639.
85. Fujihashi K, Dohi T, Rennert PD et al. Peyer's patches are required for oral tolerance to proteins. Proc Natl Aca Sci USA 2001; 98:3310-5.
86. Shroff KE, Meslin K, Cebra JJ. Commensal enteric bacteria engender a self-limiting humoral mucosal immune response while permanently colonizing the gut. Infect Immun 1995; 63:3904-3913.
87. Wannemuehler MJ, Kiyono H, Babb JL et al. Lipopolysaccharide (LPS) regulation of the immune response: LPS converts germfree mice to sensitivity to oral tolerance induction. J Immunol 1982; 129:959-965.
88. Kramer DR, Cebra JJ. Early appearance of "Natural" mucosal IgA responses and germinal centers in suckling mice developing in the absence of maternal antibodies. J Immunol 1995; 154:2051-2062.
89. Coffman RL, Lebman DA, Shrader B. Transforming growth factor β specifically enhances IgA production by lipopolysaccharide-stimulated murine B lymphocytes. J Exp Med 1989; 170:1039-1044.
90. Sonoda E, Matsumoto R, Hitoshi R, et al. Transforming growth factor β induces IgA production and acts additively with interleukin 5 for IgA production. J Exp Med 1989; 170:1415-1420.
91. Yamamoto M, Rennert PD, McGhee JR et al. An alternate mucosal immune system: organized Peyer's Patches are not required for IgA responses in the GI tract. J Immunol 2000; 164:5184-5191.
92. Viney JL, Mowat AM, O'Malley JM et al. Expanding dendritic cells in vivo enhances the induction of oral tolerance. J Immunol 1998; 160:5815-5825.

The Role of T Cells in the Intestinal Mucosa

Giovanni Monteleone and Thomas T. MacDonald

Introduction

The intestine contains the largest population of T cells in the body. This reflects the fact that the intestine has a large surface area continuously exposed to dietary antigens and microorganisms. The gut immune system is therefore fundamentally different from the systemic immune system in that specific responses to pathogens have to take place on a high background of responses to food and bacteria. Intestinal T cells occupy several distinct niches. They are abundant in the organised lymphoid tissue (tonsils, appendix, Peyer's patches) and are also present in the gut epithelium and lamina propria. Other chapters in this volume deal with Peyer's patches and their role in immunity and tolerance, and so in this section we will confine ourselves to discussion of cells at the effector arm of the mucosal immune response, the 400 m2 of intestinal mucosa. There is compelling evidence that mucosal T cells (CD4⁺T cells at least) are the progeny of Peyer's patch T cells responding to luminal antigens.

Lamina Propria T Cells

The lamina propria is the loose connective tissue between the epithelium and the muscularis mucosa. T cells normally constitute one-third of the cells in the intestinal lamina propria, the remainder being myofibroblasts, macrophages, plasma cells, nerve cells and the occasional neutrophils, mast cells or eosinophils. The proportion of CD4⁺ to CD8⁺ T cells is similar to that of peripheral blood lymphocytes, with a preponderance of CD4⁺, αβ TcR⁺ cells. Gamma δ cells are uncommon.[1-3] Lamina propria T cells have all the characteristics of antigen-experienced cells entering and lodging in the lamina propria as the progeny of Peyer's patch-derived T blasts which homed back to the lamina propria using α4β7/MAdCAM interactions to target gut vascular endothelium. The majority of CD4⁺ T lamina propria lymphocytes (LPLs) are L-selectin negative, and 66-96% of them express the CD45RO isoform of the CD45 molecule associated with memory-like T cells. However, CD4⁺ T-LPLs express no markers of resting memory cells. CD25, CD69, the 4F2 lymphocyte activation antigen and transferrin receptors are expressed at relatively high levels.[1-3] They show no evidence of local division and clonal expansion in the lamina propria. CD8⁺ T-LPLs are also CD45RO⁺ and express high levels of αEβ7, which has been shown to mediate the binding of T lymphocytes to epithelial cells.[4]

It is thus very likely that lamina propria T cells are end stage cells and do not re-enter the recirculating pool. T-LPLs express the apoptotic molecule FAS and a subpopulation of them are FAS ligand positive.[5] They exhibit an increased level of apoptosis in comparison to peripheral blood lymphocytes (PBLs) and respond to CD2 stimulation with enhanced FAS-dependent apoptosis.[6] There is moreover some evidence that T-LPL apoptosis can be related to their state

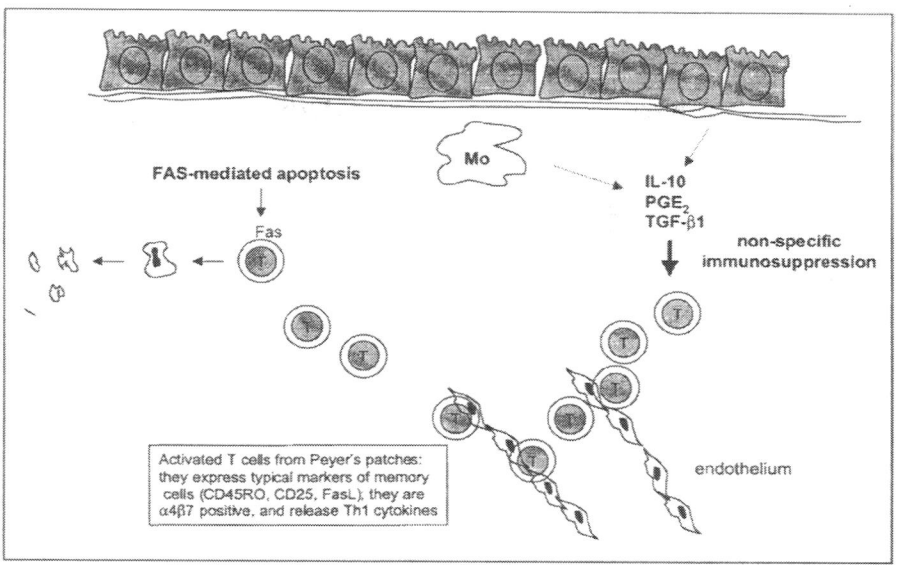

Figure 1. In normal intestine, T cell immunoblasts extravasate from the blood into the lamina propria, but once in the tissue they enter an immunosuppressive environment and die.

of anergy/hyporesponsiveness. Indeed, despite the fact that T-LPLs do not proliferate in response to IL-2, they return to a more responsive state when cultured in the presence of IL-2, a condition that is known to rescue T cells from apoptosis.[6-7] Importantly, IL-2 mediates its activities by signaling through the common γ-chain receptor family of cytokine receptors, a receptor subunit shared by other cytokines, including IL-7 and IL-15, all having been reported to decrease T-LPL apoptosis.[6,8,9]

Beside its endogenous predisposition to induce cells to undergo apoptosis, the lamina propria is a generally unresponsive environment. It is probable that the antigens that stimulate the T cells in the Peyer's patch will not be present in the lamina propria so that there will be no antigen-driven clonal expansion. Finally, there is evidence that intestinal epithelial cells produce high levels of TGF-β1 and IL-10, which could potentially downregulate lamina propria T cell activity.[10,11] Indeed targeted disruption of the TGF-β1 gene in the gut leads to inflammatory bowel disease in mice.[12,13] The fate of T cells in normal lamina propria is illustrated in Figure 1.

Despite the fact that T-LPLs are persistently stimulated, the gut has developed effective mechanisms which specifically prevent excessive inflammation and tissue injury. First, the reactivity of T-LPL to TCR/CD3 engagement is reduced when compared with peripheral blood T lymphocytes.[14-17] This state of hyporesponsiveness has been associated with the local production of suppressive molecules (e.g., IL-10, TGF-B1, PGE2), insufficient delivery of costimulatory signals, and synthesis of low molecular weight non-protein mediators with oxidative capacities.[11,18,19] Moreover, Sido et al have recently shown that proliferation of T-LPL is subject to thiol-mediated redox regulation.[20] In contrast to peripheral blood lymphocyte, resident lamina propria mononuclear cells lack the capacity to synthesise cysteine, resulting in a deficient production of glutathione, which is a prerequisite for cell cycle progression.[20]

At the intestinal level, the relationship between T cell activation and tissue injury is highlighted by studies showing that an inappropriately directed T cell-mediated immune response to food antigens (i.e., wheat gluten in celiac disease) or to unknown antigens (i.e., gut bacteria in Crohn's disease) leads to chronic tissue injury. In both diseases there is a compelling evidence that cytokines are important mediators of tissue damage.[1]

Mucosal Chemokines Which Attract and Maintain T Cells

The factors which control the migration of T cells into the gut mucosa have been a subject of intense interest in recent years. Several years ago a major role was demonstrated for $\alpha 4\beta 7^+$ cells derived from Peyer's patches recognising MAdCAM on gut vascular endothelium and delivering a post-code to extravasate in the gut.[21,22] More recently however, it has become clear that chemokines are also involved in this process. The chemokine stromal derived factor-1 (SDF-1) is highly expressed by human gut epithelial cells.[23] Gut lamina propria cells express the SDF-1 receptor CXCR4 at low levels but in culture rapidly upregulate expression.[23] T-LPLs also express the chemokine receptors CCR5, CXCR3, and CCR2 and migrate in response to I-TAC (a CXCR3 ligand) and RANTES (a CCR5 ligand).[24] More importantly all LPL express CCR9 and its ligand, thymus-expressed chemokine (TECK) is only expressed by epithelium in the small bowel but not the colon.[25] In vitro human LPL migrate towards TECK.[25] Finally, another chemokine, mucosa-associated epithelial chemokine (MEC) is highly expressed by gut epithelium. MEC can attract eosinophils and memory T cells since it is a ligand for CCR3.[26] Collectively, these results show that gut epithelial cells may secrete a distinct panel of chemokines to attract and retain cells in the gut.

Cytokine Production by Lamina Propria T Cells

As a result of their state of activation, T-LPLs spontaneously produce high levels of cytokines. Freshly isolated human T-LPLs contain a very high number of cytokine-secreting cells when compared to autologous blood T cells, and the response is dominated by interferon (IFN)-γ.[27] There are about 10-fold fewer cells spontaneously secreting IL-4, and IL-10 whereas IL-5-secreting cells are uncommon.[27] Similarly, IL-4 and IL-5 RNA transcripts are barely detectable in the human intestinal lamina propria. Experiments with CD4⁺ or CD8⁺ cell depleted suspensions indicate that CD4⁺ T-LPLs are the major source of IFN-γ and IL-4.[28] Stimulation of T-LPLs via the alternative pathways of activation (e.g., CD2 and CD28) elicits a strong cytokine response, which is again dominated by IFN-γ. Fuss and colleagues showed that CD2/CD28 activated normal human T-LPLs secrete 50,000 pg/ml IFN-γ compared to just over 100 pg/ml IL-4 and less than 50 pg/ml IL-5.[29] These results were confirmed by Targan and colleagues who showed that CD3 ligation yielded equivalent cytokine responses in T-LPLs and peripheral blood lymphocytes (PBLs), whereas CD2 stimulation induced a greater response in LPLs compared to PBLs.[15] This response, dominated by IFN-γ, was magnified further by co-ligation of the CD28 receptor. Studies on the molecular events and mechanisms involved in the regulation of IFN-γ production after CD2/CD28 stimulation revealed that activation of LPLs via CD2 induced IFN-γ mRNA expression and that CD28 stimulation enhanced mRNA stability without up-regulating the rate of gene transcription.[30] It was moreover demonstrated that activation of LPLs resulted in transactivation of multiple promoter elements regulating IFN-γ expression distinct from those in PBLs, and that in lamina propria mononuclear cells (LPMCs) there are at least two regions involved in the control of CD2-mediated trans-activation of the IFN-γ promoter. The first is a major CD2-regulatory element contained within the region -204 to -108 bp upstream of the transcriptional start site, whereas the other is a minor regulatory element residing within -108 to -40 bp of the transcriptional start site.[30]

The characteristic cytokine products of Th1 and Th2 cells are mutually inhibitory for the differentiation and effector functions of the reciprocal phenotype. IFN-γ inhibits differentiation of Th2 cells, whereas IL-10 blocks activation of Th1 cells.[31] The differentiation of Th1 or

Th2 cell subtype is influenced by other factors, including the nature of the antigen and environmental stimuli to which the cells are exposed. Intracellular bacteria, which activate macrophages, promote Th1 cell differentiation by stimulating the synthesis of IL-12, the major Th1-inducing cytokine.[32] In contrast, IL-4, produced by basophils and mast cells mostly in response to allergens and extracellular microbes, is an essential requirement for the differentiation of Th2 cells.[32]

The reason why Th1 cytokine synthesis is enhanced in response to T-LPL activation remains unclear, given that the cytokine which induce Th1 cells (e.g., IL-12, IL-18, IFN-α) are barely detectable in the intestinal lamina propria of normal subjects.[33] The most likely explanation is that T-LPLs are derived from the Peyer's patches where bacterial antigens, transported across the epithelium by M cells into the dome region, stimulate IL-12 production and Th1 cell polarisation.[34,35] Thus they might be the recent progeny of Th1 blasts driven along that pathway by the Th1 inducing micro-environment of the human Peyer's patch.

Intraepithelial Lymphocytes

Human intraepithelial T lymphocytes (IELs) are nearly all αβ or γδ T cells.[36-38] The function of γδ IELs remains obscure. The number of γδ IELs is increased in celiac disease[39] but the reason for this is unknown. IL-7 is a potent growth factor for γδ IELs[40] in mice, but its effect on human γδ IELs is unclear. Recently, human γδ cells have been shown to recognise MICA and MICB, two MHC class I molecules expressed on the surface of stressed epithelial cells.[41,42] γδIELs are predominantly CD4⁻ CD8⁻ and present at all levels of the intestine.[43] In contrast, αβIELs express different surface markers at different levels of the intestine.[43] In the jejunum, CD8⁺ αβIELs dominate although CD4⁺ αβIELs are also present. In the ileum, CD8⁺ and CD4⁺ αβIELs are present in similar numbers. In the colon, CD4⁻ CD8⁻ γδIELs and CD4⁺ αβIELs constitute two major populations, but CD8⁺ αβIELs and low numbers of B cells (CD20⁺) are also present.[43] Another IEL subset is represented by CD3-/CD7⁺ cells expressing typical natural killer cell markers (CD161, CD122).[44] Several studies have demonstrated that IELs are constitutively activated. They are HLA-DR⁺, CD45RO⁺, and CD68⁺.[43] In addition, IELs have an increased expression of FAS in comparison to peripheral blood lymphocytes, and a discrete fraction of IELs constitutively express FAS ligand (FASL).[45] All IELs express BY55, a ligand for classical and non-classical MHC class I.[46] IELs freshly isolated from different levels of the intestine express mRNA for several cytokines, suggesting that they are secreting cytokines in vivo. In both the small and large intestines, the profile of cytokines synthesised is Th1, with IFNγ predominant over IL-4 and IL-5.[47] This is consistent with the cytolytic functions of IELs.[47] In vitro studies using redirected cytolytic killing assays have revealed that IELs kill target cells by secreting perforin and/or by using the FAS/FASL pathway.[48]

A large body of evidence supports the concept that both αβ and γδ IELs are oligoclonal, which may explain the response of the intestinal mucosal immune system to a restricted set of antigens.[37,38,49,50] Sequencing of TcR gene segments used by isolated IELs shows that a large proportion of the expressed T cell Vβ receptors have identical D and J regions with the same N-region insertions, with each subject showing a unique pattern of oligoclonal expansion. Vβ regions are dominant over large sections of the intestine, even though there is considerable local variation and a Vβ dominant at one site may not be dominant at an adjacent site.[50,51] Analysis of Vβ expression in human fetal intestine also shows a considerable skewing of Vβ usage, thus indicating that factors other than luminal antigens control Vβ expression in the gut.[51] IELs and LPLs express a similar pattern of chemokine receptors, an important fact given the possible role of epithelial chemokines in attracting and retaining T cells in the gut epithelium.[23-26]

T Cells in the Inflamed Gut Mucosa

Crohn's disease and celiac disease are two important pathologies involving excessive T cell activation. The number of T cells is increased in the mucosa of Crohn's disease and celiac disease patients, as it is in the other inflammatory diseases of the gut, such as ulcerative colitis. By and large, immunophenotypic studies of T cells in inflammatory bowel disease (IBD) and celiac disease have not been particularly informative. In IBD for example, there are increased numbers of CD45RA[+] cells in the mucosa but they probably derive non-specifically from the blood.[52]

In this section, we will confine our discussion on mucosal T cells to IBD, since celiac disease is the subject of another chapter. Many studies have characterised the patterns of cytokine production in both Crohn's disease (CD) and ulcerative colitis (UC) using in situ hybridisation, immunohistochemistry, organ culture of biopsies, cytokine profiles of freshly isolated cells, and in vitro activated T cells and macrophages. A consensus has emerged from these studies. A difference in cytokine profiles between CD and UC was first highlighted by Mullin and colleagues who showed that IL-2 RNA transcripts were markedly elevated in CD but not UC.[53] This result was confirmed by several studies showing that the profile of cytokines produced in CD is polarised toward the Th1 type, and that Th1 cells are essential mediators of the tissue-damaging intestinal inflammation.[29,54-56] T-LPLs isolated from the inflamed mucosa of CD patients contain appreciable amounts of IFN-γ mRNA and spontaneously release high levels of IFN-γ in comparison to control cells.[57] Furthermore, IFN-γ-secreting cells have been demonstrated in actively inflamed CD mucosa.[27] These cells express activation markers such as CD26 and lymphocyte activation gene-3, which have been associated with the production of Th1 cytokines.[58] There is a single report that IL-4 transcripts are elevated in the early lesions of recurrent CD, but this may be a transient situation, since the biopsies were taken at the very edge of aphthoid ulcers.[59] Some immunological responses observed in CD inflamed tissues may involve Th1 cytokines. They include the increased epithelial expression of MHC class II antigens and CD98, the enhancement of ICAM-1 expression on endothelial and mononuclear cells, and the presence of multinucleated giant cells. IFN-γ can also facilitate the activation of resident macrophages and the release of pro-inflammatory cytokines, such as interleukin (IL)-1, IL-6 and TNF-α which in turn maintain and expand the local inflammatory response.[54]

In Crohn's disease, the differentiation of Th1 cells seems to depend on locally induced molecules. IFNγ production is strictly associated with the expression of IL-12.[58,60,61] RNA transcripts for both IL-12 subunits (p40 and p35) have been detected in gastric and intestinal mucosa of patients with CD using reverse transcriptase polymerase chain reaction and in situ hybridisation.[60,61] In addition, lamina propria mononuclear cells (LPMC) isolated from inflamed mucosa of CD patients release the functionally active IL-12 heterodimer, and neutralisation of IL-12 by a specific antibody results in a dramatic decrease in the number of IFN-γ-producing cells.[58,60] Consistent with these results, CD LPMCs exhibit high levels of IL-12Rβ-2 chain, the signaling component of the IL-12 receptor, and of active STAT-4, a transcription factor essential in the IL-12-dependent Th1 polarisation, in comparison to UC and control LPMCs.[62]

A growing body of evidence indicates that in CD mucosa the IL-12-induced Th1 cell polarisation is expanded by other cytokines locally induced, including IL-7, IL-15 and IL-18.[63-65] In addition, TNF-α released within the CD mucosa can enhance IFN-γ production through a mechanism independent on IL-12 and IL-18.[66]

Studies in animal models of IBD support the role of the IL-12/STAT-4 signaling pathway in the Th1 cell-mediated injury in the gut. T cells lacking STAT-4 have an impaired IFN-γ production in response to IL-12 and are unable to promote the development of colitis when transferred to immunodeficient mice.[67] Moreover, the overexpression of STAT-4 in transgenic mice results in a colitis characterised by a diffuse infiltration of the intestinal wall by IFN-γ- and TNF-α-secreting cells.[68] Finally, IL-12 antibodies abrogate the mucosal inflammation induced in mice by 2,4,6-trinitrobenzene sulfonic acid [TNBS], a model mimicking some characteristics of CD.[69]

In UC, an enhanced humoral immunity appears to predominate. Mucosal plasma cells isolated from the intestine of UC patients produce high levels of immunoglobulins (Ig), particularly IgG1.[70] In addition, a large variety of autoantibodies (i.e., anti-colon and anti-neutrophil antibodies) may be detected in the serum of these patients.[71,72] These autoantibodies are not tissue specific and seldom correlate with clinical variables of the disease, suggesting that they have no pathogenic role. The profile of regulatory T cell cytokines produced in UC is consistent with the findings mentioned above. Indeed, expression of IFN-γ is lower than that in CD and not different from that in normal controls.[29] UC T lymphocytes stimulated via the CD3/CD28 pathway release high levels of IL-5, a cytokine that may be relevant in helping antibody response. However, the same cells still produce 50 times as much IFN-γ as IL-5.[29] The idea that a Th2 type response is prevalent in UC remains unfounded. In agreement with the profile of cytokines released by T-LPLs, the production of IL-12 is small or undetectable in colonic mucosa of patients with UC, despite a massive infiltration by activated macrophages.[60] In the inflamed mucosa of patients with UC but not active CD, there is an increased production of the protein encoded by the Epstein-Barr-induced gene 3 (EBI3), a protein able to form an heterodimer with the p35 subunit.[73] This new heterodimer might function as an IL-12 antagonist and favour the downregulation of Th1 cytokines.

The factors/mechanisms that lead to the uncontrolled T cell activation in IBD are unknown. However, it has been suggested that loss of tolerance to antigens from the intestinal flora is relevant and may partly depend on an altered mucosal balance between proinflammatory (IFN-γ) and counter-regulatory molecules (TGF-β1).[74] Recent studies have demonstrated that CD mucosal T cells display a defective response to several apoptotic stimuli, in association with an increase in the ratio between the anti-apoptotic protein Bcl-2 and the pro-apoptotic molecule Bax.[75-77] The factors involved in the resistance of CD LPLs to apoptotic signals remain to be determined. However, there is evidence that activation of STAT-3 by IL-6/IL-6R interaction, activation of JAK3 by common γ-chain cytokine receptor stimulation (i.e., by IL-7 or IL-15) or IL-12/IL-12R-mediated signals can rescue T cells from apoptosis, extending their life span and eventually favouring their accumulation.[75-78] Figure 2 illustrates how increased concentrations of local cytokines can prevent T cell death in the lamina propria.

The Mechanism of Action of T Cells in Mediating Mucosal Injury

The excessive mucosal immune response in IBD is characterised by an increased synthesis of proinflammatory cytokines, including IL-1β, IL-6, IL-8, and TNF-α accompanying the influx of non-specific inflammatory cells into the mucosa.[79-81] The local injury is also probably mediated by nitric oxide and other free radicals. The cytokines activate mechanisms leading to important morphologic changes. IL-1β and TNF-α stimulate gut fibroblasts to synthesise matrix metalloproteinases (MMPs), a family of zinc-containing neutral endopeptidases which slowly replace the matrix.[82] Stromal cells of the normal lamina propria secrete low amounts of MMPs and of tissue inhibitors of MMPs (TIMPs) which act together with α-macroglobulin to prevent excess enzyme activity. IL-1β and TNF-α rapidly up-regulate MMP production without altering TIMP production.[82] The importance of this pathway is illustrated in an ex vivo model of T cell-mediated gut inflammation based on the activation by pokeweed mitogen (PWM) or anti-CD3 and IL-12 of T-LPL in explant cultures of human small intestine.[83,84] The T cell response induced in the fetal gut explants by PWM or anti-CD3 and IL-12 is strongly Th1-biased and leads within 4 days to a severe mucosal injury. Culture supernatants of explants treated with PWM or anti-CD3 and IL-12 contain increased concentrations of MMP-1 (collagenase) and MMP-3 (stromelysin-1). Importantly, MMP inhibitors prevent

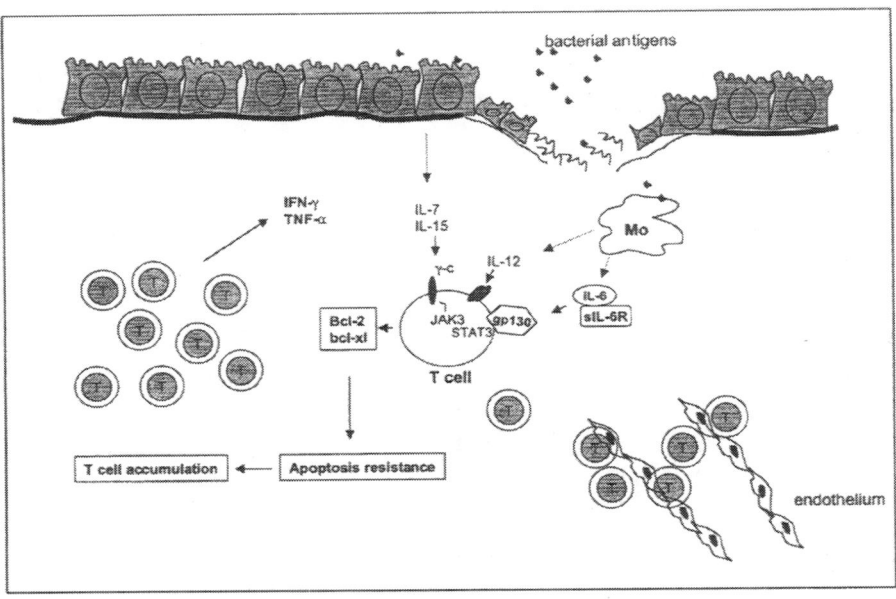

Figure 2. In inflamed intestine, T cell immunoblasts extravasate into the lamina propria from the blood, but overexpression of factors such as IL-6 and IL-12 prevent the cells from dying, so they accumulate.

tissue damage without altering T cell activation. In addition, mucosal degradation can be prevented by a p55 TNF-α receptor human IgG fusion protein also able to inhibit MMP-3 production.[85]

Stromelysin-1 is extremely potent at degrading gut mucosa. It has a broad substrate specificity, being capable of degrading proteoglycans, laminin, fibronectin, collagen core protein, and non-helical cross-linked regions of type IV collagen.[86,87] Stromelysin-1 has the potential to destroy the structure of the intestinal lamina propria, thereby removing the scaffolding on which the epithelium lies. Since enterocytes adhere to basement membrane through extracellular matrix receptors, modification and loss of the basement membrane may result in decreased adhesiveness and epithelial cell shedding.[88,89] Consistently, abundant stromelysin-1 has been found in the mucosa of patients with IBD, particularly near ulcers.[90-92]

However, it is important to remember that MMPs are not only involved in tissue injury, but also in tissue repair. We have shown that gut myofibroblasts activated through surface α4β1 integrin, whose ligands are fibronectin and VCAM-1 on macrophages, rapidly upregulate membrane type 1 (MT-1) metalloproteinase production.[93] MT-1 activates gelatinase A in the pericellular space and allows the myofibroblasts to migrate through the matrix. MT-1 may therefore be important in allowing myofibroblasts to migrate through granulation tissue in ulcer beds and help heal ulcers.[93] In IBD, MT-1 is very strongly expressed in inflamed regions, suggesting that myofibroblasts are not static in the gut wall but motile.[93]

Another pathway by which cytokines could indirectly produce changes in the gut is through stromal cell production of epithelial growth factors, such as members of the fibroblast growth factor family. One of these molecules, keratinocyte growth factor (KGF), is produced by stromal cells mainly in response to TNF-α. KGF is over-expressed in IBD and celiac disease and may be responsible for the crypt cell hyperplasia observed in these conditions.[94-95] Stimulation of human fetal gut explants with KGF enhances epithelial cell proliferation.[96] A neutralising

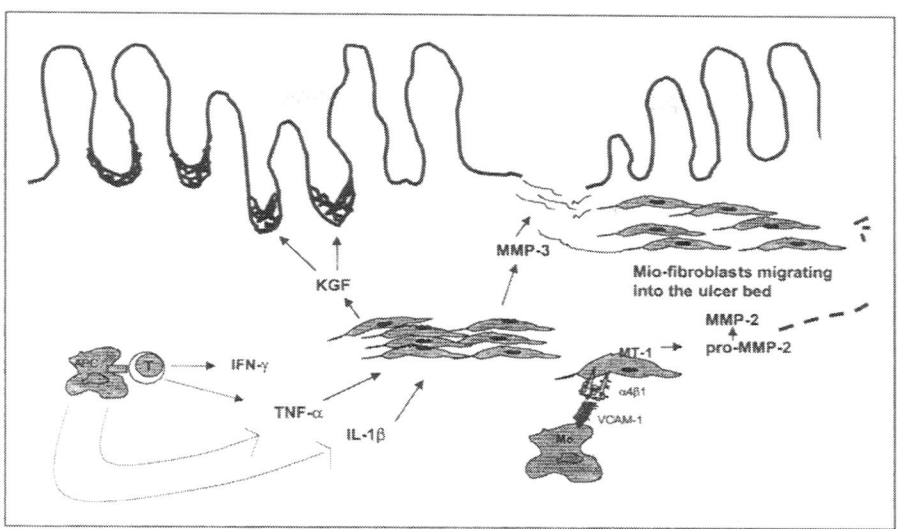

Figure 3. In inflamed intestine, overexpression of pro-inflammatory cytokines by T cells and macrophages leads to upregulation of matrix degrading enzymes and epithelial growth factors which drive the tissue damage. However, macrophages can also activate gut fibroblasts to move and migrate through ulcer beds, aiding mucosal restitution.

KGF antibody also partially inhibits the crypt cell hyperplasia induced in explant cultures of fetal gut by lamina propria $V\beta3^+$ T cell activation with *Staphylococcus aureus* enterotoxin B (SEB).[96] In this model, SEB-induced crypt hyperplasia is also associated with an enhanced expression of TGF-α, a member of the epidermal growth factor family produced by epithelial cells and able to modulate epithelial cell functions. The addition of anti-TGF-α prevents the SEB-stimulated crypt hyperplasia. Interestingly, stimulation of explants with recombinant KGF enhances TGF-α induction, suggesting a molecular cross-talk between KGF and TGF-α in T cell-mediated crypt cell hyperplasia.[96] A unifying picture of the way in which Th1 cytokines cause tissue injury and perhaps repair is shown in Figure 3.

References

1. MacDonald TT, Pender SLF. Lamina propria T cells. Chem Immunol 1998; 71:103-117.
2. Schieferdecker HL, Ullrich R, Hirseland H et al. T cell differentiation antigens on lymphocytes in the human intestinal lamina propria. Eur J Immunol 1997; 27:1774-1781.
3. Peters MG, Secrist H, Anders KR et al. Normal human intestinal lymphocytes. Increased activation compared with peripheral blood. J Clin Invest 1989; 83: 1827-1831.
4. Farstad IN, Halstensen TS, Lien B et al. Distribution of β7 integrins in human intestinal mucosa and organised gut-associated lymphoid tissue. Immunology 1996; 89:227-237.
5. DeMaria R, Boirivant M, Cifone MG et al. Functional expression of Fas and Fas ligand on human gut lamina propria T lymphocytes: A potential role for the acidic sphingomyelinase pathway in normal immunoregulation. J Clin Invest 1996; 97:316-322.
6. Boirivant M, Pica R, DeMaria R et al. Stimulated human lamina propria T cells manifest enhanced FAS-mediated apoptosis. J Clin Invest 1996; 98:2616-2622.
7. Beverly B, Kang S, Lenardo M et al. Reversal of in vitro T cell clonal anergy by IL-2 stimulation. Int Immunol 1992; 4:661-667.
8. Demoulin JB, Renauld JC. Signalling by cytokines interacting with the interleukin-2 receptor gamma chain. Cytokines Cell Mol Ther 1998; 4:243-256.

9. Nakajima H, Noguchi M, Leonard WJ. Role of the common cytokine receptor gamma chain (γc) in thymocyte selection. Immunol Today 2000; 21:88-94.

10. Panja A, Siden E, Mayer L. Synthesis and regulation of accessory/proinflammatory cytokines by intestinal epithelial cells. Clin Exp Immunol 1995; 100:298-305.

11. MacDonald TT. Effector and regulatory lymphoid cells and cytokines in mucosal sites. Curr Top Microbiol Immunol 1999; 236:113-35.

12. Christ M, McCartney-Francis NL, Kulkarni AB et al. Immune dysregulation in TGF-β1-deficient mice. J Immunol 1994; 153:1936-1946.

13. Shull MM, Ormsby I, Kier ABT et al. Targeted disruption of the mouse TGF-β1 gene results in multifocal inflammatory disease. Nature 1992; 359:693-699.

14. Qiao L, Schurmann G, Betzler M et al. Activation and signaling status of human lamina propria lymphocytes. Gastroenterology 1991; 101:1529-1536.

15. Targan SR, Deem RL, Liu M et al. Definition of lamina propria T cell responsive state. Enhanced cytokine responsiveness of T cell stimulated through the CD2 pathway. J Immunol 1995; 154:664-675.

16. Boirivant M, Fuss I, Fiocchi C et al. Hypo-proliferative human lamina propria T cell retain the capacity to secrete lymphokines when stimulated via the CD2/CD28 accessory signaling pathways. Proc Assoc Am Physicians 1996; 108:55-67.

17. De Maria R, Fais S, Silvestri M et al. Continuous in vivo activation and transient hyporesponsiveness to TcR/CD3 triggering of human gut lamina propria lymphocytes. Eur J Immunol 1993; 23:3104-3108.

18. Qiao L, Braunstein J, Golling M et al. Differential regulation of human T cell responsiveness by mucosal versus blood monocytes. Eur J Immunol 1996; 26:922-927.

19. Qiao L, Schurmann G, Autschbach F et al. Human intestinal mucosa alters T cell reactivities. Gastroenterology 1993; 105:814-819.

20. Sido B, Braunstein J, Breitkreutz R et al. Thiol-mediated redox regulation of intestinal lamina propria T lymphocytes. J Exp Med 2000; 192:907-912.

21. Parker CM, Cepek KL, Russell GJ et al. A family of β7 integrins on human mucosal lymphocytes. Proc Natl Acad Sci USA 1992; 89:1924-1928.

22. Rott LS, Rose' JR, Bass D et al. Expression of mucosal homing receptor α4β7 by circulating CD4+ cells with memory for intestinal rotavirus. J Clin Invest 1997; 100:1204-1208.

23. Agace WW, Amara A, Roberts AI et al. Constitutive expression of stromal derived factor-1 by mucosal epithelia and its role in HIV transmission and propagation. Curr Biol 2000; 10:325-328.

24. Agace WW, Roberts AI, Wu L et al. Human intestinal lamina propria and intraepithelial lympho-cytes express receptors specific for chemokines induced by inflammation. Eur J Immunol 2000; 30:819-826.

25. Kunkel EJ, Campbell JJ, Haraldsen G et al. Lymphocyte CC chemokine receptor 9 and epithelial thymus-expressed chemokine (TECK) expression distinguish the small intestinal immune compart-ment: Epithelial expression of tissue -specific chemokines as an organising principle in regional immunity. J Exp Med 2000; 192:761-768.

26. Pan J, Kunkel EJ, Gosslar U et al. A novel chemokine ligand for CCR10 and CCR3 expressed by epithelial cells in mucosal tissues. J Immunol 2000; 165:2943-2949.

27. Breese E, Braegger CP, Corrigan C J et al. Interleukin-2- and interferon-γ secreting T cells in normal and diseased human intestinal mucosa. Immunology 1993; 78:127-131.

28. Carol M, Lambrechts A, Van Gossum A et al. Spontaneous secretion of interferon-γ and interleukin 4 by human intraepithelial and lamina propria gut lymphocytes. Gut 1998; 42:643-649.

29. Fuss IJ, Neurath M, Boirivant M et al. Disparate CD4+ lamina propria (LP) lymphokine secretion profiles in inflammatory bowel disease. Crohn's disease LP cells manifest increased secretion of IFN-γ, whereas Ulcerative Colitis LP cells manifest increased secretion of IL-5. J Immunol 1996; 157:1261-1270.

30. Gonsky R, Deem RL, Bream JH et al. Mucosa-specific targets for regulation of IFN-γ expression: lamina propria T cells use different cis-elements than peripheral blood T cells to regulate transactivation of IFN-γ expression. J Immunol 2000; 164:1399-1407.

31. Romagnani S. Lymphokine production by human T cells in disease states. Annu Rev Immunol 1994; 12:227-257.

32. Abbas AK, Murphy KM, Sher A. Functional diversity of helper T lymphocytes. Nature 1996; 383:787-793.

33. Pallone F, Monteleone G. Interleukin 12 and Th1 responses in inflammatory bowel disease. Gut 1998; 43:735-736

34. Nagata S, McKenzie C, Pender SLF et al. Human Peyer's patch T cells are sensitized to dietary antigen and display a Th cell type 1 cytokine profile. J Immunol 2000; 165:5315-5321.

35. Hauer AC, Bajaj-Elliott M, Williams CB et al. An analysis of interferon γ, IL-4, IL-5 and IL-10 production by ELISPOT and quantitative reverse transcriptase-PCR in human Peyer's patches. Cytokine 1998; 10:627-634.

36. Lefrancois L, Puddington L. Extrathymic T cell development: virtual reality? Immunol Today 1995; 16:16-21.

37. Holtmeier W, Chowers Y, Lumeng A et al. The delta T cell receptor repertoire in human colon and peripheral blood oligoclonal irrespective of V region usage. J Clin Invest 1995; 96:1108-1117.

38. Chowers Y, Holtmeier W, Harwood J et al. The V delta 1 T cell receptor repertoire in human small intestine and colon. J Exp Med 1994; 180:183-190.

39. Spencer J, Isaacson PG, Diss TC et al. Expression of disulfide-linked and non-disulfide-linked forms of the T cell receptor gamma/delta heterodimer in human intestinal intraepithelial lymphocytes. Eur J Immunol 1989; 19:1335-1338.

40. Laky K, Lefrancois L, Lingenheld EG et al. Enterocyte expression of interleukin 7 induces development of gammadelta T cells and Peyer's patches. J Exp Med 2000; 191:1569-1580.

41. Griffith E, Ramsburg E, Hayday A et al. Recognition by human gut gamma delta cells of stress inducible major histocompatibility molecules on enterocytes. Gut 1998; 43:166-167.

42. Steinle A, Groh V, Spies T. Diversification, expression, and gamma delta T cell recognition of evolutionarily distant members of the MIC family of major histocompatibility complex class I-related molecules. Proc Natl Acad Sci USA 1998; 95:12510-12515.

43. Lundqvist C, Baranov V, Hammarstrom S et al. Intraepithelial lymphocytes: evidence for regional specialization and extrathymic T cell maturation in the human gut epithelium. Int Immunol 1995; 7:1473-1479.

44. Eiras P, Leon F, Camarero C et al. Intestinal intraepithelial lymphocytes contain a CD3-CD7+ subset expressing natural killer markers and a singular pattern of adhesion molecules. Scand J Immunol 2000; 52:1-6.

45. Hongo T, Morimoto Y, Iwagaki H et al. Functional expression of Fas and Fas ligand on human colonic intraepithelial T lymphocytes. J Int Med Res 2000; 28:132-142.

46. Anumanthan A, Bensussan A, Boumsell L et al. Cloning of BY55, a killer inhibitory receptor-related protein expressed on NK cells, cytolytic T lymphocytes, and intestinal intraepithelial lymphocytes. J Immunol 1998; 161:2780-2784.

47. Lundqvist C, Melgar S, Yeung M M-W et al. Intraepithelial lymphocytes in human gut have lytic potential and a cytokine profile that suggest T helper 1 and cytotoxic functions. J Immunol 1996; 157:1926-1934.

48. Guy-Grand D, Cerf-Bensussan N, Malissen B et al. Two gut intraepithelial CD8+ lymphocyte population with different T cell receptors: a role for the gut epithelium in T cell differentiation. J Exp Med 1991; 173:471-481.

49. Van Kerckhove C, Russell GJ, Deusch K et al. Oligoclonality of human intestinal intraepithelial T cells. J Exp Med 1992; 175:57-63.

50. Blumberg RS, Yockey CE, Gross GG et al. Human intestinal intraepithelial lymphocytes are derived from a limited number of T cell clones that utilize multiple VβT cell receptor genes. J Immunol 1993; 150:5144-5153.

51. Thomas R, Schurmann, Lionetti P et al. T cell receptor Vβ expression in human intestine: regional variation in postnatal intestine and biased usage in fetal gut. Gut 1996; 38:190-195.

52. Burgio VL, Fais S, Boirivant M et al. Peripheral monocyte and naive T-cell recruitment and activation in Crohn's disease. Gastroenterology 1995; 109:1029-1038.

53. Mullin GE, Lazenby AJ, Harris ML et al. Increased interleukin-2 messenger RNA in the intestinal mucosal lesions of Crohn's disease but not in ulcerative colitis. Gastroenterology 1992; 102:1620-1627.

54. MacDonald TT, Monteleone G, Pender SLF. Recent developments in the immunology of inflammatory bowel disease. Scand J Immunol 2000; 51:2-9.
55. Fiocchi C. Inflammatory Bowel Disease: Etiology and Pathogenesis. Gastroenterology 1998; 115:182-205.
56. Strober W, Ludviksson BR, Fuss IJ. The pathogenesis of mucosal inflammation in murine models of inflammatory bowel disease and Crohn's disease. Ann Intern Med 1998; 128:848-856.
57. Fais S, Capobianchi MR, Pallone F et al. Spontaneous release of interferon gamma by intestinal lamina propria lymphocytes in Crohn's disease. Kinetics of in vitro response to interferon gamma inducers. Gut 1991; 32:403-407.
58. Parronchi P, Romagnani P, Annunziato F et al Type 1 T-helper cell predominance and interleukin-12 expression in the gut of patients with Crohn's disease. Am J Pathol 1997; 150:823-832.
59. Desreumaux P, Brandt E, Gambiez L et al. Distinct cytokine patterns in early and chronic ileal lesions of Crohn's disease. Gastroenterology 1997; 113:118-126.
60. Monteleone G, Biancone L, Marasco R et al Interleukin 12 is expressed and actively released by Crohn's disease intestinal lamina propria mononuclear cells. Gastroenterology 1997; 112:1169-1178.
61. Berrebi D, Besnard M, Fromont-Hankard G et al Interleukin-12 expression is focally enhanced in the gastric mucosa of pediatric patients with Crohn's disease. Am J Pathol 1998; 152:667-672.
62. Parrello T, Monteleone G, Cucchiara S et al. Up-regulation of the IL-12 Receptor β2 Chain in Crohn's Disease. J Immunol 2000; 165:7234-7239.
63. Monteleone G, Parrello T, Luzza F et al. Response of human intestinal lamina propria T lymphocytes to interleukin 12: additive effects of interleukin 15 and 7. Gut 1998; 43:620-628.
64. Monteleone G, Trapasso F, Parrello T et al.. Bioactive interleukin-18 expression is up-regulated in Crohn's disease. J Immunol 1999; 163:143-147.
65. Pizarro TT, Michie MH, Bentz M et al. IL-18, a novel immunoregulatory cytokine, is up-regulated in Crohn's disease: expression and localization in intestinal mucosal cells. J Immunol 1999; 162:6829-6835.
66. Prehn JL, Landers CJ, Targan SR. A soluble factor produced by lamina propria mononuclear cells is required for TNF-α enhancement of IFN-γ production by T cells. J Immunol 1999; 163:4277-4283.
67. Simpson SJ, Shah S, Comiskey M et al. T cell-mediated pathology in two models of experimental colitis depends predominantly on the interleukin 12/Signal transducer and activator of transcription (Stat)-4 pathway, but is not conditional on interferon gamma expression by T cells. J Exp Med 1998; 187:1225-1234.
68. Wirtz S, Finotto S, Kanzler S et al. Chronic intestinal inflammation in STAT-4 transgenic mice: characterization of disease and adoptive transfer by TNF-plus IFN-gamma-producing CD4+ T cells that respond to bacterial antigens. J Immunol 1999; 162:1884-1888.
69. Neurath MF, Fuss I, Kelsall BL et al. Antibodies to interleukin 12 abrogate established experimental colitis in mice. J Exp Med 1995; 182:1281-1290.
70. Kett K, Rognum TO, Brandtzaeg P. Mucosal subclass distribution of immunoglobulin G-producing cells is different in ulcerative colitis and Crohn's disease of the colon. Gastroenterology 1987; 93:919-924.
71. Das KM, Dasguptaandal A, Geng X. Autoimmunity to cytoskeletal protein tropomyosin. A clue to the pathogenetic mechanism for ulcerative colitis. J Immunol 1993; 150:2487-2493.
72. Duerr RH, Targan SR, Landers CJ et al. Neutrophil cytoplasmic antibodies: A link between sclerosing cholangitis and ulcerative colitis. Gastroenterology 1991; 100:1385-1391.
73. Christ AD, Stevens AC, Koeppen H et al. An interleukin 12-related cytokine is up-regulated in ulcerative colitis but not in Crohn's disease. Gastroenterology 1998; 115:307-313.
74. Strober W, Kelsall B, Fuss I et al. Reciprocal IFN-γ and TGF-β responses regulate the occurrence of mucosal inflammation. Immunol Today 1997; 18:61-64.
75. Boirivant M, Marini M, Di Felice G et al. Lamina propria T cells in Crohn's disease and other gastrointestinal inflammation show defective CD2 pathway-induced apoptosis. Gastroenterology 1999; 116:557-565.
76. Ina K, Itoh J, Fukushima K et al. Resistance of Crohn's disease T cells to multiple apoptotic signals is associated with a Bcl-2/Bax mucosal imbalance. J Immunol 1999; 163:1081-1090.

77. Atreya R, Mudter J, Finotto S et al. Blockade of interleukin 6 trans signaling suppresses T-cell resistance against apoptosis in chronic intestinal inflammation: evidence in Crohn's disease and experimental colitis in vivo. Nat Med 2000; 6:583-588.

78. Neurath MF, Fuss I, Kelsall BL et al. Antibodies to IL-12 abrogate established experimnetal colitis in mice. J Exp Med 1995; 182:1281-1290.

79. Sartor RB. Pathogenetic and clinical relevance of cytokines in inflammatory bowel disease. Immunol Res 1991; 10:465-471.

80. Breese EJ, Michie CA, Nicholls SW et al. Tumor necrosis factor alpha-producing cells in the intestinal mucosa of children with inflammatory bowel disease. Gastroenterology 1994; 106:1455-1466.

81. van Deventer SJH. Tumour necrosis factor and Crohn's disease. Gut 1997; 40:443-448.

82. MacDonald TT, Bajaj-Elliott M, Pender SLF. T cells orchestrate intestinal mucosal shape and integrity. Immunol Today 1999; 20:505-510.

83. Pender SLF, Tickle SP, Docherty AJP et al. A major role for matrix metalloproteinases in T cell injury in the gut. J Immunol 1997; 158:1582-1590.

84. Monteleone G, MacDonald TT, Wathen NC et al. Enhancing lamina propria Th1 cell responses with interleukin 12 produces severe tissue injury. Gastroenterology 1999; 117:1069-1077.

85. Pender SLF, Fell JME, Chamow SM et al. A p55 TNF receptor immunoadhesin prevents T cell-mediated intestinal injury by inhibiting matrix metalloproteinase production. J Immunol 1998; 160:4098-4103.

86. Murphy G, Docherty AJP, Hembry RM et al. Metalloproteinases and tissue damage. Br J Rheumathol 1991; 30:25-31.

87. He CS, Wilhelm SM, Pentland AP et al. Tissue cooperation in a proteolytic cascaded activating human interstitial collagenase. Proc Natl Acad Sci USA 1989; 86:2632-2636.

88. Laurie GW, Leblond CP, Martin GR. Localization of type IV collagen, laminin, heparansulfate proteoglycan and fibronectin to the basal lamina of basement membranes. J Cell Biol 1982; 95:340-344.

89. Hann U, Stallmach A, Hahn EG et al. Basement membrane ccmponents are potent promoters of rat intestinal epithelial cell differentiation in vitro. Gastroenterology 1990; 98:322-335.

90. Heuschkel RB, MacDonald TT, Monteleone G et al. Imbalance of stromelysin-1 and TIMP-1 in mucosal lesions of children with inflammatory bowel disease. Gut 2000; 47:57-62.

91. Vaalamo M, Karjalainen-Lindsberg ML, Puolakkainen P et al. Distinct expression profiles of stromelysin-2 (MMP-10), collagenase-3 (MMP13), macrophage metalloelastase (MMP12), and tissue inhibitor of metalloproteinases-3 (TIMP-3) in intestinal ulcerations. Am J Pathol 1998; 152:1005-1014.

92. Saarialho-Kere U, Vaalamo M, Puolakkainen P et al. Enhanced expression of matrilysin, collagenase, and stromelysin-1 in gastrointestinal ulcers. Am J Pathol 1996; 148:519-526.

93. Pender SL, Salmela MT, Monteleone G et al. Ligation of alpha4β1 integrin on human intestinal mucosal mesenchymal cells selectively up-regulates membrane type-1 matrix metalloproteinase and confers a migratory phenotype. Am J Pathol 2000; 157:1955-1962.

94. Brauchle M, Madlener M, Wagner AD et al. Keratinocyte growth factor is highly overexpressed in inflammatory bowel disease. Am J Pathol 1996; 149:521-529.

95. Bajaj-Elliott M, Breese E, Poulsom R et al. Keratinocyte growth factor in inflammatory bowel disease: increased mRNA transcripts in ulcerative colitis compared to Crohn's disease in biopsies and isolated stromal cells. Am J Pathol 1997; 151:1469-1476.

96. Bajaj-Elliott M, Poulsom R, Pender SLF et al. Interactions between stromal cell-derived keratinocyte growth factor and epithelial transforming growth factor in immune-mediated crypt cell hyperplasia. J Clin Invest 1998; 102:1473-1480.

CHAPTER 5

Cytokines, Cyclooxygenases and Oral Tolerance

Olivier Morteau

Introduction

The intestinal mucosa faces a perpetual challenge: to allow the entry of minerals and nutrients from the lumen while modulating the immune responses to luminal antigens, in order to prevent mucosal inflammation. The immunosuppressive response of the mucosa to food antigens and bacteria of the normal flora is an active response defined as "oral" or mucosal tolerance.

Oral tolerance occurs through three distinct mechanisms involving mucosal T cells: T cell clonal anergy, T cell clonal deletion and secretion of immunosuppressive cytokines by regulatory T cells. Regulatory T cells are generated in Peyer's patches after antigen feeding[1-2] and subsequently migrate in the spleen. Regulatory T cells are either CD8+ (cytotoxic) or CD4+ (helper),[3] but only CD4+ T cells are required for oral tolerance, since mice genetically deficient in CD8 but not in CD4 can be rendered tolerant by antigen feeding.[4,5] CD4+ T cells are subdivided into two T helper (Th) subsets, according to their pattern in cytokine expression. Th1 cells secrete interleukin (IL)-2, interferon (IFN)γ, and tumor necrosis factor (TNF)-β and are involved in cell-mediated immunity, whereas Th2 cells secrete IL-4, IL-5, IL-6 and IL-10 and promote humoral immunity and antibody production.[6] Prior to differenciation, naive T cells located in the thymus (Th0) can secrete both Th1 or Th2 cytokines. Upon encounter with an antigen, Th0 cells become memory cells that differentiate into either Th1 or Th2 cells. Th1 and Th2 subsets suppress each other's functions[7,8] and are exclusively expressed in response to a specific antigen.[9] According to the Th1/Th2 paradigm established in mice, proinflammatory Th1 cytokines are involved in the abrogation of oral tolerance, whereas Th2 cytokines suppress the Th1 response and promote oral tolerance. In human pathologies, such as inflammatory bowel disease (IBD), the dichotomy between Th1- and Th2-type responses is usually less clearcut. IBD is a group of chronic inflammatory affections evolving through alternance of relapses and remissions, which includes ulcerative colitis (UC) and Crohn's disease (CD). The pathogenesis of IBD remains obscure but clearly involves multiple factors of genetic, immunological and environmental natures. According to the current concept developed in Chapter 8, IBD results from a lack or an abrogation of mucosal tolerance to commensal bacterial antigens in genetically susceptible individuals. The cytokine profile in CD is characterized by an increase in the expression of IL-12, TNF-α and IFN-γ expression, whereas the immune response in UC is associated with enhanced production of IL-5, but not IL-4 or IFN-γ.[10,11] Therefore, CD is commonly associated with a Th1 response, whereas the immune response in UC is closer to a Th2-type response.[12] Additional mediators to Th1- and Th2-derived cytokines are involved

Oral Tolerance: The Response of the Intestinal Mucosa to Dietary Antigens,
edited by Olivier Morteau. ©2004 Eurekah.com and Kluwer Academic / Plenum Publishers.

in the regulation of oral tolerance. They include the immunosuppressive cytokine tumor growth factor (TGF)-β, the chemokine monocyte chemoattractant protein (MCP)-1 and the prostaglandins produced by the action of the enzymes cyclooxygenase (COX)-1 and COX-2.

This Chapter will review the main mediators (Th1 and Th2 cytokines, chemokines and cyclooxygenases) involved in oral tolerance or the abrogation of oral tolerance. Based on the properties of these mediators, we will emphasize the links between oral tolerance and colitis prevention, and between abrogation of tolerance and mucosal inflammation.

IL-4 and IL-10 in Oral Tolerance

IL-4 and IL-10 can promote the differentiation of Th0 cells into Th2. The high basal levels of IL-4 and IL-10 expression in the intestinal mucosa are up-regulated shortly after oral administration of antigen.[13] IL-4 plays a critical role in the induction of tolerance by anti-CD2 plus anti-CD3 monoclonal antibodies[14] (Table 1) and oral tolerance to collagen can be reversed by an anti-IL-4 antibody in an arthritis model.[15] In addition, IL-4 plays a conditional but limited role in a model of transplantation tolerance.[16] Administration of IL-10 can restore tolerance to indigenous flora in mice with colitis.[17] In addition, IL-10 production can be increased in association with IL-4 upregulation in mice tolerized with an oral antigen.[17-22]

However, conflicting results were obtained by different groups.[23-25] Moreover, oral tolerance to both low and high doses of antigen develops normally in the absence of Th2 cells in mice genetically deficient in IL-4[26,27] and in mice treated with neutralizing anti-IL-4 antibodies.[28] Similar conclusions were made in other models of peripheral tolerance.[29] Similarly, oral tolerance can occur normally in mice treated with anti-IL-10 antibodies.[30] Therefore, the importance of IL-4 and IL-10 in oral tolerance depends largely on the model investigated.

These results were confirmed in mice genetically deficient in signal transducer and activator of transcription (STAT)-6.[31] STATs are a family of DNA-binding proteins involved in the responses of lymphocytes to signaling via cytokines. STAT-6 is activated only in response to IL-4[32] and mice in which the STAT-6 gene has been inactivated are deficient in the functional differentiation of Th2 cells.[33-35] Shi et al[31] have reported that both cell-mediated and humoral peripheral tolerance to oral ovalbumin (OVA) is maintained in absence of Th1 cells in STAT-6-/- mice. In addition, oral tolerance can occur in mice genetically deficient in the Th2 cytokines IL-5 or IL-6.[31]

Taken together, these observations demonstrate that Th2 cytokines have a specific and limited role in the development of oral tolerance.

Antiinflammatory Properties of IL-10

Mice genetically deficient in IL-10 spontaneously develop a chronic enterocolitis[36] which involves the cecum and colon in three-week old mice and can extend to the rectum and small intestine in older mice (Table 2).[37] Anti-IFN-γ treatment reduces the severity of the disease in young IL-10-/- mice[37] while IL-10 treatment prevents colitis in young IL-10-/- mice and reverses it in adult IL-10-/- mice. These observations suggest that the intestinal inflammation in IL-10 deficient mice results from the absence of inhibition by IL-10 of proinflammatory cytokine production by macrophages and Th1 cells.[37] A severe colitis can be induced in recombinase-activating gene (RAG) -2 deficient mice that lack functional T or B cells by transfer of T cell-enriched lamina propria lymphocytes or intraepithelial lymphocytes from IL-10-/- mice.[38] This confirms the involvement of T cells in the pathogenesis of IL-10-/- spontaneous colitis. In addition, a susceptibility to bacterial antigens of the normal flora is involved in the pathogenesis of this disease, since IL-10-/- mice maintained in specific pathogen-free conditions exhibit a less severe form of colitis.[36]

Table 1. Roles of cytokines and COX-2 in various tolerance model

Mediator	Role in Tolerance	Murine Tolerance Model
IL-4	Promotes	Oral tolerance in collagen-induced arthritis[15]
	Not involved	Cardiac transplantation tolerance[14,16]
		Oral tolerance in IL-4 knockouts[26,27]
		Anti-IL-4 treatment and intranasal tolerance[28]
IL-10	Promotes	Oral tolerance[17]
	Not involved	Anti-IL-10 treatment and oral tolerance[30]
TGF-β	Promotes	Oral tolerance[96]
		Oral tolerance in EAE[18,97]
IL-12	Abrogates	Oral tolerance[17]
		Intranasal tetanus toxoid[57]
		T cell anergy in vivo[58]
	Not involved	Oral tolerance in IL-12 knockouts[59,60]
IFN-γ	Promotes	Oral tolerance in IFN-γ-/- mice[75,78]
	Not involved	Oral tolerance in IFN- γ -/- mice[27,60,76,78]
MCP-1	Promotes	Oral tolerance in EAE[117]
COX-2	Promotes	Oral tolerance[171]

Table 2. Roles of cytokines and COX-2 in experimental intestinal inflammation

Mediator	Role in Colitis	Colitis Model
IL-10	Protects	IL-10-/- mice[38]
		IL-10-/- T cell transfer[38]
		CD45RB[hi] T cell transfer[43]
		PG-PS in rats[45]
TGF-β	Protects	TGF-β-/- mice[106]
		CD45RB[hi] CD4[+] T cell transfer[8,105]
		TNBs in mice[21,101,103]
IL-12	Mediates	CD45RB[hi] CD4[+] T cell transfer[67]
		BMC transfer[65]
		IL-10-/- mice[64]
		IL-2-/- mice[63]
		TNBs in mice[61]
		DSS in mice[69]
IFN-γ	Mediates	IFN-γ -/- T cell transfer[80]
	Not involved	TNBs in mice[81]
COX-2	Protects	TNBs in rats[164]
		DSS in COX-2-/- mice[170]

Transfer of CD4⁺ T cells expressing high levels of the CD45RB antigen (CD45RB^hi) into CB.17 SCID mice can evoke a wasting syndrome and a severe transmural colitis that develop 7 to 10 weeks after transfer.[39-42] Conversely, transfer of CD4⁺ T cells expressing low levels of CD45RB (CD45RB^lo), alone or with CD4⁺ CD45RB^hi T cells, can prevent the development of colitis in the recipient mice. C.B-17 SCID mice treated with IL-10 following reconstitution with CD45RB^hi T cells are protected from colitis, and this effect is correlated with a reduction in IFN-γ and TNF-α expression in the colon.[43] Another model of colitis is based on the intramural injection of streptococcal peptidoglycan-polysaccharides (PG-PS) in the intestine of rats.[44] Both resistant Fisher and susceptible Lewis rats develop a transient stage of acute colitis, but Lewis rats further relapse and develop a chronic granulomatous colitis. IL-10 treatment can attenuate the acute stage of the disease and abolish the chronic stage of colitis.[45] In PG-PS-treated rats, IL-10 may act directly or through the induction of IL-1 receptor antagonist (IL-ra), a cytokine that was reported to attenuate colitis in that model.[44]

In vitro, IL-10 suppresses T cell-mediated injury in cultures of human fetal small intestine explants.[46] Clinical IL-10 treatment of patients with CD gave promising results.[47] Recently, Steidler et al[48] partly abrogated murine colitis by administration of genetically engineered IL-10-secreting *Lactococcus lactis*, a nonpathogenic Gram-positive bacterium used to produce fermented food, allowing the prospect of a new therapeutic approach for CD.

IL-12 and STAT-4 in the Abrogation of Oral Tolerance

IL-12 has been reported to drive Th1 differentiation and IFN-γ production.[49,50] Induction of IFN-γ expression in Th1 cells is dependent on the activity of STAT-4, which mediate signals via the IL-12 receptor.[51-55]

Using a model of oral tolerance in OVA-TCR transgenic mice, Marth et al[17] have shown that the immunosuppression associated with a strong mucosal TGF-β response is enhanced when oral administration of antigen is accompanied by systemic administration of anti-IL-12 antibodies blocking Th1 cell differentiation and IFN-γ production. This increase in oral tolerance by IL-12 neutralization is associated with an increase in Fas-mediated apoptosis of peripheral T cells.[56] This observation agrees with other reports that exogenous IL-12 can prevent the induction of tolerance and act as a mucosal adjuvant[57] and can also partially reverse T cell anergy in vivo after parenteral administration of soluble peptide.[58] However, it has been shown that genetic absence of IL-12 does not influence oral tolerance to high doses of keyhole limpet hemocyanin (KLH)[59] or to OVA[60] in IL-12-/- mice. A similar conclusion was reached in a study using tolerance to OVA in STAT-4-/- mice lacking IL-12 signalling.[31]

Treatment with monoclonal anti-IL-12 antibodies abrogates colitis induced by intracolonic administration of 2,4,6-trinitrobenzene sulfonic acid (TNBs) in mice,[61] through induction of Fas-mediated apoptosis.[62] Spontaneous colitis in IL-2-/-[63] and IL-10-/- mice[64] can also be abolished by administration of anti-IL-12 antibodies. Anti-IL-12 treatment also decreases the severity of colitis induced by bone marrow cell (BMC) reconstitution in T cell- NK- cell-deficient (Tgε26) mice,[65] a model in which recipient Tgε26 mice develop after 4 to 6 weeks a wasting syndrome and a severe inflammation of the colonic mucosa which correlates with the expansion of activated peripheral and intestinal T cells.[66] In addition, the impact of colitis induced either by BMC transfer into Tgε26 mice or by CD45RB^hi CD4⁺ T cells transfer into CB.17 SCID mice is dramatically reduced when the transferred cells originate from STAT-4-/- mice.[65] Immunization of STAT-4 transgenic mice with KLH evokes an increase in STAT-4 expression in lamina propria CD4⁺ T cells associated with the development of chronic transmural colitis.[67] Colitis can be induced in SCID mice by reconstitution with STAT-4 transgenic activated spleen cells or LPMC.[67] Exogenous IL-12 increases Th1 cytokine expression, leading to mucosal injury in intestinal fetal explants[68] and to an increase in severity in the colitis induced by dextran sodium sulfate in mice.[69]

IFN-γ in Oral Tolerance and Colitis

Studies have reported an increase in the Th1 cytokine IFN-γ in the gut-associated lymphoid tissue (GALT) following oral administration of antigen to mice[17,22,24,70-73] and a reversal of tolerance after IFN-γ depletion.[74] IFN-γ was shown to mediate the induction of oral tolerance, and B cell responses were fully restored and T cell responses partly restored in IFN-γ deficient mice fed OVA.[75] However, other studies reported that oral tolerance can occur normally in IFN-γ-/- mice[27,60,76] and in STAT-4-/- mice that exhibit impaired Th1 responses.[31] In one study, oral tolerance to OVA occurred normally in mice depleted in IFN-γ, in IFN-γ-/- mice and in IL-12-/- mice.[60] Very recently, the role of IFN-γ in oral tolerance was investigated using a model in which OVA-specific CD4⁺ T cells from TCR transgenic mice were transferred into wild type Balb/C recipient mice.[77] Following OVA feeding, IFN-γ production was increased in intestinal lymphoid tissues of T cell recipient mice and T cell responses were down-regulated in the periphery.[78] The authors suggested that the induction of IFN-γ may enhance intestinal immune responses while impairing the expression of homing molecules needed for CD4⁺ T cells to participate in peripheral immune responses.[78] Anti-IFN-γ treatment in OVA-fed recipient mice abrogated oral tolerance as measured by delayed-type hypersensitivity responses but not as measured by antibody responses,[78] which suggests that B cell responses are much more affected than T cell responses by the absence of IFN-γ and explains partly the discrepancies between previous studies.[79]

The transfer of in vitro activated CD4⁺ T cells from wild type mice induces a lethal colitis in the recipient SCID mice.[80] The disease is less severe when the CD4⁺ T cells originate from IFN-γ-/- mice. Colitis reduction is associated with a 2-3 fold increase in IL-4-positive lamina propria T cells as measured by intracellular cytokine staining.[80] MHC class II antigen expression was strongly regulated in the colonic epithelial cells of SCID mice that received wild type CD4⁺ T cells when compared with SCID mice recipient for IFN-γ-/- CD4⁺ T cells. These observations suggest that IFN-γ is an important proinflammatory factor in colitis. However, the severity of TNBs-induced colitis was similar in wild type and in IFN-γ-/- mice.[81] Thus, the role of IFN-γ in the development of experimental colitis clearly depends on the model used, and more studies will be needed in order to establish the importance of this cytokine in IBD.

TGF-β and the Promotion of Oral Tolerance

TGF-β is secreted by various mucosal cell types including T cells, enterocytes and macrophages and exerts anti-inflammatory and immunosuppressive actions in numerous cells.[82-84] TGF-β1 in particular can suppress macrophage functions in vitro,[85] reduce MHC class II expression[86] and diminish the induction of cytotoxic lymphocytes.[87] TGF-β promotes both B cell activation[88] and IgA isotype switching.[89-94] TGF-β1 may also have a role in T cell trafficking, since it can induce in vitro the expression of the mucosal homing receptor $\alpha_E\beta_7$ integrin in human T cells.[95]

The involvement of TGF-β in oral tolerance has been demonstrated[96] in vivo and in vitro.[18,97] Two specific subtypes of TGF-β-secreting CD4⁺ T cells have been reported to play an important role in oral tolerance: Th3 cells and Tr1 cells. Th3 cells were isolated and cloned from Peyer's patches and mesenteric lymph nodes of tolerized mice.[18,98] Th3 cells share similarities with Th2 cells, including the ability to produce Th2 cytokines such as IL-4 and IL-10, but also secrete TGF-β. TGF-β can stimulate the differentiation of Th3 cells, a process potentiated by IL-10 or anti-IL-12.[99] Tr1 cells were cloned by expanding TcR transgenic T cells in the presence of IL-10.[8] Tr1 cells have the ability to produce both IL-10 and TGF-β, to suppress the function of CD4⁺ effector cells in vitro and to inhibit colitis in vivo. Tr1 immunosuppressive properties are largely dependent on TGF-β.[8]

TGF-β-producing Tr1 cells can prevent the induction of colitis by transfer of CD4[+] CD45RB[hi] T cells in SCID mice.[8] Intrarectal administration of TNBs in mice generates severe granulomatous inflammatory lesions of the colonic mucosa associated with an increase in Th1 cytokine secretion.[61,100] Interestingly, TNBs-induced colitis can be prevented by oral administration of TNP-haptenated colonic protein.[21] This suppression is associated with the generation of mucosal T cells producing TGF-β and can be abrogated by anti-TGF-β antibody treatment.[21] Ingested proteins evoke in the mucosal follicles of nondiseased mice an IFN-γ-driven Th1 type response that is counter-regulated by induction of T-cell anergy/deletion.[17,72] If this Th1 response is inhibited, an active immunosuppression occurs through generation of TGF-β-secreting T cells.

Multiple intraperitoneal administrations of TGF-β plasmid DNA ameliorate TNBs-induced colitis[101] and intranasal administration of naked TGF-β DNA displays immunosuppressive effects associated with long-term expression of TGF-β in various tissues.[102] Based on these findings, Strober's group recently prevented and reversed TNBs-induced colitis in mice using a single intranasal administration of TGF-β1 plasmid and reported the expression of TGF-β1 in mucosal tissues.[103] In that model, TGF-β1 down-regulates IL-12 receptor expression and enhances the secretion of IL-10 which in turn inhibits IL-12 and TNF-α production.[103] Both TGF-β and IL-10 can be secreted by the Tr1 subset[8] and intranasal administration of TGF-β or IL-10 DNA has immunosuppressive effects.[102,104] As reported above, genetic or pharmacologic neutralization of TGF-β or IL-10 results in the development of colitis in the TNBs model and the CD45RB T cell transfer model, respectively,[105] showing that both TGF-β and IL-10 can prevent intestinal mucosal inflammation. Based on these observations, it was suggested that IL-10 may be necessary for the development of TGF-β-producing T cells or for TGF-β secretion and that conversely, TGF-β may be necessary for the development of IL-10-producing cells or for IL-10 secretion.[103]

The absence of TGF-β1 gene expression in TGF-β1-/- mice[106] induces a wasting syndrome that generates high mortality rates and is associated with multifocal inflammatory disease in many tissues. The overexpression of MHC class I and II antigens and the overproduction of Igs suggest an autoimmune etiology.[106] The authors reported elevated IgE levels, excess of complement-binding IgG and IgM and lack of antiinflammatory IgA in serum and external secretions, due to an abberrant production of Igs in both the systemic and mucosal compartments.[107] These uncontrolled B cell responses were associated with an increased production of Th2 cytokines. The authors have postulated that the impairment of mucosal immunity in TGF-β1-/- mice may contribute to the pulmonary and gastrointestinal mucosal lesions observed.[107]

MCP-1: A Chemokine Promoting Oral Tolerance

Monocyte chemoattractant protein 1 (MCP-1) is a CC chemokine that attracts monocytes, memory T cells and natural killer cells in vitro.[108-112] MCP-1 is a potential actor in the intestinal mucosal inflammatory response. In inflamed intestinal specimens from patients with IBD, MCP-1 mRNA expression is dramatically increased[113-115] and specifically located in macrophages, smooth-muscle cells and endothelial cells.[114,115] Infection of human colon epithelial cell lines (Caco-2 and HT-29) with *Salmonella dublin* induces an upregulation of the expression of MCP-1 and other chemokines.[116] MCP-1 mRNA expression is upregulated by proinflammatory IL-1 in freshly isolated normal epithelial cells and Caco-2 cells.[115] However, the mechanism of action of MCP-1 in the mucosal inflammatory responses of the intestine has not been yet established.

MCP-1 has been reported to promote oral tolerance in a murine model of experimental autoimmune encephalomyelitis (EAE).[117] In that model, immunization of SJL/J mice with proteolipid protein (PLP)[118] induces a progressive ascending clinical paralysis followed by periods of remission and subsequent relapses.[119] Oral administration of PLP inhibits the development of EAE and induces clonal anergy associated with a decrease in antigen-specific IL-2 and IFN-γ production in the absence of measurable TGF-β production.[120] In tolerized mice, MCP-1 expression is increased in the intestinal mucosa, Peyer's patches and mesenteric lymph nodes.[117] Moreover, the administration of anti-MCP-1 antibody inhibits oral tolerance and increases the production of IL-12 in the intestinal mucosa.[117] Three distinct mechanisms could explain the regulation of oral tolerance by MCP-1 in that model. The first is a direct upregulation of IL-4 expression, potentiating the differentiation of Th2 cells. The second is a direct downregulation of IL-12 production, inducing a block of peripheral Th1 differentiation and/or an increase in mucosal TGF-β production. The third is the induction of T cell infiltration into the mucosal immune tissues in response to a chemotactic gradient, followed by the migration of these activated T cells to the central nervous system.

MCP-1 is associated with the development of polarized Th2 responses[121,122] and stimulates T cell-induced IL-4 secretion.[117,123] A recent study showed that MCP-1-/- mice[121] do not accomplish the immunoglobulin subclass switching characteristic of Th2 responses.[124] MCP-1-/- mice exhibit a dramatic decrease in the ratio of total serum IgG1 to IgG2α that persists after immunization with TNP-derivatized OVA. Lymph node cells from immunized MCP-1-/- secrete very little IL-4, IL-5 and IL-10 but normal levels of IL-12, Il-2 and IFN-γ. Moreover, MCP-1-/- mice are unable to develop a Th2 response in a model of footpad swelling generated by the parasite *Leishmania major*. These observations imply that MCP-1 is required for Th2 polarization and acts by a direct mechanism that does not involve abnormal cell migration, since the trafficking of naive T cells is undisturbed in MCP-1 deficient mice.[124] The authors point out that their findings are at odds with the observation that mice deficient in CCR2 (the only receptor to MCP-1 identified so far) show a defect in Th1 response.[125,126] The existence of two other ligands (MCP-3 and MCP-5) for CCR2 could explain this discrepancy.

Taken together, these data suggest that MCP-1 promotes oral tolerance in the murine EAE model through potentiation of a Th2 response rather than by regulating T cell infiltration in secondary lymphoid organs. Whether MCP-1 acts through the regulation of IL-4 or IL-12 expression remains to be determined.

Prostaglandins and Protection of the Intestinal Mucosa

The homodimeric enzyme cyclooxygenase (COX) (or prostaglandin H synthase) catalyzes the synthesis of prostaglandins (PGs) through a two-step process. A di-oxygenase activity first cyclizes and oxygenates arachidonic acid into PGG_2. Then, a peroxidase activity catalyzes the reduction of PGG_2 into PGH_2. PGH_2 is the precursor of PGD_2, PGE_2, $PGF_{2\alpha}$, PGI_2 and thromboxane A_2 which are synthesized via cell-specific synthases. Two 70 kDa isoforms of COX (COX-1 and COX-2) encoded by two distinct genes have been identified.[127-132] Importantly, COX-1 is constitutively expressed in most organs, while COX-2 expression is only constitutive in a few tissues and is generally inducible by a variety of mitogens, tumor promoters and proinflammatory stimuli, including bacterial factors and cytokines (reviewed in ref. 133).

Prostaglandins are pro-inflammatory in most organs. They mediate fever, hyperalgesia, increase in vascular permeability and edema, and are involved in a number of inflammatory conditions and diseases including arthritis,[134] skin inflammation[135] and asthma.[136] Classical nonsteroidal anti-inflammatory drugs (NSAIDs), such as indomethacin or aspirin, exert anti-inflammatory, analgesic and antipyretic effects[137] through inhibition of both COX-1 and COX-2 enzymatic activities.

In the gastrointestinal mucosa, PGs exert a cytoprotective, anti-inflammatory action.[138] Experimental colitis can be attenuated by pretreatment with exogenous PGs.[139,140] PGE_2

mediates the regeneration of the epithelial crypts following intestinal damage induced in mice by radiation[141] and by the chemical dextran sodium sulfate (DSS).[142] In genetically susceptible rats, inhibition of PG synthesis by the NSAID indomethacin induces acute and chronic enterocolitis.[143] Similarly, active or passive immunization with PGE_2, PGE_1 and prostacyclin (PGI_2) induces gastrointestinal ulcers in rabbits.[144,145] Moreover, NSAIDs display severe gastrointestinal side effects including gastroduodenal perforations and massive hemorrhage, which are partly attributed to the inhibition of PG synthesis in the gastrointestinal mucosa.[146-149]

COX-1, COX-2 and Intestinal Mucosal Inflammation

COX-1 is constitutively expressed in most organs and its expression is unaffected by anti-inflammatory treatment by glucocorticoids. In the gastrointestinal mucosa, COX-1 is thought to maintain physiological homeostasis. On the other hand, COX-2 expression is inducible by a variety of proinflammatory factors and cytokines and can be inhibited by glucocorticoids.[150-152] The induction of COX-2 expression by TNF-α in colonic epithelial cells is mediated by the activation of the nuclear factor NF-κB,[153] a major transcription factor for cytokines. Based on these observations, the antiinflammatory properties of NSAIDs were attributed to the inhibition of proinflammatory COX-2, whereas their ulcerogenic actions were attributed to the inhibition of a constitutive pool of COX-1-derived protective PGs.[154-157] Selective inhibitors of COX-2 activity were reported to display equivalent anti-inflammatory and analgesic efficacy than classic NSAIDs without causing any gastrointestinal injury, when used in animal models of inflammation[158,159] and in patients with osteoarthritis or rheumatoid arthritis.[160-163]

The beneficial role of COX-2 in gastrointestinal inflammation was demonstrated in rodent models of experimental colitis. The selective COX-2 inhibitor etodolac exacerbates the severity of TNBs-induced colitis in rats[164] and the selective COX-2 inhibitor NS-398 delays the healing of acetic acid-induced gastric ulcers in mice.[165] In addition, selective COX-2 inhibitors delay gastric ulcer healing[166] and increase the severity of stress-induced gastric ulcers[167] in rats. As a complement to these pharmacologic studies, the impact of DSS-induced colitis was investigated in mice genetically deficient in either COX-1[168] or COX-2[169] isoform.[170] In the absence of DSS treatment, no spontaneous intestinal inflammation occurs in any of the naive COX-1 or COX-2 deficient mice, even in absence of detectable intestinal levels of PGE2 in COX-1 knockouts. However, DSS-induced colitis is exacerbated in both COX-1 and COX-2 knockouts and more severely in the COX-2 deficient mice.[170] Thus, both COX-1 and COX-2 isoforms play a protective role during intestinal inflammation, although none of the isoforms alone is sufficient to maintain mucosal homeostasis in the absence of intestinal injury.

COX-2, Prostaglandins and Immunosuppression

COX-2 was shown to mediate oral immunologic tolerance to a dietary antigen in T cell receptor (TCR) mutant mice.[171] Oral administration of a specific dietary antigen to TCR transgenic mice resulted in no intestinal pathology, while coadministration of the antigen and of selective COX-2 inhibitors induced an intestinal inflammation characterized by villus erosion, crypt expansion and proliferation of lamina propria mononuclear cells (LPMNCs).[171] Furthermore, LPMNCs from COX-2 deficient mice produced less than 1% of the PGE2 produced by LPMNCs from wild-type or COX-1 knockouts, which demonstrates that the high levels of PGE2 produced by LPMNCs during oral tolerance depend on COX-2 but not COX-1 activity.[171] This study suggests that COX-2 may promote intestinal mucosal protection by suppressing pathogenic cellular immune responses to luminal bacterial antigens which perpetuate intestinal inflammation.[172]

Prostaglandins display immunosuppressive properties. PGE$_2$ inhibits the secretion of the proinflammatory cytokines IL-1 and TNF-α by stimulated human[173] and murine[174] monocytes in vitro and the inflamed colons of DSS-treated COX-2-/- mice produce increased levels of IL-1β.[170] PGs have the ability to promote the Th2 cytokine pathway. PGE2 can suppress IL-2 and IFN-γ production by Th1 cells, but not IL-4 and IL-5 production by Th2 cells.[175] PGE2 can inhibit IFN-γ production by mice splenocytes in vitro[176] and in vivo administration of the COX-2 inhibitor NS-398 to mice enhances IFN-γ production but not IL-4 production by activated splenocytes.[176] In the differentiation phase of naive T cells, PGE2 inhibits the differentiation of Th1 and IL-12R expression via cAMP accumulation.[177,178] PGE2 enhances LPS-induced IL-10 production and decreases IL-12 production by APCs.[179] IL-12 and PGE2 derived from APCs determine the IFN-γ level of activated human CD4+T cells.[180] PGE2 increases IgE production by IL-4- and LPS-stimulated B cells in vitro.[181] Recent studies show that COX-1[182] and COX-2[182-184] are expressed in human T cells and that COX-2 expression and PGD2 production are preferentially induced in Th2 cell lines.[185] COX-2 inhibition by NS-398 or Celecoxib induces a decrease in T cell proliferation associated with an inhibition in IL-2, TNF-α and IFN-γ production.[183] These data seem to disagree with the property of PGs to promote the Th2 pathway. However the effects of COX-2 inhibitors on T cell-derived cytokine production might be unrelated to the inhibition of PGs.[183]

Conclusion

Although the Th2-derived cytokines IL-4 and IL-10 have been associated with the induction of oral tolerance, their role is limited to specific experimental models. Nevertheless, IL-10 is an important factor in the prevention and reversal of the mucosal inflammatory response, both in experimental colitis and in IBD. The immunosuppressive cytokine TGF-β shares many antiinflammatory and immunosuppressive properties with IL-10. TGF-β is a critical mediator of oral tolerance that exerts antiinflammatory actions in the intestinal mucosa.

By contrast, IL-12 is an important promoter of Th1 differentiation and IFN-γ production whose role in the abrogation of oral tolerance has been demonstrated in some but not all models of oral tolerance. In addition, IL-12 clearly promotes the inflammatory response in the intestinal mucosa. The role of the Th1 cytokine IFN-γ in the abrogation of oral tolerance and the establishment of colitis remains controversial.

MCP-1 is the only chemokine so far involved in oral tolerance in a model of experimental autoimmune encephalomyelitis in mice. MCP-1 may promote oral tolerance via stimulation of Th2 differentiation and might influence the production of IL-4 or IL-12.

Prostaglandins produced by the action of COX-1 and COX-2 are important anti-inflammatory mediators in the intestinal mucosa and COX-2 can promote oral tolerance in a specific model. Although their mechanisms of action are unclear, PGs might act through downregulation of proinflammatory cytokines and promotion of the Th2 cytokine pathway.

In conclusion, the involvement of Th1 and Th2 cytokines in oral tolerance and its abrogation critically depends on the experimental model considered. Nevertheless, TGF-β, IL-10 and COX-2 are usually associated with oral tolerance and colitis prevention, whereas IL-12 is involved in the abrogation of tolerance and the development of intestinal inflammation. Although the link between oral tolerance and prevention of colitis remains loose, the mediators of oral tolerance may constitute promising tools in the treatment of IBD.

Acknowledgements

Supported in part by NIH grants HL63645 and AI41851.

References

1. Asherson GL, Zembala M, Perera MACC et al. Production of immunity and unresponsiveness in the mouse by feeding contact sensitizing agents and the role of suppressor cells in the Peyer's patches, mesenteric lymph nodes and other lymphoid tissues. Cell Immunol 1977; 33:145-155.
2. Mattingly JA and Walksman BH. Immunologic suppression after oral administration of antigen. I. Specific suppressor cells formed in rat Peyer's patches after oral administration of sheep erythrocytes and their systemic migration. J Immunol 1978; 121:1878-1882.
3. Faria AMC, Weiner HL. Oral tolerance: mechanisms and therapeutic applications. In: Dixon FJ, ed. Advances in Immunology, Vol. 73. Academic Press, 1999:153-264.
4. Desvignes C, Bour H, Nicolas JF et al. Lack of oral tolerance but oral priming for contact sensitivity to dinitrofluorobenzene in major histocompatibility complex class II-deficient mice and in CD4⁺ T-cell-depleted mice. Eur J Immunol 1996; 26:1756-1761.
5. Tada Y, Ho DR, Mak TW. Collagen-induced arthritis in CD4- or CD8-deficient mice. CD8-T-cells play a role in initiation and regulate recovery phase of collagen-induced arthritis. J Immunol 1996; 156:4520-4526.
6. Mosmann TR, Coffman RL. Th1 and Th2 cells: different patterns of lymphokine secretion lead to different functional properties. Annu Rev Immunol 1989; 7:145-173.
7. Adachi M, Oda N, Kokubu F et al. IL-10 induces a Th2 cell tolerance in allergic asthma. Int Arch Allergy Immunol 1999; 118:391-394.
8. Groux H, O'Garra A, Bigler M et al. A CD4⁺ T cell subset inhibits antigen specific T cell responses and prevents colitis. Nature 1997; 389:737-742.
9. Ferrara JLM. Cytokines and regulation of oral tolerance. J Clin Invest 2000; 105:1043-1044.
10. Fuss IJ, Neurath M, Boirivant M et al. Disparate CD4⁺ lamina propria (LP) lymphokine secretion profiles in inflammatory bowel disease. Crohn's disease manifest increased secretion of IFN-gamma, whereas ulcerative colitis LP cells manifest increased secretion of IL-5. J Immunol 1996; 157:1261-1270.
11. Monteleone G, Biancone L, Marasco R et al. Interleukin 12 is expressed and actively released by Crohn's disease intestinal lamina propria mononuclear cells. Gastroenterology 1997; 112:1169-1178.
12. Papadakis KA, Targan SR. Role of cytokines in the pathogenesis of inflammatory bowel disease. Ann Rev 2000; 51:289-296.
13. Gonnella PA, Chen Y, Inobe JI et al. In situ immune response in gut associated lymphoid tissue (GALT) following oral antigen in TcR transgenic mice. J Immunol 1998; 160:4708-4718.
14. Punch J, Tono T, Qun L et al. Tolerance induction by anti-CD2 plus anti-CD3 monoclonal antibodies: evidence for an IL-4 requirement. J Immunol 1998; 161:1156-1162.
15. Yoshino S. Treatment with an anti-IL-4 antibody blocks suppression of collagen-induced arthritis in mice by oral administration of type II collagen. J Immunol 1998; 160:3067-3071.
16. Bushell A, Niimi M, Morris P et al. Evidence for immune regulation in the induction of transplantation tolerance: a conditional but limited role for IL-4. J Immunol 1999; 162:1359-1366.
17. Marth T, Strober W, Kelsall BL. High dose oral tolerance in ovalbumin TcR-transgenic mice: systemic neutralisation of interleukin 12 augments TGFβ secretion and T cell apoptosis. J Immunol 1996; 157:2348-2357.
18. Chen Y, Kuchroo VK, Inobe JI et al. Regulatory T cell clones induced by oral tolerance: suppression of autoimmune encephalomyelitis. Science 1994; 265:1237-1240.
19. Chen Y, Inobe JI, Weiner HL. Induction of oral tolerance to myelin basic protein in CD8-depleted mice: both CD4⁺ and CD8⁺ cells mediate active suppression. J Immunol 1995; 155:910-916.
20. Chen Y, Inobe JI, Kuchroo VK et al. Oral tolerance in myelin basic protein T-cell receptor transgenic mice: suppression of autoimmune encephalomyelitis and dose-dependent induction of regulatory cells. Proc Natl Acad Sci USA 1996; 93:388-391.
21. Neurath MF, Fuss I, Kelsall BL et al. Experimental granulomatous colitis in mice is abrogated by induction of TGF-β-mediated oral tolerance. J Exp Med 1996; 183:2605-2616.
22. Chen Y, Inobe JI, Weiner HL. Inductive events in oral tolerance in the TcR transgenic adoptive transfer model. Cell Immunol 1997; 178:62-68.
23. Garside P, Steel M, Worthey EA et al. Th2 cells are subject to high dose oral tolerance and are not essential for its induction. J Immunol 1995; 154:5649-5655.

24. Hoyne GF, Callow MG, Kuhlman J et al. T-cell lymphokine response to orally administered proteins during priming and unresponsiveness. Immunology 1993; 78:534-540.
25. Wang ZY, Link H, Ljungdahl A et al. Induction of interferon-γ, interleukin-4 and transforming growth factor-β in rats orally tolerized against autoimmune myasthenia gravis. Cell Immunol 1994; 157:353-368.
26. Garside P, Steel M, Worthey E et al. T helper cells are subject to high dose oral tolerance and are not essential for its induction. J Immunol 1995; 154:5649-5655.
27. Lycke N, Bromander A, Ekman L et al. The use of knockout mice in studies of induction and regulation of gut mucosal immunity. Mucosal Immunol Update 1995; 3:1-8.
28. Wolvers DAW, van der Cammen MJF, Kraal G. Mucosal tolerance is associated with, but independent of, upregulation of Th2 responses. Immunology 1997; 92:328-333.
29. Geury JC, Galbiati F, Smiroldo S et al. Selective development of T helper (Th)2 cells induced by continuous administration of low dose soluble proteins to normal and β2-microglobulin-deficient BALB/C mice. J Exp Med 1996; 183:485-497.
30. Aroeira LS, Cardillo F, De-Albuquerque D et al. Anti-IL-10 treatment does not block either the induction or the maintenance of orally induced tolerance to OVA. Scand J Immunol 1995; 44:319-323.
31. Shi HN, Grusby MJ, Nagler-Anderson C. Orally induced peripheral nonresponsiveness is maintained in the absence of functional Th1 and Th2 cells. J Immunol 1999; 162:5143-5148.
32. O'Shea JJ. Jaks, STATs, cytokine transduction and immuno-regulation: are we there yet? Immunity 1997; 7:1-11.
33. Kaplan MH, Schindler U, Smiley ST et al. Stat 6 is required for mediating responses to IL-4 and for the development of Th2 cells. Immunity 1996; 4:313-319.
34. Takeda K, Tanaka T, Shi W et al. Essential role of STAT6 in IL-4 signalling. Nature 1996; 380:627-630.
35. Shimoda K, van Deursen J, Sangster MY et al. Lack of IL-4 induced Th2 response and IgE switching in mice with disrupted Stat 6 gene. Nature 1996; 380:630-633.
36. Kuhn R, Lohier J, Rennick D et al. Interleukin-10 deficient mice develop chronic enterocolitis. Cell 1993; 75:263-274.
37. Berg DJ, Davidson N, Kuhn R et al. Enterocolitis and colon cancer in interleukin-10-deficient mice are associated with aberrant cytokine production and CD4+ Th1-like responses. J Clin Invest 1996; 98:1010-1020.
38. Davidson NJ, Leach MW, Fort MM et al. T helper cell 1-type CD4+ T cells, but not B cells, mediate colitis in interleukin 10-deficient mice. J Exp Med 1996;184:241-251.
39. Morrissey PJ, Charrier K, Braddy S et al. CD4+ T cells that express high levels of CD45RB induce wasting disease when transferred into congenic severe combined immunodeficient mice: Disease development is prevented by cotransfer of purified CD4+ T cells. J Exp Med 1993; 178:237-244.
40. Powrie F, Leach MW, Mauze S et al. Phenotypically distinct subsets of CD4+ T cells induce or protect from chronic intestinal inflammation in C.B-17 scid mice. Int Immunol 1993; 5:1461-1467.
41. Powrie F, Correa-Olivieira R, Mauze S et al. Regulatory interactions between CD45RBhigh and CD45RBlow CD4+ T cells are important for the balance between protective and pathogenic cell-mediated immunity. J Exp Med 1994; 179:589-600.
42. Powrie F. T cells in inflammatory bowel disease: Protective and pathogenic roles. Immunity 1995; 3:171-174.
43. Powrie F, Leach MW, Mauze S et al. Inhibition of Th1 responses prevents inflammatory bowel disease in SCID mice reconstituted with CD45RBhi CD4+ T cells. Immunity 1994; 1:553-562.
44. McCall RD, Haskill S, Zimmerman EM et al. Tissue interleukin-1 and interleukin-1 receptor antagonist expression in enterocolitis in resistant and susceptible rats. Gastroenterology 1994; 10:960-972.
45. Herfarth HH, Mohanty SP, Rath HC et al. Interleukin 10 suppresses experimental chronic granulomatous inflammation induced by bacterial cell wall polymers. Gut 1996; 39:836-845.
46. Pender SLF, Breese EJ, Günther U et al. Suppression of T cell-mediated injury in human gut by interleukin 10: role of matrix metalloproteinases. Gastroenterology 1998; 115:573-583.
47. van Deventer SJ, Elson CO, Fedorak RN. Multiple doses of intravenous interleukin 10 in steroid-refractory Crohn's disease. Crohn's disease study group. Gastroenterology 1997; 113:383-389.

48. Steidler L, Hans W, Schotte L et al. Treatment of murine colitis by Lactococcus lactis secreting interleukin 10. Science 2000; 289:1352-1355.

49. Trinchieri G. Interleukin 12: a cytokine produced by antigen-presenting cells with immunoregulatory functions in the generation of T-helper cells type 1 and cytotoxic lymphocytes. Blood 1994; 84:4008.

50. Magram J, Connaughton SE, Warrier RR et al. IL-12-deficient mice are defective in IFNγ production and type 1 cytokine responses. Immunity 1996; 4:471-481.

51. Cho SS, Bacon CM, SudarshanC et al. Activation of STAT4 by IL-12 and IFN-α: evidence for the involvement of ligand-induced tyrosine and serine phosphorylation. J Immunol 1996; 157:4781-4789.

52. Bacon CM, Petricoin EFR, Ortaldo JR et al. Interleukin 12 induces tyrosine phosphorylation and activation of STAT4 in human lymphocytes. Proc Natl Acad Sci USA 1995; 92:7307-7311.

53. Ihle JN. STATs: signal transducers and activators of transcription. Cell 1996; 84:331-334.

54. Jacobson NG, Szabo SJ, Weber-Nordt RM et al. Interleukin 12 signalling in T helper 1 (Th1) cells involves tyrosine phosphorylation of signal transducer and activator of transcription (Stat)3 and Stat4. J Exp Med 1995; 181:1755-1762.

55. Thierfelder WE, van Deursen JM, Yamamoto K et al. Requirement for Stat-4 in interleukin-12-mediated responses of natural killer and T cells. Nature 1996; 332:171-174.

56. Marth T, Zeitz M, Ludviksson BR et al. Extinction of IL-12 signalling promotes Fas-mediated apoptosis of antigen-specific T cells. J Immunol 1999; 162:7233-7240.

57. Boyaka P, Marinaro M, Jackson RJ et al. IL-12 is an effective adjuvant for induction of mucosal immunity. J Immunol 1999; 162:122-128.

58. van Parijs L, Perez VL, Biuckians A et al. Role of interleukin 12 and costimulators in T cell anergy in vivo. J Exp Med 1997; 186:1119-1128.

59. Grdic D, Smith RE, Donachie AM et al. the mucosal adjuvant effect of cholera toxin and ISCOMS differ in their requirement for IL-12, indicating different pathways of action. Eur J Immunol 1999; 29:1774-1784.

60. Mowat AM, Steel M, Leishman A et al. Normal induction of oral tolerance in the absence of a functional IL-12-dependent IFN-γ signalling pathway. J Immunol 1999; 163:4728-4736.

61. Neurath MF, Fuss I, Kelsall BL et al. Antibodies to IL-12 abrogate established experimental colitis in mice. J Exp Med 1995; 182:1281-1290.

62. Fuss I, Marth T, Neurath MF et al. Anti-interleukin 12 treatment regulates apoptosis of Th1 T cells in experimental colitis. Gastroenterology 1999; 117:1078-1088.

63. Ehrhardt RO, Ludviksson BR, Gray B et al. Induction and prevention of colonic inflammation in IL-2 deficient mice. J Immunol 1997; 158:566-573.

64. Davidson NJ, Hudak SA, Lesley RE et al. IL-12, but not IFN-γ, plays a major role in sustaining the chronic phase of colitis in IL-10-deficient mice. J Immunol 1998; 161:3143-3149.

65. Simpson SJ, Shah S, Comiskey M et al. T cell-mediated pathology in two models of experimental colitis depends predominantly on the interleukin 12/signal transducer and activator of transcription (Stat)-4 pathway, but is not conditional on interferon γ expression by T cells. J Exp Med 1998; 187:1225-1234.

66. Hollander GA, Simpson SJ, Mizoguchi E et al. Severe colitis in mice with aberrant thymic selection. Immunity 1995; 3:27-38.

67. Wirtz S, Finotto S, Kanzler S et al. Cutting edge: chronic intestinal inflammation in STAT-4 transgenic mice: characterization of disease and adoptive transfer by TNF- plus IFN-γ-producing CD4⁺ T cells that respond to bacterial antigens. J Immunol 1999; 162:1884-1888.

68. Monteleone G, MacDonald TT, Wathen NC et al. Enhancing lamina propria Th1 cell responses with interleukin 12 produces severe tissue injury. Gastroenterology 1999; 117:1069-1077.

69. Hans H, Scholmerich J, Gross V et al. Interleukin-12 induced interferon-gamma increases inflammation in acute dextran sulfate sodium induced colitis in mice. Eur Cytokine Netw 2000; 11:67-74.

70. Gautam SC, Chikkala NF, Battisto JR. Oral administration of the contact sensitizer trinitrochloro benzene: initial sensitization and subsequent appearance of a suppressor population. Cell Immunol 1990; 125:437-448.

71. Hoyne GF, Thomas WR. T-cell responses to orally administered antigens. Study of the kinetics of lymphokine production after single and multiple feeding. Immunology 1995; 84:304-309.

72. Strober W, Kelsall B, Fuss I et al. Reciprocal IFN-γ and TGF-β responses regulate the occurrence of mucosal inflammation. Immunol Today 1997; 18:61-64.

73. Spiekermann GM, Nagler-Anderson C. Oral administration of the bacterial superantigen staphylococcal enterotoxin B induces activation and cytokine production by T cells in murine gut-associated lymphoid tissue. J Immunol 1998; 161:5825-5831.

74. Liu Y, Janeway CA. Interferon γ plays a critical role in induced cell death of effector cells: A possible third mechanism of self-tolerance. J Exp Med 1990; 172:1735-1739.

75. Kweon M-N, Fujihashi K, VanCott JL et al. Lack of orally induced systemic unresponsiveness in IFN-γ knockout mice. J Immunol 1998; 160:1687-1693.

76. Kjerrulf M, Grdic D, Ekman L et al. Interferon-gamma receptor-deficient mice exhibit impaired gut mucosal immune responses but intact oral tolerance. Immunology 1997; 92:60-68.

77. Kearney ER, Pape KA, Loh DY et al. Visualization of peptide-specific T cell immunity and peripheral tolerance induction in vivo. Immunity 1994; 1:327-339.

78. Lee H-O, Miller SD, Hurst SD et al. Interferon gamma induction during oral tolerance reduces T-cell migration to sites of inflammation. Gastroenterology 2000; 119:129-138.

79. Whitacre C. New insights into oral tolerance. Gastroenterology 2000; 119:260-262.

80. Bregenholt S, Brimnes J, Nissen MH et al. In vitro activated CD4⁺ T cells from interferon-gamma (IFN-gamma)-deficient mice induce intestinal inflammation in immunodeficient hosts. Clin Exp Immunol 1999; 118:228-234.

81. Camoglio L, te Velde AA, de Boer A et al. Hapten-induced colitis associated with maintained Th1 and inflammatory responses in IFN-gamma receptor-deficient mice. Eur J Immunol 2000; 30:1486-1495.

82. Roberts A, Sporn M. Physiological actions and clinical applications of transforming growth factor β (TGFβ). Growth Factors 1993; 8:1-9.

83. McCartney-Francis NL, Wahl SM. Transforming growth factor β: A matter of life and death. J Leukocyte Biol 1994: 55:401-409.

84. Wahl SM. Transforming growth factor β: The good, the bad and the ugly. J Exp Med 1994; 180:1587-1590.

85. Tsunakawi S, Sporn M, Ding A et al. Deactivation of macrophages by transforming growth factor β. Nature 1988: 334:260-262.

86. Czarniecki CW, Chui HH, Wong GHW et al. Transforming growth factor-β1 modulates the expression of class II histocompatibility antigens on human cells. J Immunol 1988; 140: 4217-4223.

87. Wahl SM, Hunt DA, Wong HL et al. Transforming growth factor β is a potent immunosuppressive agent that inhibits IL-1-dependent lymphocyte proliferation. J Immunol 1988; 140:3026-3032.

88. Smeland EB, Blomhoff HK, Holte H et al. Transforming growth factor β (TGF-β) inhibits G₁ to S transition, but not activation of human B lymphocytes. Exp Cell Res 1987; 171:213-222.

89. Ehrhardt RO, Strober W, Harriman GR. Effect of transforming growth factor (TGF-β) β1 on IgA isotype expression: TGF-β1 induces a small increase in sIgA+ B cells regardless of the method of B cell activation. J Immunol 1992; 148:3830-3836.

90. McIntyre TM, Kehry MR, Snapper CM. Novel in vitro model for high-rate IgA class switching. J Immunol 1995; 154:3156-3161.

91. Stavnezer J. Regulation of antibody production and class switching by TGF-β. J Immunol 1995; 154:1647-1651.

92. Matsuoka M, Yoshida K, Maeda T et al. Switch circular DNA formed in cytokine-treated mouse splenocytes: evidence for intramolecular DNA deletion in immunoglobulin class switching. Cell 1990; 62:135-142.

93. Lebman DA, Nomura DY, Coffman RL et al. Molecular characterization of germ-line immunoglobulin A transcripts produced during transforming growth factor type β-isotype switching. Proc Natl Acad Sci USA 1990; 87:3962-3966.

94. Kim PH, Kagnoff MF. Transforming growth factor-β1 is a costimulator for IgA production. J Immunol 1990; 144:3411-3416.

95. Swain SL, Huston G, Tonkonogy S et al. Transforming growth factor-β and IL-4 cause helper T cell precursor to develop onto distinct effector helper cells that differ in lymphokine secretion pattern and cell surface phenotype. J Immunol 1991; 147:2991-3000.

96. Miller A, Lider O, Weiner HL. Antigen-driven bystander suppression following oral administration of antigens. J Exp Med 1991; 174:791-798.
97. Al-Sabbagh A, Miller A, Santos LMB et al. Antigen-driven tissue-specific suppression following oral tolerance: Orally administered myelin basic protein suppresses proteolipid protein-induced experimental autoimmune encephalomyelitis in the SJL mouse. Eur J Immunol 1994; 24:2104-2109.
98. Weiner HL. Oral tolerance: immune mechanisms and treatment of autoimmune disease. Immunol Today 1997; 18:335-343.
99. Seder RA, Marth T, Sieve MC et al. Factors involved in the differentiation of TGF-β-producing cells from naive CD4⁺ T cells: IL-4 and IFN-γ gave opposing effects, while TGF-β positively regulates its own production. J Immunol 1998; 160:5719-5728.
100. Dohi T, Fujihashi K, Rennert PD et al. Hapten-induced colitis is associated with colonic patch hypertrophy and T helper cell2-type responses. J Exp Med 1999; 189:1169-1180.
101. Giladi E, Raz E, Karmeli F et al. Transforming growth factor-β gene therapy ameliorates experimental colitis in rats. Eur J Gastroenterol Hepatol 1995; 7:341-347.
102. Kuklin NA, Daheshia M, Chun S et al. Immunomodulation by mucosal gene transfer using TGF-β DNA. J Clin Invest 1998; 102:438-444.
103. Kitani A, Fuss IJ, Nakamura K et al. Treatment of experimental (trinitrobenzene sulfonic acid) colitis by intranasal administration of transforming growth factor (TGF)-β1 plasmid: TGF-β1-mediated suppression of T helper cell type 1 response occurs by interleukin (IL)-10 induction and IL-12 receptor β2 chain downregulation. J Exp Med 2000; 1:41-52.
104. Chun S, Daheshia M, Lee S et al. Distribution fate and mechanism of immune modulation following mucosal delivery of plasmid DNA encoding IL-10. J Immunol 1999; 163:2393-2402.
105. Asseman C, Mauze S, Leach MW et al. An essential role for interleukin 10 in the function of regulatory T cells that inhibit intestinal inflammation. J Exp Med 1999; 190:995-1004.
106. Kulkarni AB, Ward JM, Yaswen L et al. Transforming growth factor-β1 null mice: an animal model for inflammatory disorders. Am J Pathol 1995; 146:264-275.
107. van Ginkel FW, Wahl SM, Kearney JF et al. Partial IgA-deficiency with increased Th2-type cytokines in TGF-β1 knockout mice. J Immunol 1999; 163:1951-1957.
108. Matsushima K, Larsen CG, DuBois GC et al. Purification and characterization of a novel monocyte chemotactic and activating factor produced by a human myelomonocytic cell line. J Exp Med 1989; 169:1485-1490.
109. Yoshimura T et al. Purification and amino acid analysis of two human glioma-derived monocyte chemoattractants. J Exp Med 1989; 169:1449-1459.
110. Carr MW, Roth SJ, Luther E et al. Monocyte chemoattractant protein 1 acts as a T-lymphocyte chemoattractant. Proc Natl Acad Sci USA 1994; 91:3652-3656.
111. Allavena P et al. Induction of natural killer cell migration by monocyte chemotactic protein-1, -2 and -3. Eur J Immunol 1994; 24:3233-3236.
112. Maghazachi AA, al-Aoukaty A, Schall TJ. Chemokines induce the chemotaxis of NK and IL-2-activated NK cells. Role for G proteins. J Immunol 1994; 153:4969-4977.
113. Reinecker HC, Loh EY, Ringler DJ et al. Monocyte-chemoattractant protein 1 gene expression in intestinal epithelial cells and inflammatory bowel disease mucosa. gastroenterology 1995; 108:40-50.
114. Grimm MS, Elsbury SKO, Pavli P et al. Enhanced expression and production of monocyte chemoattractant protein-1 in inflammatory bowel disease mucosa. J Leukoc Biol 1996; 56:804-812.
115. Mazzucchelli L, Hauser C, Z'graggen K et al. Differential in situ expression of the genes encoding the chemokines MCP-1 and RANTES in human inflammatory bowel disease. J Pathol 1996; 178:201-206.
116. Yang SK, Eckmann L, Panja A et al. Differential and regulated expression of CXC, CC, and C-chemokines by human colon epithelial cells. Gastroenterology 1997; 113:1214-1223.
117. Karpus WJ, Kennedy KJ, Kunkel SL et al. Monocyte chemotactic protein 1 regulates oral tolerance induction by inhibition of T helper cell 1-related cytokines. J Exp Med 1998; 187:733-741.
118. Tuohy VK, Sobel RA, Lu RA et al. Myelin proteolipid protein: minimum sequence requirements for active induction of autoimmune encephalomyelitis in SWR/J and SJL/J mice. J Neuroimmunol 1992; 39:67-74.

119. McRae BL, Kennedy MK, Tan LJ et al. Induction of active and adoptive chronic-relapsing experimental autoimmune encephalomyelitis (EAE) using an encephalitogenic epitope of proteolipid protein. J Neuroimmunol 1992; 38:229-240.

120. Karpus WJ, Kennedy KJ, Smith WS et al. Inhibition of relapsing experimental autoimmune encephalomyelitis in SJL mice by feeding the immunodominant PLP139-151 peptide. J Neurosci Res 1996; 45:4602-4608.

121. Lu B, Rutledge BJ, Gu L et al. Abnormalities in monocyte recruitment and cytokine expression in monocyte chemoattractant protein 1-deficient mice. J Exp Med 1998; 187:601-608.

122. Chensue SW et al. Monocyte chemoattractant protein expression during schistosome egg granuloma formation. Sequence of production, localization, contribution, and regulation. Am J Pathol 1995; 146:130-138.

123. Karpus WJ, Juckacs NW, Kennedy KJ et al. Differential CC chemokine-induced enhancement of T helper cell cytokine production. J Immunol 1997; 158:4129-4136.

124. Gu L, Tseng S, Horner RM et al. Control of Th2 polarization by the chemokine monocyte chemoattractant protein-1. Nature 2000; 404:407-411.

125. Boring L, Gosling J, Chensue SW et al. Impaired monocyte migration and reduced type 1 (Th1) cytokine responses in C-C chemokine receptor 2 knockout mice. J Clin Invest 1997; 100:2552-2561.

126. Warmington KS. Effect of C-C chemokine receptor 2 (CCR2) knockout on type-2 (schistosomal antigen-elicited) pulmonary granuloma formation: analysis of cellular recruitment and cytokine responses. Am J Pathol 1999; 154:1407-1416.

127. Yokoyama C, Tanabe T. Cloning of human gene encoding prostaglandin endoperoxide synthase and primary structure of the enzyme. Biochem Biophys Res Commun 1989; 165:888-894.

128. Kraemer SA, Meade EA, Dewitt DL. Prostaglandin endoperoxide synthase gene structure: identification of the transcriptional start site and 5′-flanking regulatory sequences. Arch Biochem Biophys 1992; 293:391-400.

129. Xie WL, Chipman JG, Robertson DL et al. Expression of a mitogen-responsive gene encoding prostaglandin synthase is regulated by mRNA splicing. Proc Natl Acad Sci USA 1991; 88:2692-2696.

130. Kujubu DA, Fletcher BS, Varnum BC et al. TIS10, a phorbol ester tumor promoter-inducible mRNA from Swiss 3T3 cells, encodes a novel prostaglandin synthase/cyclooxygenase homologue. J Biol Chem 1991; 266:12866-12872.

131. O'Banion MK, Sadowski HB, Winn V et al. A serum- and glucocorticoid-regulated 4-kilobase mRNA encodes a cyclooxygenase-related protein. J Biol Chem 1991; 266:23261-23267.

132. Wen PZ, Warden C, Fletcher Bset al. Chromosomal organization of the inducible and constitutive prostaglandin synthase/cyclooxygenase genes in mouse. Genomics 1993; 15:458-460.

133. Herschman HR. Prostaglandin synthase 2. Biochim Biophys Acta 1996; 1299:125-140.

134. Crofford LJ. COX-2 in synovial tissues. Osteoarthritis Cartilage 1999; 7:406-408.

135. Greaves MW, Camp RD. Prostaglandins, leukotrienes, phopholipase, platelet activating factor, and cytokines: an integrated approach to inflammation of human skin. Arch Dermatol Res 1988; 280(Suppl.):S33-S41.

136. Henderson WJ Jr. Eicosanoids and platelet-activating factor in allergic respiratory diseases. Am Rev Respir Dis 1991; 143:S86-S90.

137. Abramson S. Therapy with and mechanisms of nonsteroidal anti-inflammatory drugs. Curr Opin Rheumatol 1991; 3:336-340.

138. Hoult JRS, Moore PK. Sulphasalazine is a potent inhibitor of prostaglandin 15 hydroxydehydrogenase: possible basis for therapeutic action in ulcerative colitis. Br J Pharmacol 1978; 64:6-8.

139. Allgayer H, Deschryver K, Stenson WF. Treatment with 16,16′-dimethyl PGE2 before and after induction of colitis with trinitrobenzene sulfonic acid in rats decreases inflammation. Gastroenterology 1989; 96:1290-1300.

140. Fedorak RN, Empey LR, MacArthur C, Jewell LD. Misoprostol provides a colonic mucosal protective effect during acetic acid-induced colitis in rats. Gastroenterology 1990; 98:615-625.

141. Cohn SM, Schloeman S, Tessner T et al. Crypt stem cell survival in the mouse intestinal epithelium is regulated by prostaglandins synthesized through cyclooxygenase-1. J Clin Invest 1997; 99:1367-1379.

142. Tessner TG, Cohn SM, Schloeman et al. Prostaglandins prevent decreased epithelial cell proliferation associated with dextran sodium sulfate injury in mice. Gastroenterology 1998; 115:874-882.
143. Yamada T, Deitch E, Specian RD et al. Mechanisms of acute and chronic intestinal inflammation induced by indomethacin. Inflammation 1993; 17:641-662.
144. Redfern JS, Blair AJ, Lee E, Feldman M. Gastroinetstinal ulcer formation in rabbits immunized with prostaglandin E_2. Gastroenterology 1987; 93:744-752.
145. Olson GA, Leffler CW, Fletcher AM. Gastroduodenal ulceration in rabbits producing antibodies to prostaglandins. Prostaglandins 1985; 29:475-480.
146. Raskin JB. Gastrointestinal effects of nonsteroidal anti-inflammatory therapy. Am J Med 1999; 106:3S-12S.
147. Kauffman HJ, Taubin HL. Nonsteroidal anti-inflammatory drugs activate quiescent inflammatory bowel disease. Ann Intern Med 1987; 107:513-516.
148. Bjarnason I, Hayllar J, MacPherson AJ et al. Side effects of nonsteroidal anti-inflammatory drugs on the small and large intestine in humans. Gastroenterology 1993; 104:1832-1847.
149. Bjarnason I, MacPherson A. The changing gastrointestinal side effect profile of non-steroidal anti-inflammatory drugs. A new approach for the prevention of a new problem. Scand J Gastroenterol 1989; 163(Suppl.):56-64.
150. Raz A, Wyche A, Needleman P. Temporal and pharmacological division of fibroblast cyclooxygenase expression into transcriptional and translational phases. Proc Natl Acad Sci USA 1989; 86:1657-1661.
151. Masferrer JL, Seibert K, Zweifel BS et al. Endogenous glucocorticoids regulate an inducible cyclooxygenase enzyme. Proc Natl Acad Sci USA 1992; 89:917-3921.
152. Kujubu DA, Herschman H. Dexamethasone inhibits mitogen induction of the TIS10 prostaglandin synthase/cyclooxygenase gene. J Biol Chem 1992; 267:7991-7994.
153. Jobin C, Morteau O, Han DS et al. Specific NF-kappa B blockade selectively inhibits tumour necrosis factor-alpha-induced COX-2 but not constitutive COX-1 gene expression in HT-29 cells. Immunology 1998; 95:537-543.
154. Dewitt DL, Meade EA, Smith WL. PGH synthase isoenzyme selectivity : the potential for safer nonsteroidal antiinflammatory drugs. Am J Med 1993; 95:40S-44S.
155. Seibert K, Masferrer JL. Role of inducible cyclooxygenase (COX-2) in inflammation. Receptor 1994; 4:17-23.
156. Seibert K, Masferrer JL, Zhang Y et al. Mediation of inflammation by cyclooxygenase-2. Agents Actions 1995; 46(Suppl.):41-50.
157. Meade EA, Smith WL, Dewitt DL. Differential inhibition of prostaglandin endoperoxide synthase (cyclooxygenase) by aspirin and other non-steroidal anti-inflammatory drugs. J Biol Chem 1993; 268:6610-6614.
158. Masferrer JL, Zweifel BS, Manning PT et al. Selective inhibition of inducible cyclooxygenase. Proc Natl Acad Sci USA 1994; 91:3228-3232.
159. Seibert K, Zhang Y, Leahy K et al. Pharmacological and biochemical demonstartion of the role of cyclooxygenase in inflammation and pain. Proc Natl Acad Sci USA 1994; 91:12013-12017.
160. Laine L, Harper S, Simon T et al. A randomized trial comparing the effect of rofecoxib, a cyclooxygenase 2-specific inhibitor, with that of ibuprofen on the gastroduodenal mucosa of patients with osteoarthritis. Gastroenterology 1999; 117:776-783.
161. Langman MJ, Jensen DM, Watson DJ et al. Adverse upper gastrointestinal effects of rofecoxib compared with NSAIDs. JAMA 1999; 282:1929-1933.
162. Goldenberg MM Celecoxib, a selective cyclooxygenase-2 inhibitor for the treatment of rheumatoid arthritis and osteoarthritis. Clin Ther 1999; 21:1497-1513.
163. Simon LS, Weaver AL, Graham DY et al. Anti-inflammatory and upper gastrointestinal effects of celecoxib in rheumatoid arthritis : a randomized controlled trial. JAMA 1999; 282:1921-1928.
164. Reuter BK, Asfaha S, Buret A et al. Exacerbation of inflammation-associated colonic injury in rat through inhibition of cyclooxygenase-2. J Clin Invest 1996; 98:2076-2085.
165. Mizuno H, Sakamoto C, Matsuda K et al. Induction of cyclooxygenase 2 in gastric mucosal lesions and its inhibition by the specific antagonist delays healing in mice. Gastroenterology 1997; 112:645-648.
166. Shigeta J, Takahashi S, Okabe S. Role of cyclooxygenase-2 in the healing of gastric ulcers in rats. J Pharmacol Exp Ther 1998; 286:1383-1390.

167. Nakattsugi S, Terada N, Yoshimura T et al. Effects of nimesulide, a preferential cyclooxygenase-2 inhibitor, on carrageenan-induced pleurisy and stress-induced gastric lesions in rats. Prostaglandins Leukot Essent Fatty Acids 1996; 55:395-402.

168. Langenbach R, Morham SG, Tiano HF et al. Prostaglandin synthase 1 gene disruption in mice reduces arachidonic acid-induced inflammation and indomethacin-induced gastric ulceration. Cell 1995; 83:483-492.

169. Morham SG, Langenbach R, Loftin CD et al. Prostaglandin synthase 2 gene disruption causes severe renal pathology in the mouse. Cell 1995; 83:473-482.

170. Morteau O, Morham SG, Sellon R et al. Impaired mucosal defense to acute colonic injury in mice lacking cyclooxygenase-1 or cyclooxygenase-2. J Clin Invest 2000; 105:469-478.

171. Newberry RD, Stenson WF, Lorenz RG. Cyclooxygenase-2-dependent arachidonic acid metabolites are essential modulators of the intestinal immune response to dietary antigen. Nat Med 1999; 5:900-906.

172. Morteau O. COX-2: promoting tolerance. Nat Med 1999; 5:867-868.

173. Knudsen PJ, Dinarello CA, Strom TB. Prostaglandins posttranscriptionally inhibit monocyte expression of interleukin 1 activity by increasing intracellular cyclic adenosine monophosphate. J Immunol 1986; 137:3189-3194.

174. Kunkel SL, Chensue SW, Phan SH. Prostaglandins as endogenous mediators of interleukin-1 production. J Immunol 1986; 136:186-192.

175. Snijdewint FGM, Kalinski P, Wierenga EA et al. Prostaglandin E2 differentially modulate cytokine secretion profiles of human T helper lymphocytes. J Immunol 1993; 150:5321-5329.

176. Kuroda E, Sugiura T, Zeki K et al. Sensitivity difference to the suppressive effect of prostaglandin E2 among mouse strains: a possible mechanism to polarize Th2 type response in BALB/C mice. J Immunol 2000; 164:2386-2395.

177. Katamura K, Shintaku N, Yamauchi Y et al. Prostaglandin E2 at priming of naive CD4+ T cells inhibits acquisition of ability to produce IFN-γ and IL-2, but not IL-4 and IL-5. J Immunol 1995; 155:4604-4612.

178. Wu CY, Wang K, McDyer JF et al. Prostaglandin E2 and dexamethasone inhibit IL-12 receptor expression and IL-12 responsiveness. J Immunol 1998; 161:2723-2730.

179. van der Pouw Kraan TC, Boeije LC, Smeenk RJ et al. Prostaglandin-E2 is a potent inhibitor of interleukin 12 production. J Exp Med 1995; 181:775-779.

180. Hilkens CM, Snijders A, Vermeulen H et al. Accessory cell-derived IL-12 and prostaglandin E2 determine the IFN-γ level of activated human CD4+ T cells. J Immunol 1996; 156:1722-1727.

181. Fedyk ER, Phipps RP. Prostaglandin E2 receptors of the EP_2 and EP_4 subtypes regulate activation and differentiation of mouse B lymphocytes to IgE-secreting cells. Proc Natl acad Sci USA 1996; 93:10978-10983.

182. Pablos JL, Santiago B, Carreira PE et al. Cyclooxygenase-1 and -2 are expressed by human T cells. Clin Exp Immunol 1999; 115:86-90.

183. Iniguez MA, Punzon C, Fresno M. Induction of cyclooxygenase-2 on activated T lymphocytes: regulation of T cell activation by cyclooxygenase-2 inhibitors. J Immunol 1999; 163:111-119.

184. Iniguez MA, Martinez-Martinez S, Punzon C et al. An essential role of NFAT in the regulation of the expression of cyclooxygenase-2 gene in human T lymphocytes. J Biol Chem 2000; 275:23627-23635.

185. Tanaka K, Ogawa K, Sugamura K et al. Cutting edge: differential production of prostaglandin D2 by human helper T cell subsets. J Immunol 2000; 164:2277-2280.

CHAPTER 6

IgA and Mucosal Homeostasis

Jesper Reinholdt and Steffen Husby

Mucosal surfaces represent the major interface between host and environment. They constitute the point of entry of most infectious pathogens, and are in contact with potentially injurious antigens present in the normal mucosal microflora and in ingested or inhaled substances. To deal appropriately with this challenge, the host immune system rely on both cell-mediated and humoral responses. Whereas cell-mediated responses involve a range of different effector cells,[1,2] the humoral immune defense at mucosal level is mediated predominantly by antibodies of the immunoglobulin (Ig) A isotype. The mucosal immune system contains more than 80% of all Ig-producing cells in the body, and the major product of these cells in normal individuals is IgA.[3] In the circulation, IgA is the second most abundant Ig class, its concentration (~2 mg/ml) being surpassed only by that of IgG (~12 mg/ml). Considering the distribution in various body fluids of the major Ig isotypes and their catabolic rates, IgA is clearly synthesized in quantities (~66 mg/kg body weight/day) that exceed by far the combined daily synthesis of all other isotypes.[4,5]

The mucosal immune system has a unique anatomical and functional organisation. IgA is present in several molecular forms and displays biological properties not shared by other immunoglobulin classes. IgA antibodies perform their protective functions discretely without interfering with the physiological activities of mucosal membranes. Moreover, IgA is believed to mitigate, when appropriate, the activity of phlogistic, potentially injurious immune defence mechanisms and to contribute in this way to mucosal homeostasis. However, a major question in mucosal immunity remains: how does IgA, and the mucosal immune system in general, discriminate between innocuous dietary components or commensal bacteria, and pathogens that represent a threat to the individual's health.

Mucosal IgA antibody responses have been comprehensively studied, particularly with respect to a potential exploitation for immune prophylaxis. Less is known of the immune-modulating properties of IgA, and few studies have directly addressed the relationship of IgA antibodies to the concept of oral (or mucosal) tolerance. In this chapter, we will describe fundamental aspects of the mucosal IgA system and discuss current conceptions regarding the biological functions of IgA antibodies. A final section will review briefly some aspects of oral tolerance related to B cell reactions and IgA antibody responses.

Structure of IgA

IgA is the most heterogeneous immunoglobulin isotype. It is present in a variety of molecular forms, subclasses and allotypes, with patterns of heterogeneity that vary between different species of mammals and birds.[6] Early studies revealed that the variation in molecular form is intimately related to the fact that IgA is not only present in the circulation and tissues, but is

Oral Tolerance: The Response of the Intestinal Mucosa to Dietary Antigens, edited by Olivier Morteau. ©2004 Eurekah.com and Kluwer Academic / Plenum Publishers.

also the predominant immunoglobulin in external secretions, in the form of secretory IgA (S-IgA).[7,8] Secretory IgA exerts biological activities different from those of IgA in the circulation and tissues. The functional significance of structural variation in terms of IgA subclasses and allotypes, however, is poorly understood.

In the serum of adults, IgA is found in concentrations ranging from 0.7 to 3.4 mg/ml,[9] and is mainly present (> 80%) in the form of monomeric IgA (mIgA) composed of two α (M_r ~53,000) and two κ or λ (M_r ~22,500) chains. Human α chains are glycoproteins (6 to 10% carbohydrate) consisting of one variable and three constant domains. The remaining part of serum IgA is in a polymeric, mainly dimeric form, with monomers connected by disulphide bonds and linked to an additional polypeptide called J chain (M_r ~16,000; 8% carbohydrate). The J chain is present also in IgM (pentameric) and appears to play a regulatory -though not indispensable- role in the polymerisation of these isotypes.[10]

S-IgA is a molecule of dual cellular origin. It consists of a polymeric, J chain-containing IgA disulphide-linked to another glycoprotein, secretory component (SC; M_r ~70,000). Whereas polymeric IgA is produced by local plasma cells, SC originates from secretory epithelial cells. SC consists of five immunoglobulin-like domains and is highly glycosylated (22 %). It is a fragment of the polyimmunoglobulin receptor (pIgR), which serves as a vehicle for the transport of polymeric, J chain-containing immunoglobulins (polymeric IgA and IgM) through the polarized epithelial cells that line mucosal surfaces and constitute the secretory cells of mucosal glands. pIgR-mediated IgM transport is quantitatively insignificant in normal, IgA-producing individuals. In most IgA-deficient individuals, though, secretory IgM (S-IgM) substitutes for S-IgA in the secretions, which may explain why many IgA-deficient individuals remain healthy.[11]

The perpetual regulated transfer of pIgR through secretory epithelial cells is a key element of humoral mucosal immunity (for review, see ref. 12). Briefly, pIgR, synthesized as an integral membrane protein in the rough endoplasmic reticulum, is delivered to the baso-lateral surface of the epithelial cell where it binds pIgA produced by the plasma cell in the underlying lamina propria. pIgR is endocytosed and travels by vesicular transport to the apical plasma membrane. There, the extracellular ligand-binding portion of pIgR (the future SC) is cleaved off and released with its potential Ig ligand. The binding of pIgR (and SC) to immunoglobulins appears to depend on the presence of the J chain, although SC and J-chain are not mutually linked by covalent bonds (both polypeptides are disulphide-attached to the C-terminal half of the α chain). In addition to its role in IgA secretion, SC confers functional advantages to the S-IgA molecule.

Secretions collected at some mucosal surfaces, particularly the airways and the female genital tract, contain significant proportions of mIgA.[13,14] Like other systemic immunoglobulins, mIgA reach the secretion by passive transudation, which reflects the degree of mucosal inflammation.

IgA Subclasses and Allotypes

In humans, hominoid primates, and lagomorphs (including rabbits), several IgA subclasses have been described on the basis of their α chain isotype. Within a given species, the α chains belonging to each subclass are highly homologous in amino acid sequence. Two subclasses, IgA1 and IgA2, have been identified in human serum and secretions. A major difference between the two subclasses is found in the hinge region: IgA2 molecules lack a 13 amino acid segment, which is present in the hinge region of IgA1 and consists exclusively of prolyl, seryl, and threonyl residues. Four to five of the seryl and threonyl residues carry O-linked glycans.[15,16] This extended hinge region confers greater segmental flexibility on IgA1 molecules, but renders this isotype susceptible to the activity of certain post-proline endopeptidases, called IgA1 proteases, which are produced by bacterial pathogens and commensals colonizing the mucosa (see below). These enzymes, by their ability to cleave IgA1 molecules into intact Fc (or Fc.SC) and monovalent Fab fragments, seem to constitute means of evading IgA antibody-mediated defence (reviewed by Kilian et al[17]). For this particular reason, IgA2 has been hypothesized to be the phylogenetically youngest of the IgA subclasses, selected for its resistance to bacterial IgA1 protease activity. This hypothesis, however, was proven wrong when phylogenetical studies of the IgA subclasses in hominoid primates and humans demonstrated that IgA1 evolved subsequently to IgA2 through events of gene-duplication and conversion.[18] The human IgA subclasses also differ at 14 amino acid positions in the α chain sequence, and in N-linked glycans.

The two IgA subclasses are unequally distributed in the systemic and mucosal lymphoid compartments. IgA1 is vastly predominant in the serum (>85%), consistently with a similar predominance of IgA1-producing cells in the bone marrow, where most serum IgA is produced.[19,20,21] In secretions, however, proportions of IgA2 vary from 10% in the upper respiratory tract secretions, to 30-40% in the saliva and the small intestine, and more than 50% in the secretions of the large intestine and female genital tract, reflecting the subclass distribution of IgA-producing plasma cells in the local mucosa.[19,21,22] The local distribution of IgA1- and IgA2-producing cells may be the result of subclass-specific clonal expansion induced by certain types of antigens.[10,23] However, the factors that determine the subclass of IgA antibodies are still partly unknown.[24]

The human IgA2 subclass exists in two allotypic forms designated A2m(1) and A2m(2).[25,26] The A2m(1) allotype is unconventional in that the heavy (H) and light (L) chains are not covalently linked, and therefore can be separated by non-reducing dissociating agents. Population studies of the IgA2 allotypes have revealed a characteristic racial and ethnic distribution. The A2m(1) allotype is highly predominant in caucasians whereas A2m(2) dominates in people of African origin.[25,26]

Glycan Moiety

The glycan moiety of α chains, which is of significance to the function of IgA antibodies, has been analysed in detail. In addition to the contrasting presence of glycans in the α1 and α2 hinge regions mentioned above, early studies reviewed by Mestecky et al[10] found a N-glycosylation at two Asn residues located in CH2 and in the very C-terminal "tail-piece" of IgA1 and IgA2. In IgA2, two or three additional sites of N-glycosylation have been identified in the Fc. A recent study reported considerable O- and N-glycosylation in Fab of polyclonal serum IgA1.[16] While the short O-linked glycans in the hinge of IgA1 contain GalNAc, Gal, and frequently terminal NeuNAc, N-linked glycans in Fc of IgA are of the complex, multiantennary type. Unlike the corresponding N-linked glycans in IgG1, confined to the space between the two heavy chains, those of IgA are directed away from the protein backbones and are highly sialylated.[16] With this make up, the glycans presumably confer hydrophilicity and negative net charge to the IgA molecule. Also at variance with the situation for IgG, IgA glycans are not involved in interactions with the isotype-specific Fc receptor (CD89 in the case of IgA) that triggers IgA-mediated defence reactions in granulocytes and macrophages.[16,27,28] N-linked glycans of the high-mannose type have been identified in both IgA subclasses. IgA molecules carrying such glycans may interact through their terminal mannose residues with corresponding receptors (type 1 fimbriae) on certain bacteria and inhibit their adherence to epithelial cells.[29,30]

The total carbohydrate content of S-IgA is considerably higher than that of serum IgA because both J chain and SC are rich in carbohydrates. Moreover, glycans of both components are sialylated.[31,32] Accordingly, these components can be expected to add significantly to the negative charge and hydrophilicity of S-IgA molecules.

Induction of IgA Responses

Antigen Handling and Reactions in Mucosa-Associated Lymphoid Tissue (MALT)

Any site on mucosal membranes may under various circumstances permit the entry of exogenous material, including potential immunogens. Nevertheless, mucosal membranes are equipped with lymphoepithelial structures specialized in the sampling of microbial and molecular antigens by way of particular epithelial cells highly efficient in transcytosis (microfold or M cells). In these structures, collectively denoted mucosa-associated lymphoid tissue (MALT), the sampled material is immediately brought into contact with the cells and molecular environment required for an appropriate immune response. The lymphoepithelial structures of MALT are distributed strategically at multiple mucosal sites. In the gut-associated lymphoid tissue (GALT), they are the Peyer's patches, which contain several lymphoid follicles. Analogous small solitary follicles are dispersed throughout the intestine in humans and some other species.[33] In the airways, bronchus-associated lymphoid tissue (BALT) has a similar architecture and function. BALT is not constitutively present but develops in response to infections by respiratory pathogens and to persisting allergic reactions. MALT also includes the organized lymphoid tissues of the Waldeyer's pharyngeal ring, which includes the palatine tonsils and the nasal-associated lymphoid tissue (NALT), such as the adenoids.

In response to an antigen uptake by the elements of MALT, germinal centers develop in the follicles, triggering the affinity maturation of antibodies and the development of memory cells, much like during parenteral antigen challenge in the lymph nodes and spleen. Unlike these organs, however, MALT provides a unique microenvironment that promotes the development of B cells producing antibodies in the form of dimeric, J chain-containing IgA, although switching to other non-IgM isotypes also occurs.[34] Apparently, the induction of IgA antibody responses at these sites occurs irrespectively of the local Th1/Th2 balance, which may vary depending on the activity of mucosal adjuvants, such as substances derived from the mucosal microflora.[35] The mechanisms responsible for the preferential expression of IgA are not clear, but the effects of specialized antigen-presenting cells (APC), such as dendritic cells,[36,37] and the local expression of cytokines, such as transforming growth factor-β (TGF-β),[38] appear to be important. A cytokine-independent factor, activation-induced cytidine deaminase, has also been implicated as a regulator of switching from IgM to IgA.[39] Studies of Peyer's patches indicate that TGF-β and cytokines that regulate subsequent differentiation of B cells into antibody-secreting plasma cells (IL-5, IL-15, IL-6, IL-10) may be produced by several cell types including T cells, epithelial cells, and dendritic cells.[40,41] The mechanisms that regulate the differentiation of human B cells into IgA1- or IgA2-producing cells have only been sparsely elucidated.[42]

Mucosal Lymphocyte Trafficking in MALT

Contrary to other peripheral lymphoid tissues, the immune induction sites of MALT lack afferent lymphatics, but do have efferent lymphatics. Naive B and T lymphocytes enter MALT through high endothelial venules. Upon stimulation they exit as lymphoblasts via efferent lymphatics to regional lymph nodes, where they may undergo further division and differentiation.[43] From there, the cells travel via the thoracic duct to the blood stream, and subsequently migrate extensively to the lamina propria of the inductive and the remote mucosal membranes and glands, where they terminate as effector cells. A small fraction of the stimulated IgA-producing effector cells also migrate to the systemic compartment, including the bone marrow.[24] The preferential migration (homing) of mucosally stimulated lymphocytes to the mucosal compartment may be linked to the expression of adhesion molecules that are complementary to endothelial addressins specifically expressed within mucosal tissues.[44] Accordingly, stimulation of e.g., GALT B cells (Fig. 1) by an intestinal antigen may lead to the presence of IgA antibodies in intestinal secretions, and also in the secretions of the respiratory tract and the lacrimal, salivary, and lactating mammary glands. In contrast, antibodies of any isotype are barely detectable in serum. Thus, through functional specialization of its afferent and efferent limbs, MALT is partially independent of the systemic immune apparatus. This integrated common mucosal immune system (CMIS) was originally reported in rodents, and convincingly documented in humans.[45-47] Production and transport of S-IgA represent a major physiological investment. In humans, the intestine alone receives 3 to 5 g of S-IgA each day, testifying to the biological significance of this system.

Recent studies indicate a partial compartmentalization within the mucosal immune system, especially a dichotomy between the gut and the upper respiratory and digestive tracts with respect to migration of stimulated B cells (Fig. 2).[46,48,49] The mechanisms involved in the preferential homing to selected mucosal effector sites have not been revealed, but tissue-specific homing receptors or local chemotactic factors are probably critical. The patterns of migration have important implications for the design of vaccine protocols that could provide protective immunity at mucosal surfaces.

Uptake and Handling of Antigens by Enterocytes

Whereas stratified epithelia, present in the oral cavity, oesophagus, and vagina, are impermeable to molecules larger than ~40,000 Da,[50] the polarized cells of the pseudostratified, simple epithelia lining the small and large intestines (enterocytes) actively sample luminal macromolecules by endocytosis. Although most endosomal constituents are sorted for the degradative pathway,[51,52] enterocytes have been shown to transport small amounts of intact proteins and peptides across the epithelium by transcytosis.[53] This mechanism probably explains why dietary proteins can be detected in the circulation after a protein-rich meal.[54,55] Low levels of antibodies to dietary substances are found in the secretions (S-IgA) and the circulation (IgG and IgA) of most healthy individuals (reviewed by Husby[56]). How and where these antibodies are induced is not clear. IgA responses in particular may involve priming in the organized GALT, followed by restimulation of primed B cells in the lamina propria by antigens transferred through intestinal epithelial cells.[24] The capacity of M cells to bind and take up innocuous dietary antigens is a matter of controversy, mainly because experimental feeding with such antigens without adjuvant generally results in low and transient secretory and systemic responses, if any at all.[57,58] The remarkably low levels of antibodies generally found against ubiquitous food substances[59,56] are likely to reflect a downregulation of responses by the mechanisms of oral tolerance, as discussed below.

Enterocytes may display antigen-presenting properties under specific circumstances in vitro.[60,61] However, there is no evidence that they exhibit similar properties in vivo.

Role of the Mucosal Microflora in the Development and Function of the Mucosal Immune System

The alimentary tract (particularly the proximal and distal parts), upper respiratory tract, and distal female reproductive tract are permanently colonized by communities of commensal organisms. There is considerable site-dependent variation in the load and composition of the commensal flora, presumably due to the selective effects of local ecological factors, such as supply of nutrients, spectrum of mucosal receptors for microbial adhesins, and synergistic versus antagonistic intermicrobial and commensal-host relationships.[62-66] Selected in this way, communities of commensal bacteria are stable in terms of the species (though not necessarily the individual clones) represented, and may interfere efficiently with the colonization by pathogens.[67]

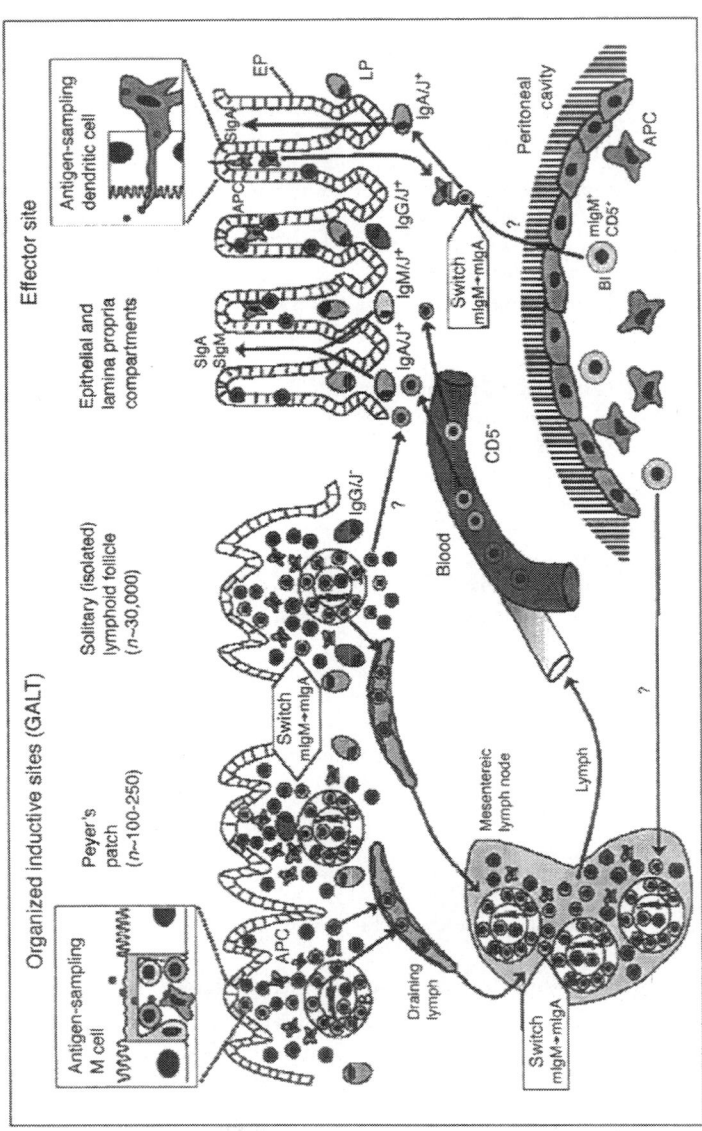

Figure 1. Antigen-sampling and B cell-switching sites for induction of intestinal IgA responses. The classical inductive sites are constituted by GALT, which is equipped with antigen-sampling M cells, T cell areas (T), B cell follicles (B) and antigen-presenting cells (APCs). Class switching from IgM to IgA occurs in GALT and mesenteric lymph nodes (MLN); from here primed B and T cells home to the lamina propria (LP) via lymph and blood. Primed B cells may also migrate from solitary follicles directly into the LP. The IgA+ cells differentiate into plasma cells that produce dimeric IgA with J chain ((IgA/J+), which becomes secretory IgA (S-IgA). Bone marrow-derived IgM+ B2 cells (CD5-) may give rise to pentameric IgM (IgM/J+) and S-IgM. B1 cells (here indicated as CD5+) from the peritoneal cavity reach LP by an unknown route, perhaps via MLNs. These IgM+ cells may switch to IgA within the LP under the influence of APCs that have sampled luminal antigen as dendritic cells within the epithelium (EP). Subsequently, they may differentiate to plasma cells that provide S-IgA. Dots denote antigen. (Adapted from: Brandtzaeg et al. Nature Immunology 2001; 2: 1093-4, with permission)

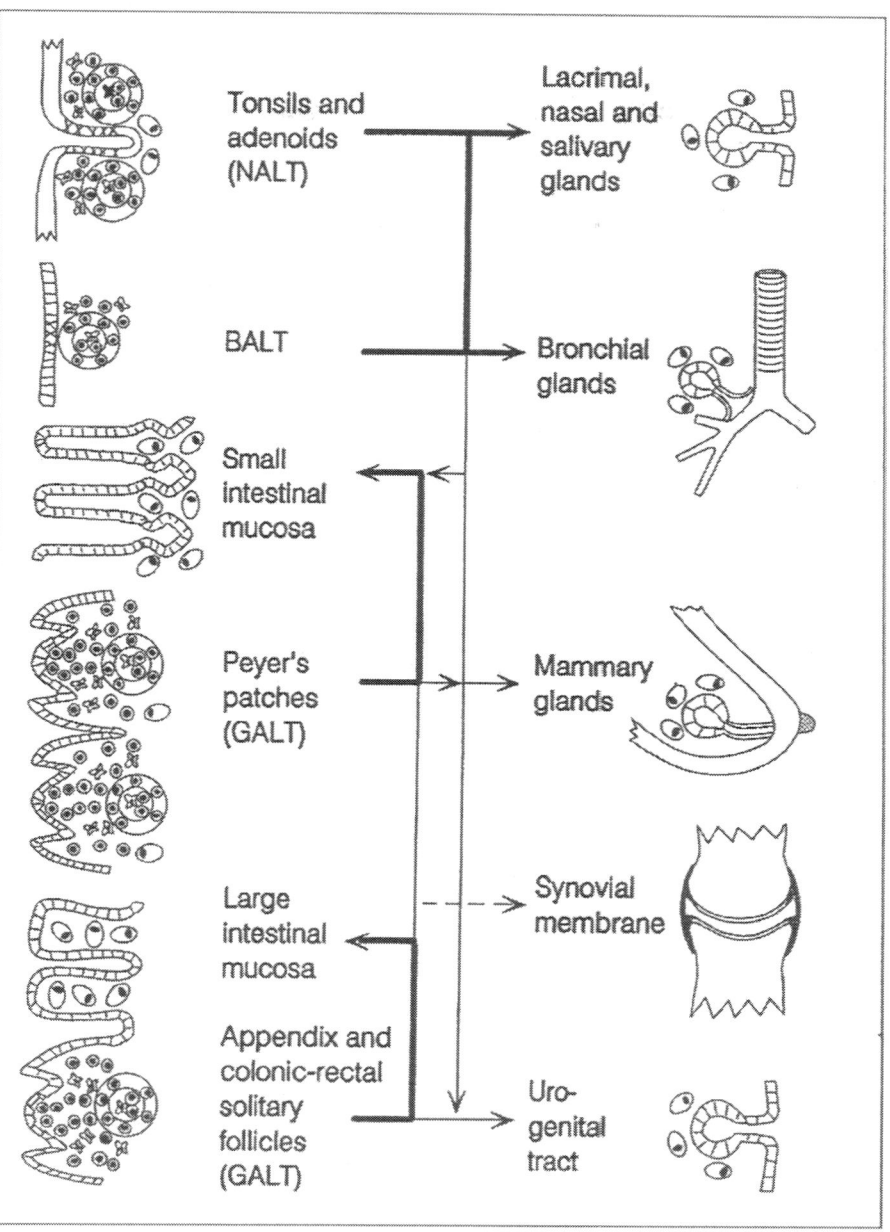

Figure 2. Model for migration of primed lymphoid cells from inductive sites to effector sites in the integrated common mucosal immune system (CMIS). Putative compartmentalization is indicated, the heavier arrows representing preferential communication pathways. (Adapted from: Brandtzaeg P, Farstad, IN. pp 439-468; in Ogra, PL et al. ed.. Mucosal Immunology. Academic Press, 1999, with permission).

At the same time, however, the commensal flora represents an enormous antigenic challenge to the mucosal immune system. It has been estimated that the number of microbial cells in the body (most of them in the large intestine) exceeds by far the total number of cells of the body.[68] The large number of plasma cells and other stimulated immune cells permanently present throughout the intestine and in the tonsils, indicate that the mucosal immune system is in a constant state of stimulation, which some investigators interpreted as a state of physiological inflammation. Exactly how the immune system deals with the load of microbial antigens is not clear, but observations in humans,[70,71] and comparisons between germ-free and conventionally reared animals (reviewed by Cebra et al[69]) have revealed essential elements of this interaction, two of which will be discussed here.

(*i*) The establishment of the mucosal flora after birth represents a major developmental and functional stimulus to the immune system.[72] Accordingly, germ-free neonates show a profound hypotrophy of mucosal and systemic lymphoid tissues and respond poorly to most antigens.[73,74] In animals maintained germ-free through adulthood, systemic responses are normalized but mucosal lymphoid tissues are poorly developed and IgA responses to mucosal antigens remain weak.[75] Germ-free animals kept on a hydrolyzed "antigen-free" diet display only limited additional hypotrophy of intestinal lymphoid tissues,[69] indicating that non microbial antigens in food and drink are not a major stimulus to the immune system. Interestingly, the repertoire as well as the level of mucosal immune responses in formerly germ-free animals may be normalized by colonization with selected bacterial taxa belonging to the intestinal commensal flora.[69,76-78] The mechanisms by which the mucosal flora stimulates the development and reactivity of the immune system in the early stages of lymphocyte development may involve specific bacterial components, such as lipopolysaccharides.[69] The local load of microorganisms is also important, as indicated by the poor development of BALT compared to GALT in the absence of respiratory infections. Interestingly, the commensal flora may also influence the immune reactions to mucosally applied antigens that lead to a state of mucosal tolerance (see below). Thus, interactions with the commensal flora seem to be a fundamental element of mucosal immune homeostasis.

(*ii*) Specific immune responses to the commensal flora, including IgA antibody production, do not normally eliminate the target organisms. Colonization by commensals starts right after birth by transfer of bacteria, particularly from the mother. Nevertheless, breast-feeding does not significantly interfere with the establishment of the commensal flora, although the mother's early milk contains abundant S-IgA, including antibodies that may inhibit the adherence of the relevant bacteria in vitro.[6] Individual clones of commensal bacteria may persist for years at mucosal sites in immunocompetent infants and adults,[70,71,79,80] apparently unaffected by local clone-reactive S-IgA antibodies (Reinholdt et al, unpublished data). While some studies suggest that the generation of IgA antibodies to commensal bacteria is driven by specific responses involving organized MALT,[81] others, involving natural transfer of oral bacteria into gnotobiotic animals, demonstrate that IgA antibodies are present at low levels even prior to acquisition of the bacteria.[82,83] These conflicting data remain unexplained. However, the latter result, along with observations that S-IgA antibodies against individual commensal bacteria are maintained at constant and relatively low levels in secretions,[84] corroborates the hypothesis that S-IgA antibodies reacting with the commensal flora derive largely from the B1 category of B cells believed to be a major source of so-called natural antibodies.[85-88]

IgA Produced by B1 cells

In mammals, B cells are physiologically heterogenous,[89] and their ontogeny seems to reflect their evolution. The B cells generated from progenitors in the liver and the omentum during fetal and early postnatal life display certain characteristics of B cells in lower vertebrates.

This early B variant, denoted B1, is maintained lifelong as a subset distinct from the population of conventional B cells (B2) that expand to predominance through infancy and adulthood (for reviews, see [90-92]). B1 and B2 cells differ in the expression of several markers, e.g., contrary to B2, some but not all B1 cells are CD5+.[91]

The early B1 cells express mainly self-reactive, germ-line encoded, low-affinity antibodies, many of which show high interconnectivity and anti-idiotype activity.[93] B1 network interactions largely determine the B1 repertoire[94] and may, together with an additional mechanism of B1 feedback regulation around the time of weaning,[95] explain that the B1 population from infancy throughout life consists of a restricted and fixed set of clones. Contrary to B2 cells, which are continuously replenished by the progeny of stem cells in the bone marrow, B1 cells persist as a self-renewing population not appreciably augmented by immigrants from the bone marrow.[96] This is possible because B1 cells constitutively display partly activated, yet tightly controlled intracellular signalling pathways, allowing them to be maintained, and even secrete small amounts of antibodies, in response to low affinity engagement of their antigen receptors with self epitopes.[97-100] Thus, the autologous immunoglobulins of the fetus and the newborn, mainly IgM but also IgA and IgG, are the products of B1 cells.[101]

After birth, despite their reactivity with self epitopes, B1 antibodies contribute to the defence against exogenous antigens. Studies of B1 antibodies produced by hybridoma technique showed that individual B1 monoclonals frequently reacted with several apparently unrelated epitopes, including epitopes of ubiquitous microorganisms (polyreactivity or multispecificity).[93,102-104] Microbial and self epitopes identified as targets of the B1 antibody repertoire are listed in reviews.[105,106] The phenomenon of polyreactivity may be explained by structural characteristics of the antibody CDR3 region.[107-109]

Although B1 cells, like other lymphocytes, are maintained by moderate signalling through their antigen receptors, extensive cross-linking of their receptors leads to apoptosis.[110-114] This explains why the mere presence of autoreactive B1 cells does not normally lead to autoimmune disease. If stimulated by antigens in combination with polyclonal activators (LPS) or certain cytokines, B1 cells can conversely be driven into differentiation and increased antibody secretion.[115] V-region somatic mutations leading to affinity maturation may also occur.[106] Because of the controlled signalling in B1 cells, however, their response to stimulation may differ from that of B2 cells. Apparently, B1 cells may increase antibody production without dividing, without becoming permanently committed to antibody production, and without losing their self-renewal capacity, i.e., their future capacity to reconstitute a portion of the B1 repertoire.[91] Stimulated B1 responses are suspected to cause certain autoimmune conditions.[116,117] Nevertheless, B1 antibodies are normally not pathogenic, and may even inhibit the effect of pathogenic autoantibodies via anti-idiotype activity.[118,119]

B1 cells produce a large proportion of the "natural" low-affinity antibodies (mainly IgM, but also IgA and IgG) that are present lifelong in normal individuals and have been detected in small amounts also in germ-free and antigen-free animals.[120-123] It seems that B1 cells have evolved to recognize mainly a limited spectrum of common (phylogenetically conserved) microbial and self structures with the characteristics of T-independent epitopes.[124] Such epitopes seem distinct from virulence-associated, genetically variable microbial structures such as the ligand-binding domains of microbial adhesins.[125] B1 cells express MHC class II and B7.1, but their maturation into antibody-secreting cells does not require cognitive T cell help. Accordingly, stimulation may occur outside the follicles of organized lymphoid tissues and does not generate classical B cell memory. B1 cells, together with marginal zone B cells, appear to be largely responsible for the initial T-independent phase of systemic IgM antibody responses to invading pathogens, which play an important role in the early phase of a protective antimicrobial immune response.[126-128] Notably, complement-activating IgM antibodies produced by B1 cells may also facilitate the induction of T-mediated responses, as demonstrated in the case of hapten-induced contact sensitivity.[129] The capacity of B1 cells for T-independent stimulation and isotype switch recombination may explain why athymic (nude, nu/nu) mice are only partially deficient in cells producing IgA and some other non-IgM isotypes.[130]

B1 cells, together with marginal zone B cells, γδ T cells, and certain NK cells, represent a phylogenetically old strategy of innate immune recognition distinct from adaptive lymphocyte responses. They are probably involved in the elimination of damaged tissue and in antimicrobial defence.[124] The physiology and functional significance of B1 and other B cell subsets have been recently reviewed.[124,131,132]

In adult animals, B1 cells are present in the pleural and peritoneal cavities and rarely in follicular lymphoid tissues such as pheripheral lymph nodes, spleen, and Peyer's patches.[133,134] B1 cells migrate from the cavities to mucosal membranes via regional lymph nodes while maturing into antibody-producing cells (Fig.1). In the case of the peritoneal cavity, this process is stimulated by the intestinal flora.[87,122] Studies in an irradiated, Ig-allotype-chimeric mouse model have shown that a fraction of peritoneal B1 cells seed to the gut lamina propria where they produce IgA antibodies reacting with the intestinal flora, as B2 cells do upon stimulation in the lymphoid follicles of MALT.[85,87,135,136] In a transgenic mouse model, the migration and stimulation of peritoneal B1 cells involved non-cognitive help from locally activated γδ T cells,i.e.,another innate-type lymphocyte.[137] Interestingly, γδ T cell receptor knock-out mice display a partial deficiency in mucosal IgA and mucosal IgA responses to antigens.[138] Whether this deficiency selectively affects B1-derived IgA is unknown. Further support for a dual origin of mucosal IgA antibodies comes from observations that the presence of IgA-producing B1 cells in the gut, contrary to IgA-producing B2 cells, depends largely on IL-5 and IL-15.[112,134,139] Recent studies suggested that T-independent priming of mouse B cells (presumably B1), and subsequent switch to the IgA isotype can take place in the gut lamina propria without involvement of Peyer's patches or solitary lymphoid follicles, the appropriate mediators being delivered by local stromal or dendritic cells.[140-142]

A study involving TCRβ[-/-]δ[-/-] mice suggested that B1 cells produce 20-30% of intestinal IgA antibodies to normal flora in a T-independent fashion, and that these antibodies cover a range of antimicrobial specificities similar to that of intestinal IgA in normal animals.[88] This suggests that B1-derived intestinal IgA have biological effects on the flora similar to those of IgA antibodies from B2 cells stimulated in mucosal follicles. However, this interpretation has been questioned.[143] Studies in various mouse models, some of which involved IgA-producing B1 cell back-pack tumors (see below), suggested that B2-derived IgA antibodies were more effective than B1-derived IgA antibodies in excluding intestinal commensals and opportunistic pathogens from the mucosal tissues.[87] A difference in the roles of B1 and B2 cells was also suggested by a study of immunity to influenza virus,[144] and by the observation that B2, but not B1 cells in reconstituted SCID mice may contribute to the defence against rotavirus by specific IgA antibody production and cooperation with CD4+ T cells.[145]

In mice, B1 cells are a source of mucosal IgA distinct from B2 cells, which are stimulated in lymphoid follicles of the common mucosal immune system (CMIS). B1 cells are believed to constitute a CMIS-independent source of IgA antibody induction.[134] A validation of this term should take into account that B cells able to produce polyreactive IgA antibodies have been isolated from Peyer's patches,[146,147] and that receptors for homing to mucosal membranes have been detected on peritoneal B1 cells.[148]

In humans, the significance of B1 cells is less clear. B1 is the major B cell subset in umbilical cord blood and constitutes 20-35% of the total B cell population in late adolescence.[148,149] The CD5+ subset of B1 cells is present mostly in the peritoneal cavity,[148] and only sparsely in the gut lamina propria.[150] However, B1-like antibodies apparently account for a significant part of salivary S-IgA antibodies to the oral microflora.[151] Antigens of non-microbial origin (e.g., foodstuffs, and allergens) seem to be inefficiently taken up by the M cells of follicle-associated epithelium.[152] The extent to which human B1 cells are responsible for IgA antibodies against these innocuous antigens is unknown. The subclass distribution of B1- versus B2-derived IgA antibodies in humans also remains to be examined.

IgA Antibody Functions

The presence of antibodies in external secretions was first suggested by the detection of local (not serum-derived) immunity in animals orally immunized with intestinal pathogens (reviewed by Mestecky et al[153]). This observation stimulated intensive research in mucosal immunity to infection, with the prospect of exploiting this mechanism for vaccination. Thus, experimental studies of mucosal immune responses to microbial antigens, often involving potent adjuvants such as cholera toxin, have contributed largely to the current knowledge of IgA biological activities. The significance of IgA responses to natural infections, and to innocuous antigens from the commensal flora, has received less attention.

Because immune responses to microbial antigens are heterogeneous, experiments involving passive immunization with purified poly- or monoclonal antibodies have been designed to identify the specific activities of IgA versus those of other Ig classes. Antibodies have been delivered either directly, often mixed with the infectious inoculum, or indirectly as in the elegant "back-pack" tumor model. In this model, hybridoma cells producing a relevant monoclonal IgA antibody in a polymeric form are injected subcutaneously in the back of a mouse. As the tumor enlarges, the IgA antibody appears in both plasma and gut mucosal secretions due to efficient transport of polymeric IgA from the circulation into the bile in this species.[154] Other activities have been ascribed to IgA mainly on the basis of observations in simplified models in vitro. Presumably, evaluation of such activities may require the involvement of gene knockout animal models to control for effects of other factors that may obscure IgA-mediated effects in vivo.

In addition to being the major Ig at mucosal surfaces, IgA is also abundant in the circulation and tissues, including the lamina propria. The host defense problems in these two compartments are by nature essentially different. The presence of a microorganism in the blood or tissues represents a potentially life-threatening invasion, which must be met with a forceful reaction. By contrast, S-IgA and the mucosal immune system in general must keep a balance with the normal microbiota, while maintaining the ability to respond vigorously to potential pathogens. Mucosal immune reactions, irrespective of the nature of the antigen, should not result in inflammatory reactions that might jeopardize the physiological functions of the mucosal membranes. The two forms of IgA, functioning in their respective compartments, appear to meet these requirements.[6,155]

Functions of IgA in Relation to Mucosal Membranes

IgA functions in mucosal membranes are often defined collectively as "immune exclusion". Whereas systemic defence aim at the ultimate destruction of intruding antigens, mucosal IgA prevent the attachment and penetration of microorganisms and molecular antigens, blocking their potential effects on the host. In secretions, S-IgA antibodies are well suited to these tasks because of their molecular characteristics. Their four or more antigen binding sites allow them to block adherence determinants, including microbial,[156-158] neutralize microbial enzymes and toxins, and agglutinate microorganisms,[159] thereby facilitating their disposal by muco-ciliary flow or peristalsis. The abundant and outward directed glycans of the Fc.Sc part of the S-IgA molecule contribute to these effects by conferring hydrophilicity and negative charge to the resulting immune complex.[160] The glycans of the highly glycosylated SC component are largely responsible for the marked resistance of S-IgA to degradation by nonspecific microbial and digestive proteases.[161,162] Structural elements of the Fc.SC part also facilitate the entrapment of immune complexes containing S-IgA in the mucus blanket covering mucosal surfaces, which leads to their disposal.[163-165] Elegant experiments have recently shown that entrapment in the mouse airways mucus depends largely on SC glycans.[164] In the human female genital tract, Ig affinity to secretory leukocyte proteinase inhibitor, a nonspecific defence protein present in most external secretions, seems to be important.[166] The capacity of bacterial IgA1 proteases to cleave IgA (including S-IgA) molecules in the hinge region has been exploited to analyse the defence mechanisms mediated by the Fc (or Fc.SC) part of IgA antibodies.[17]

Support for the notion that IgA antibodies inhibit the penetration of antigens comes from studies involving passive or active immunization,[167,169,170] and observations that IgA- and pIgR-deficient individuals often have elevated plasma levels of dietary antigen-containing immune complexes.[55,171] A report of allergen-specific IgA antibody deficiency in type 1 allergic patients is frequently cited in this context,[172] but was never confirmed. Allergy seems to be associated with elevated levels of allergen-reactive antibodies of not only IgE, but also IgG and IgA (including S-IgA) classes, whereas such antibodies are barely detectable in nonallergic individuals.[173-176] The reason for the apparent functional impairment of allergen-specific S-IgA in allergic individuals is unknown, and may involve an IgE-mediated uptake of allergens by the mucosal epithelial cells in these individuals.[177-179]

S-IgA antibodies were found to inhibit also the uptake of microbial antigens through the specialized epithelium that cover mucosal lymphoid follicles.[180] This might explain the self-limiting nature of S-IgA responses to intestinal bacteria observed in certain animal experiments.[81] However, other studies suggest that coating of antigens with enteric S-IgA antibodies facilitates their uptake through M cells.[181,182] Receptor-mediated uptake of S-IgA by dendritic cells has also been observed.[183,184] The potential consequences of S-IgA coating for the quality of the immune reactions induced, if any, are unknown. This might be a rewarding topic for research, particularly in the view of recent reports of reduced immune responsiveness to microbial antigens in IgA-deficient animals.[185]

The protective functions of mucosal IgA antibodies are not restricted to the activities of S-IgA antibodies in secretions. In vitro studies have shown that immune complexes containing polymeric IgA (pIgA) antibodies can be transported intact across polarized epithelial cell monolayers expressing pIgR, according to the same process that allows free pIgA to migrate to the apical surface.[186] As an in vivo correlate, pIgA mediate the excretion by liver cells of antigens into the bile in mice (though not significantly in humans).[187] This excretion also takes place over the intestinal epithelium.[188] Furthermore, there is evidence that pIgA antibodies during transfer through the epithelium may neutralize viruses by interfering specifically with the viral life cycle.[189] Thus, polymeric IgA antibodies, acting in concert during epithelial transfer and in the secretions, can provide for the neutralization and exclusion of potentially harmful substances without disturbing the mucosal physiology.[190]

Functions of IgA in Tissues

The two distinct environments in which IgA antibodies operate differ with respect to the presence or absence of ancillary factors. In the mucosal secretions, there is no evidence of a biologically active complement system or of significant numbers of live phagocytes. Conversely, in the circulation and tissues, both of these components are prominent defense factors.

The question remains of whether or not IgA activates complement.[6] Clearly, IgA is unable to activate complement by the classical pathway.[191] To the contrary, IgA antibodies to capsular polysaccharides may inhibit IgG or IgM antibody-dependent complement-mediated lysis of meningococci under specific circumstances,[192] and similar effects have been observed for IgA antibodies in vitro.[193,194] However, IgA molecules denatured by various procedures, including partial deglycosylation by streptococcal glycosidases, activate complement by the alternative pathway.[195] This may explain why IgA antibodies to the capsule of glycosidase-producing pneumococci mediate opsonophagocytosis by resting human phagocytes only in the presence of complement.[196] Purified human serum IgA immobilized on plastic surfaces is capable of activating complement by the mannan-binding lectin pathway.[197] However, this capacity may be restricted to IgA molecules rich in the high-mannose type of *N*-linked glycans (Reinholdt and Jensenius, unpublished data). Overall, it seems that human IgA antibodies have a poor or no complement-activating ability when bound physiologically to antigens, except for some degree of alternative pathway activation when the IgA is abnormally glycosylated or otherwise denatured.

Early studies indicated that IgA antibodies were relatively inefficient mediators of opsonophagocytosis when compared to IgG.[198] IgA was also reported to inhibit the mobilization of phagocytes,[199-201] and the release of inflammatory cytokines by LPS-stimulated human monocytes.[202] It is now clear that these results do not reflect the full potential of IgA cooperation with phagocytes. An Fc-specific IgA receptor (FcαR, designated CD89) is variably expressed on human granulocytes and monocytes/macrophages.[203,204] Several groups have shown that neutrophils activated by treatment with inflammatory cytokines display an enhanced phagocytosis of IgA-coated particles consistent with an enhanced surface expression of FcαR.[27,205-207] FcαR binds both subclasses of IgA and S-IgA, but pIgA is generally more effective than mIgA in mediating phagocytosis. Eosinophils also express cytokine-regulated FcαR, and easily degranulate upon reaction with pIgA-containing immune complexes.[208] Eosinophils also express a receptor for SC, which may explain why immobilized S-IgA are particularly efficient in eosinophil degranulation.[209,210] Whereas IgA-mediated degranulation of eosinophils may be important in the defense against parasites, it is suspected to contribute to the detrimental effects of eosinophils during the late phase of atopic reactions in the respiratory mucosa.[174,210] Conversely, IgA has been found to inhibit induced IgE-mediated hypersensitivity.[211] Taking into account the elevated levels of allergen-reactive IgA antibodies in most allergic individuals, and the inconclusive body of published data on the prevalence of allergy in IgA-deficient versus normal humans,[212-215] the overall effect of allergen-reactive IgA antibodies in relation to atopy remains unknown.

In the view of this information, the plasma and tissue forms of IgA appear to be biomolecules of high functional adaptability, able to function according to local demands. In the absence of invading pathogens, IgA antibodies may modulate the inflammatory responses to complement and phagocytic cell activation, and possibly the IgE-mediated reactions. Conversely, in reaction to alarm signals from microorganisms and the innate immune system, IgA antibodies may promote a forceful inflammatory response.

Mucosal Tolerance

Mucosal (or oral) tolerance is the suppression or down-regulation of immune effector cell responses (T and B) to an antigen by prior administration of the antigen by mucosal (e.g., oral) route. Mucosal tolerance probably evolved in order to prevent irrelevant and potentially injurious reactions to food substances and other harmless antigens encountered at mucosal surfaces. By reference to the IgA activities discussed above, mucosal tolerance may be viewed as a collaborator of IgA in the maintenance of mucosal homeostasis through peaceful neutralisation of innocuous antigens. Like other forms of immunological tolerance, mucosal tolerance also provides mechanisms to suppress pathologic reactivity against self.[216,217]

Oral tolerance has raised considerable research interest over the last 20 years, but it has been difficult to reach definite mechanistic explanations. Essential inductive events can be

i.   the development of regulatory T cells, which mediate active suppression,
ii. the inactivation of T cells (Th-1, Th-2, T-CTL), that may be brought about by cellular anergy or clonal deletion,
iii. the generation of antibodies which mediate suppression, possibly as part of an anti-idiotype network.

Generally, several tolerance mechanisms such as suppression and anergy may operate sequentially or simultaneously (for reviews, see refs. 217,218).

Mucosal tolerance, even when it involves clonal anergy or deletion, represents an active immune response and not a simple absence of antigen recognition.[218-220] Accordingly, the induction of tolerogenic reactions depends largely on the properties of the antigen-presenting cells (APC) involved. Whereas several types of mucosal cells may display antigen-presenting capacity, certain phenotypes of dendritic cells (DC) in mucosal tissues and the draining lymph nodes seem to be particularly significant in the induction of tolerogenic reactions.[221-228] The performance of DC and other APC is highly dependent on the quality of the signals received through Toll-like and other receptors.[229] These signals are mediated largely by molecular components of the mucosal flora. As mentioned, the development of a commensal flora not only represents a physiological stimulus to the immune system, but also conditions the mucosal immune system for the induction of tolerogenic reactions, which suggests that the commensal flora and the immune system have evolved to cooperate in the maintenance of mucosal homeostasis. Thus, germ-free mice develop short-lived tolerance and no tolerance at all, when fed with ovalbumin and sheep red blood cells, respectively.[230-232] The capacity for development of oral tolerance to certain antigens may be reconstituted in germ-free animals by treatment with LPS, a prominent cell wall component of gram-negative bacteria,[232,233] whereas in antigen-fed conventionally reared animals LPS may promote immune responses.[69,234,235] The tolerization of IgE antibody responses to mucosal allergens is also deficient in germ-free mice.[236] Interestingly, this deficiency can be reversed by neonatal colonization of the animals with *Bifidobacterium infantis*, a gram-positive bacterium of value as an intestinal probiotic in human.[236,237] Remarkably, immune responses to the commensal flora appear to be down-regulated by certain mechanisms of mucosal tolerance in healthy individuals.[238-240] However, the hyporesponsive, yet activated state of the immune system towards the commensal flora may break down in some individuals, in which case strong T cell-mediated and humoral responses against a subset of bacterial antigens may develop, much like a response against pathogenic bacteria. Such breakdown possibly underlies inflammatory bowel diseases such as Crohn's disease and ulcerative colitis.[238,240,241] Furthermore, changes in the flora caused by mucosal infection with certain pathogens may adversely affect the induction of tolerance to non-microbial substances like dietary antigens and allergens.[242,243] As an exploitation of this principle, administration of antigens to mucosal surfaces together with cholera toxin as an adjuvant prevents the induction of tolerance and triggers systemic as well as mucosal immune responses.[244] The contrasting effects of pathogens versus commensals on mucosal immune regulation probably reflect a different quality of alarm signals to APCs, either directly[245] or via cytokines produced by the mucosal epithelium.[64-66] The distinct effects of different mucosal bacteria on the immune system may explain why mechanisms of mucosal tolerance identified in inbred animals kept under pathogen-free conditions do not always apply in humans.[35,246]

The dose of mucosally applied antigen influences the type of tolerogenic mechanism involved.[247] High doses of antigen (10-100 mg in repeated doses in mice) induced anergy.[248,249] The antigens cross the mucosa in significant amounts, circulate either in a native form or as immune aggregates, and presumably anergize antigen-specific T cells by reacting with the cells under conditions different from those required for T cell activation.[228] Anergy in T cells is characterized by an induced defect in IL-2 transcription, while the expression of IL-2 receptor is preserved.[250] High dose mucosal tolerance may be detected 1-2 days after antigen is fed to the animal.[251] It is not clear whether persistence of antigen is required for maintenance of tolerance, but repeated tolerogenic stimuli cause a reduction in T cell responses.[252]

The immune responses to common dietary antigens appear to be controlled by mechanisms of oral tolerance that involve T cell anergy, as shown in a comprehensive study of humoral and cellular immunity to common antigens in healthy humans.[253] Consistent with the inactivation of T cells, serum levels of both IgG and IgA antibodies to individual antigens were low. Within each of these two isotypes, individuals with higher titers of antibodies to one kind of antigen had higher titers of antibodies of the same isotype to other dietary antigens. In contrast, antibodies of the T-independent IgM isotype were present at slightly higher levels, with no correlation between antigens.[253]

Low doses of antigen applied to mucosal surfaces may lead to active suppression.[254-256] Antigen-specific regulatory T cells develop after presentation by APC in organized lymphoid follicles or in the epithelium. Studies in experimental allergic encephalomyelitis with myelin-basic protein (MBP) as a model antigen[257] identified CD8+ T cells as the major regulatory cells, acting primarily via secretion of TGF-β.[258] The same research group observed that when ovalbumin feeding is followed by parenteral immunization with ovalbumin together with MBP and adjuvant, there is a suppression of responses not only to ovalbumin but also to MBP.[259] This effect, denoted antigen-driven bystander suppression, involves the secretion of antigen-nonspecific suppressive cytokines by regulatory cells stimulated by the oral antigen. Subsequent studies indicated that T cells stimulated by distinct suppressor epitopes of a protein mediate epitope-driven bystander suppression of responses to non-suppressor epitopes within the same protein.[260] The fact that tolerogenic reactions to fed antigens/epitopes may induce bystander suppression of concurrent pathogenic, or beneficial responses to other antigens/epitopes is of potential clinical and therapeutical relevance.[261] Several studies have suggested that certain phenotypic variants of CD4+ T cells, some of which may be in a state of anergy, are important regulatory cells in mucosal tolerance to fed proteins and commensal flora antigens.[227,240,262-265] Further complexity arises from observations that γδ T cells, as a result of interactions with mucosal epithelial cells, may suppress certain immune reactions, notably IgE responses, to low doses of mucosal antigen.[266,267]

B Cells and Antibodies in Mucosal Tolerance

Stimulated B cells are one of several types of APC involved in the induction of mucosal immune responses.[268] Conversely, resting B cells, which express MHC class II but no costimulatory molecules, do not activate naive T cells and can mediate T cell anergy and tolerance.[269,270] However, B cells are not essential for the development of peripheral T cell tolerance by parenterally administered antigens.[271] The same seems to apply to oral tolerance, since genetically B cell deficient mice are still able to develop T cell tolerance upon oral administration of a single high dose or repeated low doses of a protein antigen.[272] These mice, as a corollary of their genetic defect, have involuted Peyer's patches, which suggests that these structures are not obligatory for the induction of oral tolerance. However, other investigators found that B cells[273] and Peyer's patches[274] were of significance for tolerance induction, at least against low oral doses of protein antigens. Furthermore, oral tolerance cannot be induced in mice lacking both Peyer's patches and mesenteric lymph nodes.[275,276]

Early studies indicated that B cells can be involved in the induction of oral tolerance by way of antibody production. Ad libitum feeding of sheep red blood cells to mice resulted in specific suppression of IgM, IgG, and IgA responses upon subsequent parenteral immunization with that antigen, and the suppressive effect could be transferred across MHC barriers by a serum Ig factor or antigen-antibody complexes from fed animals.[277,278] The transfer of the factor did not result in suppression of delayed-type hypersensitivity in the recipient.[279] The factor (IgG or IgA) could not always be absorbed with the fed antigen.[278] Such tolerance-mediating antibodies may be part of an anti-idiotype regulatory network,[278,280,281] and appear not to be involved in the induction of oral tolerance by feeding highly T-dependent protein antigens such as ovalbumin.[235,282] However, there is evidence that rodent mothers may transfer IgE-suppressive IgG antibodies to their offspring transplacentally or by milk.[283] It is possible that such presumably anti-idiotypic antibodies confer tolerance to the neonate at a time when susceptibility to atopic priming is high. No similar allergy-preventive role of maternal IgG antibodies was observed in human infants at risk of allergy development.[284] Human neonates may take up small amounts of maternal S-IgA from colostrum in the immediate neonatal period.[285] The physiological significance of this, if any, is not known.

Conceivably, mucosal IgA antibodies, either passively acquired by the neonate or actively produced by children and adults, may prevent or arrest immune responses by excluding mucosal antigens from the tissues. Indirect support for this assumption comes from the observation that polyimmunoglobulin receptor-deficient mice, which lack S-IgA and S-IgM, show signs of mucosal inflammation suggesting an undue triggering of systemic immunity.[171] In addition, as mentioned before, IgA-deficiency has been associated with an increased prevalence of atopic diseases. However, apart from the documented protection by S-IgA antibodies against certain pathogens (discussed earlier), the role of mucosal IgA-mediated immune exclusion in the limitation of immune responses in normal individuals is not clear. The presence of low levels of systemic and mucosal antibodies reacting with innocuous environmental antigens in healthy subjects does not necessarily reflect a previous failure by mucosal antibodies to prevent the presence and immune recognition of these antigens in the tissues. Theoretically, the antibodies represent cross- or polyreactive antibodies mainly of B1 origin. On the other hand, antigen-exclusion by mucosal IgA must be limited in time or space because a state of immunological tolerance to dietary antigens and other ubiquitous antigens seems to be present in healthy individuals, reflecting previous handling of the antigens by cells of the immune system. Particular attention has been paid to the possibility that colostral S-IgA antibodies might reduce the risk of atopic priming of the newborn to environmental antigens. Increased prevalence of cow's milk allergy was found in children who were formula-fed, as compared to breast-fed, as neonates.[286,287] However, extensive studies involving additional colostral components indicated that not S-IgA antibodies, but TGF-β and certain fatty acids in colostrum were responsible for the allergy-prophylactic effect of breast feeding.[288,289] Yet other studies provided inconsistent data on the role of breast-feeding in prevention of allergies and asthma.[290] Disturbance of S-IgA-mediated immune exclusion by IgA1 protease-producing mucosal bacteria has been suggested to be a possible factor for the development or perpetuation of atopy in infancy.[291,292] However, subsequent observations suggested that IgA1 protease-producing nasopharyngeal bacteria, if present, do not cause widespread cleavage of S-IgA1 molecules in the mucosal secretion.[13,176] Future studies on the significance of mucosal IgA in immune regulation should take into account the role of M cells and dendritic cells in receptor-mediated uptake of S-IgA immune complexes,[181-184] and the possible consequences of S-IgA binding for the stimulatory or tolerogenic reactions induced.

Early experiments indicated that the B cell system was more difficult to tolerize by primary oral administration of antigen than the T cell system.[293,294] Once antibody responses had been established, B cells were also more difficult to tolerize than T cells, and they recovered more rapidly.[295,296] An exception to this pattern seems to be IgE responses, which in rodents are exquisitely sensitive to oral tolerance.[283] As mentioned above, oral tolerization of mouse IgE antibodies (and other Th2-dependent products such as IgG1 and IL-4), is conditioned by postnatal colonization by commensal bacteria.[236] Since this does not apply to Th1-assisted antibody responses including IgG2a,[236] and because Th1 and Th2 cells appear to be equally susceptible to oral tolerance in conventionally reared mice,[262] there is no clear implication of the mucosal flora in the differential susceptibility of T cell and non-IgE B cell responses to oral tolerization.

The differential susceptibility of T- versus B cell responses to tolerization by mucosally administered antigens was confirmed by two studies in humans.[297,298] Short term feeding of healthy adults with keyhole limpet hemocyanin (KLH) followed by parenteral challenge with KLH induced the development of tolerance only in the T cell system (skin test reactivity, proliferation assay). Serum antibodies and antibody producing cells as determined by ELISPOT were of IgG, IgM, and IgA classes, and B cell priming by feeding was demonstrated by an accelerated response in the orally fed study group. Furthermore, IgA antibody responses were prominent in saliva and in intestinal secretions.[297] Similar results were obtained in parallel experiments involving intranasal instead of oral administration of KLH, except that serum IgA and IgG antibody responses were suppressed.[298]

Mucosal IgA Antibody Responses As Targets of Mucosal Tolerance

Pioneering studies suggested that oral tolerance is accompanied by mucosal IgA responses.[251,254] Conventionally, the induction of tolerance by antigen feeding has been examined by secondary challenge with an antigen injected subcutaneously with an adjuvant. This protocol cannot reveal a potential suppression of mucosal immunity because subcutaneously induced IgA responses do not generally involve S-IgA.[24] Studies involving secondary challenge by mucosal or intraperitoneal routes, however, have shown that mucosal IgA responses, like systemic responses, are sensitive to oral tolerance.[244,299-304] A few studies on the tolerogenic mechanism indicate the involvement of regulatory T cells, sometimes identified as CD8+.[299,302,303] The induction of oral tolerance in the mucosal IgA system is abrogated if innocuous antigens are fed together with cholera toxin as an adjuvant.[244,302,303]

In two studies, antigen feeding was reported to suppress S-IgA responses to intraperitoneal challenge with antigen and adjuvant.[244,301] Because intraperitoneal injection of antigen stimulates the B1 cell population, the suppression observed in these studies suggests that the differentiation of peritoneal B1 cells into IgA-producing cells in the gut wall is controlled by regulatory T cells. T cell-mediated regulation of B1 cells is suggested by additional observations.[105] It should be stressed, however, that the mechanisms involved in the stimulation and control of B1 cells in vivo have been poorly explored.[131]

The susceptibility of the mucosal IgA system to oral tolerance seems to be at odds with the presence of S-IgA antibodies to dietary antigens in most healthy humans.[253,305,306] In one study, the saliva levels of S-IgA antibodies to individual dietary antigens (bovine γ-globulin, or casein) were estimated at 0.02—0.46 % of total salivary S-IgA, four to nine fold higher than serum IgA to the same antigens.[253] This might indicate a less profound tolerization of mucosal IgA than serum IgA in response to dietary antigens. The maintenance of moderate levels of mucosal IgA antibodies to otherwise tolerogenic dietary antigens may involve complex molecular factors.[307] One group has suggested that the phenomenon may result from an interplay between mucosal epithelial cells and two types of intraepithelial T cells, i.e., γδ T cells that interfere with the induction of tolerance, and αβ T cells that provide B cell help.[308,309] If so, the apparent variability of this mechanism in different experimental settings needs to be explained.

The susceptibility of the mucosal IgA system to tolerization is relevant to what is known of the biological effects of IgA antibodies. On one hand, IgA is the largest Ig class produced. On the other hand, many IgA-deficient individuals remain healthy. This paradox illustrates the complexity of the issue. Whereas the protective potential of mucosal IgA antibody responses towards pathogenic microorganisms is established, the significance of the interaction of mucosal and systemic IgA antibodies with the commensal flora and innocuous non-living antigens is unclear.[6] Hypothetically, IgA against the latter targets might occur at sub-protective concentrations, due to tolerization. This is conceivable in the case of potentially harmful molecular antigens, such as allergens. Concerning commensals, however, the inhibition of bacterial adherence by purified S-IgA antibodies at concentrations within physiological range was reported in vitro.[310,157,158] These observations may not reflect the significance of the antibodies in vivo, where other specific or nonspecific factors may substitute for, interfere with, or potentiate the functions of IgA antibodies.[311,312] However, oral and intestinal bacteria of healthy individuals were found to be coated with IgA antibodies.[313,314] Since this coating does not seem to eliminate the commensals, it remains an attractive, yet unconfirmed hypothesis that the antibodies to beneficial commensals do not block essential colonization determinants and belong to the restricted B1 repertoire.[85]

The ability to evade host immune defence is a characteristic of successful pathogens as well as commensals. Among the strategies for evading mucosal immunity, IgA1 protease activity has received most attention.[17] A hypothesis for IgA1 protease-facilitated infection by the pathogens producing these enzymes was published, based on clinical findings and the effect of potential enzyme-neutralizing antibodies.[315] However, because additional non-IgA substrates to IgA1 proteases have been identified, it is not clear to which extent these enzymes impair the protective potential of IgA at mucosal membranes.[316-318]

Clinical Aspects of IgA Antibodies

The possible clinical significance of systemic antibodies to dietary antigens is a matter of concern. Serum antibodies have been detected in the major immunoglobulin classes IgM, IgG and IgA in the majority of healthy children[319] and adults.[320] The levels of serum antibodies, but not S-IgA antibodies, seem to decline during adult age.[305, 321,322] The levels of serum IgG or IgA antibodies to dietary proteins are increased in infants and children with food allergy, but there is considerable overlap between patients and healthy individuals.[323] These antibodies may be byproducts rather than mediators of food allergy. However, the presence of serum IgA antibody to gliadin is of diagnostic value in the screening for coeliac disease.[324] Serum IgA antibodies against dietary antigens such as gliadin belong predominantly to the IgA1 subclass.[325,326]

Concluding Remarks

The human body produces IgA in amounts greater than the amounts of all other Ig classes combined. Still, in spite of considerable research efforts, the benefits of this physiological investment are only partly understood. Remarkably, many individuals with IgA deficiency, the most prevalent immunodeficiency of all, remain healthy.

Mechanisms by which S-IgA antibodies neutralize pathogens and molecular antigens at mucosal surfaces have been documented in vitro, and in several cases in vivo. The previously enigmatic functions of IgA antibodies in the circulation and tissues are now better understood. It appears that systemic IgA antibodies may adapt functionally to the quality of the actual target, functioning as powerful opsonins towards pathogens, as opposed to mediating the discrete non-inflammatory neutralization of harmless antigens such as mucosal commensals. The regulation of Fcα receptor expression on phagocytes by inflammatory cytokines seems to be an important determinant of systemic IgA functions. By their functions, S-IgA and systemic IgA antibodies help maintain mucosal homeostasis.

Maintenance of mucosal homeostasis is probably the major evolutionary argument also for the down-regulation of potentially injurious immune responses via mucosal tolerance. In this view, it is remarkable that mucosal as well as systemic IgA antibody responses to innocuous antigens became subject to tolerization by mucosally applied antigens. Nevertheless, mucosal IgA antibodies to innocuous molecular antigens are produced at moderate levels in healthy individuals, as are IgA antibodies to commensal bacteria. The cellular origin, B1 versus B2, and physiological significance of these IgA antibodies are not known. Notably, mucosal IgA responses to pathogenic bacteria, or to innocuous antigens in combination with mucosal adjuvants such as cholera toxin, are not suppressed by mucosal tolerance, presumably testifying to the importance of mucosal IgA antibodies in the protection against pathogens.

Acknowledgements

The authors are grateful to Charles O. Elson for discussions and advice concerning the structure of the manuscript, to Mogens Kilian for discussions, careful reading of the manuscript, and suggestions for its improvement, and to Per Brandtzaeg for providing the two illustrations.

References

1. Fujihashi K, Ernst PB. A mucosal internet. Epithelial cell-immune cell interactions. In: Ogra PL et al, eds. Mucosal Immunology. Academic Press, 1999:619-630.
2. London SD, Rubin, DH. Functional role of mucosal cytotoxic lymphocytes. In: Ogra PL et al, eds. Mucosal Immunology. Academic Press, 1999:643-653.
3. Brandtzaeg P, Farstad IN. The human mucosal B-cell system. In: Ogra PL et al, eds. Mucosal Immunology. Academic Press, 1999:439-468.
4. Mestecky J, Russell MW, Jackson S et al. The human IgA system: A reassessment. Clin Immunol Immunopathol 1986; 40:105-114.
5. Conley ME, Delacroix DL. Intravascular and mucosal immunoglobulin A: Two separate but related systems of immune defense? Ann Intern Med 1987; 106:892-899.
6. Russell MW, Kilian M, Lamm ME. Biological activities of IgA. In: Ogra PL et al, eds. Mucosal Immunology. Academic Press, 1999:225-240.
7. Hanson LA Comparative immunological studies of the immunoglobulin of human milk and blood serum. Int Arch Allergy Appl Immunol 1961; 18:227-241.
8. Tomasi TB Jr, Tan EM et al. Characteristics of an immune system common to certain external secretions. J Exp Med 1965; 121:101-124.
9. Heremans JF. Immunoglobulin A. In: Sela M, ed. The Antigens. Academic Press, 1974:365-522.
10. Mestecky J, Moro I, Underdown BJ. Mucosal immunoglobulins. In: Ogra PL et al, eds. Mucosal Immunology. Academic Press, 1999:133-552.
11. Brandtzaeg P, Karlsson G, Hansson G et al. The clinical condition of IgA-deficient patients is related to the proportion of IgD- and IgM-producing cells in their nasal mucosa. Clin Exp Immunol 1987; 67:626-636.
12. Mostov K, Kaetzel C. Immunoglobulin transport and the polymeric immunoglobulin receptor. In: Ogra PL et al, eds. Mucosal Immunology. Academic Press, 1999:181-211.
13. Kirkeby L, Rasmussen TT, Reinholdt J et al. Immunoglobulins in nasal secretions of healthy humans: Structural integrity of secretory immunoglobulin A1 (IgA1) and occurrence of neutralizing antibodies to IgA1 proteases of nasal bacteria. Clin Diagn Lab Immunol 2000; 7:31-39.
14. Kutteh WH, Mestecky J. Secretory immunity in the female reproductive tract. Am J Reprod Immunol 1994; 31:40-46.
15. Baenziger J, Kornfeld S. Structure of the carbohydrate units of IgA1 immunoglobulin. II. Structure of the O-glycosidically linked oligosaccharide units. J Biol Chem 1974; 249:7270-7281.
16. Mattu TS, Pleass RJ, Willis AC et al. The glycosylation and structure of human serum IgA1, Fab, and Fc regions and the role of N-glycosylation on Fc alpha receptor interactions. J Biol Chem 1998; 273:2260-2272.
17. Kilian M, Reinholdt J, Lomholt H et al. Biological significance of IgA1 proteases in bacterial colonization and pathogenesis: Critical evaluation of experimental evidence. APMIS 1996; 104:321-338.
18. Kawamura S, Saitou N, Ueda S. Concerted evolution of the primate immunoglobulin alpha-gene through gene conversion. J Biol Chem 1992; 267:7359-7367.
19. Crago SS, Kutteh WH, Moro et al. Distribution of IgA1-, IgA2-, and J chain-containing cells in human tissues. J Immunol 1984; 132:16-18.

20. Skvaril F, Morell A. Distribution of IgA subclasses in sera and bone marrow plasma cells of 21 normal individuals. Adv Exp Med Biol 1974; 45:433-435.
21. Kett K, Brandtzaeg P, Radl J et al. Different subclass distribution of IgA-producing cells in human lymphoid organs and various secretory tissues. J Immunol 1986; 136:3631-3635.
22. Kutteh WH, Hatch KD, Blackwell RE et al. Secretory immune system of the female reproductive tract: I. Immunoglobulin and secretory component-containing cells. Obstet Gynecol 1988; 71:56-60.
23. Mestecky J, Russell MW. IgA subclasses. Monogr Allergy 1986; 19:277-301.
24. Russell MW, Lue C, van den Wall Bake AW et al. Molecular heterogeneity of human IgA antibodies during an immune response. Clin Exp Immunol 1992; 87:1-6.
25. Wang AC, Fudenberg HH. Genetics and evolution of human immunoglobulin A. Adv Exp Med Biol 1974; 45:161-165.
26. van Loghem E, Biewenga J. Allotypic and isotypic aspects of human immunoglobulin A Mol Immunol 1983; 20:1001-1007.
27. van Egmond M, Damen CA, van Spriel AB et al. IgA and the IgA Fc receptor. Trends Immunol 2001; 22:205-211.
28. Nose M, Wigzell H. Biological significance of carbohydrate chains on monoclonal antibodies. Proc Natl Acad Sci USA 1983; 80:6632.
29. Wold AE, Mestecky J, Tomana M et al. Secretory immunoglobulin A carries oligosaccharide receptors for Escherichia coli type 1 fimbrial lectin. Infect Immun 1990; 58:3073-3077.
30. Adlerberth I, Ahrne S, Johansson ML et al. A mannose-specific adherence mechanism in Lactobacillus plantarum conferring binding to the human colonic cell line HT-29. Appl Environ Microbiol 1996; 62:2244-2251.
31. Niedermeier W, Tomana M, Mestecky J. The carbohydrate composition of J chain from human serum and secretory IgA. Biochim Biophys Acta 1972; 257:527-530.
32. Mizoguchi A, Mizuochi T, Kobata A. Structures of the carbohydrate moieties of secretory component purified from human milk. J Biol Chem 1982; 257:9612-9621.
33. Cornes JS. Peyer's patches in the human gut. Proc R Soc Med 1965; 58:716.
34. Craig SW, Cebra JJ. Peyer's patches: an enriched source of precursors for IgA-producing immunocytes in the rabbit. J Exp Med 1971; 134:188-200.
35. MacDonald TT, Monteleone G. IL-12 and Th1 immune responses in human Peyer's patches. Trends Immunol 2001; 22:244-247.
36. Spalding DM, Williamson SI, Koopman WJ et al. Preferential induction of polyclonal IgA secretion by murine Peyer's patch dendritic cell-T cell mixtures. J Exp Med 1984; 160:941-946.
37. Iwasaki A, Kelsall BL. Freshly isolated Peyer's patch, but not spleen, dendritic cells produce interleukin 10 and induce the differentiation of T helper type 2 cells. J Exp Med 1999; 190:229-239.
38. Coffman RL, Lebman DA, Shrader B. Transforming growth factor beta specifically enhances IgA production by lipopolysaccharide-stimulated murine B lymphocytes. J Exp Med 1989; 170:1039-1044.
39. Muramatsu M, Kinoshita K, Fagarasan S et al. Class switch recombination and hypermutation require activation-induced cytidine deaminase (AID), a potential RNA editing enzyme. Cell 2000; 102:553-563.
40. Kelsall BL, Strober W. Gut-associated lymphoid tissue: antigen handling and T-lymphocyte responses. In: Ogra PL et al, eds. Mucosal Immunology. Academic Press, 1999:293-317.
41. McIntyre TM, Strober W. Gut-associated lymphoid tissue: Regulation of IgA B-cell development. In: Ogra PL et al, eds. Mucosal Immunology. Academic Press, 1999:319-356.
42. Fayette J, Dubois B, Vandenabeele S et al. Human dendritic cells skew isotype switching of CD40-activated naive B cells towards IgA1 and IgA2. J Exp Med 1997; 185:1909-1918.
43. Scicchitano R, Husband AJ, Clancy RL. Contribution of intraperitoneal immunization to the local immune response in the respiratory tract of sheep. Immunology 1984; 53:375-384.
44. Salmi M, Jalkanen S. Regulation of lymphocyte traffic to mucosa-associated lymphatic tissues. Gastroenterol Clin North Am 1991; 20:495-510.
45. Mestecky J, McGhee JR, Michalek SM et al. Concept of the local and common mucosal immune response. Adv Exp Med Biol 1978; 107:185-192.
46. Moldoveanu Z, Russell MW, Wu HY et al. Compartmentalization within the common mucosal immune system. Adv Exp Med Biol 1995; 371A:97-101

47. Czerkinsky C, Quiding M, Eriksson K et al. Induction of specific immunity at mucosal surfaces: prospects for vaccine development. Adv Exp Med Biol 1995; 371B:1409-416.

48. Quiding-Jabrink M, Nordstrom I, Granstrom G et al. Differential expression of tissue-specific adhesion molecules on human circulating antibody-forming cells after systemic, enteric, and nasal immunizations. A molecular basis for the compartmentalization of effector B cell responses. J Clin Invest 1997; 99:1281-1286.

49. Wu HY, Russell MW. Nasal lymphoid tissue, intranasal immunization, and compartmentalization of the common mucosal immune system. Immunol Res 1997; 16:187-201.

50. Squier CA, Hall BK. The permeability of skin and oral mucosa to water and horseradish peroxidase as related to the thickness of the permeability barrier. J Invest Dermatol 1985; 84:176-179.

51. Fujita M, Reinhart F, Neutra M. Convergence of apical and basolateral endocytic pathways at apical late endosomes in absorptive cells of suckling rat ileum in vivo. J Cell Sci 1990; 97(Pt 2):385-394.

52. Matter K, Mellman I. Mechanisms of cell polarity: Sorting and transport in epithelial cells. Curr Opin Cell Biol 1994; 6:545-554.

53. Neutra MR, Kraehenbuhl JP. Transepithelial transport of proteins by intestinal epithelial cells. In: Audus KL, Raub TJ, eds. Biological Barriers to Protein Delivery. Vol. 4. Plenum, 1993:107-129.

54. Husby S, Jensenius JC, Svehag SE. Passage of undegraded dietary antigen into the blood of healthy adults. Quantification, estimation of size distribution, and relation of uptake to levels of specific antibodies. Scand J Immunol 1985; 22:83-92.

55. Cunningham-Rundles C. Analysis of the gastrointestinal secretory immune barrier in IgA deficiency. Ann Allergy 1986; 57:31-35.

56. Husby S. Dietary antigens: Uptake and humoral immunity in man. APMIS Suppl 1988; 1:1-40.

57. Dahlgren UI, Wold AE, Hanson LA et al. Secretory antibody response against bacterial antigens and food proteins. Immunol Res 1991; 10:437-440.

58. McGhee JR, Mestecky J, Dertzbaugh MT et al. The mucosal immune system: From fundamental concepts to vaccine development. Vaccine 1992; 10:75-88.

59. Korenblat PE, Rothberg RM, Minden P et al. Immune responses of human adults after oral and parenteral exposure to bovine serum albumin. J Allergy 1968; 41:226-235.

60. Strobel S, Mowat AM. Immune responses to dietary antigens: oral tolerance. Immunol Today 1998; 19:173-181.

61. Hershberg RM, Mayer LF. Antigen processing and presentation by intestinal epithelial cells—Polarity and complexity. Immunol Today 2000; 21:123-128.

62. Freter R, Jones GW. Models for studying the role of bacterial attachment in virulence and pathogenesis. Rev Infect Dis 1983; 5 Suppl 4:S647-S658.

63. Bowden GH, Hamilton IR. Survival of oral bacteria. Crit Rev Oral Biol Med 1998; 9:54-85.

64. Henderson B, Wilson M. Commensal communism and the oral cavity. J Dent Res 1998; 77:1674-1683.

65. Hooper LV, Gordon JI. Commensal host-bacterial relationships in the gut. Science 2001; 292:1115-1118.

66. Neish AS. The gut microflora and intestinal epithelial cells: A continuing dialogue. Microbes Infect 2002; 4:309-317.

67. van der Waaij, D. Colonization resistance of the digestive tract—Mechanism and clinical consequences. Nahrung 1987; 31:507-517.

68. Savage DC. Gastrointestinal microflora in mammalian nutrition. Annu Rev Nutr 1986; 6:155-178.

69. Cebra JJ, Jiang HQ, Sterzl J et al. The role of mucosal microbiota in the development and maintenance of the mucosal immune system. In: Ogra PLeal, ed. Mucosal Immunology. Academic Press, 1999:267-280.

70. Caugant DA, Levin BR, Selander RK. Genetic diversity and temporal variation in the E. coli population of a human host. Genetics 1981; 98:467-90.

71. Hohwy J, Reinholdt J, Kilian M. Population dynamics of Streptococcus mitis in its natural habitat. Infect Immun 2001; 69:6055-6063.

72. Crabbe PA, Bazin H, Eyssen H et al. The normal microbial flora as a major stimulus for proliferation of plasma cells synthesizing IgA in the gut. The germ-free intestinal tract. Int Arch Allergy Appl Immunol 1968; 34:362-375.

73. MacDonald TT, Carter PB. Requirement for a bacterial flora before mice generate cells capable of mediating the delayed hypersensitivity reaction to sheep red blood cells. J Immunol 1979; 122:2624-2629.

74. Tlaskalova-Hogenova H, Sterzl J, Stepankova R et al. Development of immunological capacity under germfree and conventional conditions. Ann NY Acad Sci 1983; 409:96-113.

75. Parrott DM, MacDonald TT. The ontogeny of the mucosal immune system in rodents. In: MacDonald TT, ed. Ontogeny of the Immune System of the Gut. CRC Press, 1990:51-67.

76. Moreau MC, Ducluzeau R, Guy-Grand D et al. Increase in the population of duodenal immuno-globulin A plasmocytes in axenic mice associated with different living or dead bacterial strains of intestinal origin. Infect Immun 1978; 21:532-539.

77. Klaasen HL, Van der Heijden PJ, Stok W et al. Apathogenic, intestinal, segmented, filamentous bacteria stimulate the mucosal immune system of mice. Infect Immun 1993; 61:303-306.

78. Talham GL, Jiang HQ, Bos NA et al. Segmented filamentous bacteria are potent stimuli of a physiologically normal state of the murine gut mucosal immune system. Infect Immun 1999; 67:1992-2000.

79. Alaluusua S, Alaluusua SJ, Karjalainen J et al. The demonstration by ribotyping of the stability of oral Streptococcus mutans infection over 5 to 7 years in children. Arch Oral Biol 1994; 39:467-471.

80. Caufield PW, Cutter GR, Dasanayake AP. Initial acquisition of mutans streptococci by infants: Evidence for a discrete window of infectivity. J Dent Res 1993; 72:37-45.

81. Shroff KE, Meslin K, Cebra JJ. Commensal enteric bacteria engender a self-limiting humoral mucosal immune response while permanently colonizing the gut. Infect Immun 1995; 63:3904-3913.

82. Cole MF, Hsu SD, Sheridan MJ et al. Natural transmission of Streptococcus sobrinus in rats: Saliva and serum antibody responses to colonization. Infect Immun 1992; 60:778-783.

83. Cole MF, Bryan S, Evans MK et al. Humoral immunity to commensal oral bacteria in human infants: salivary secretory immunoglobulin A antibodies reactive with Streptococcus mitis biovar 1, Streptococcus oralis, Streptococcus mutans, and Enterococcus faecalis during the first two years of life. Infect Immun 1999; 67:1878-886.

84. Riviere GR, Wagoner MA, Freeman IL. Chronic peroral immunization of conventional laboratory rats with mutans streptococci leads to stable acquired suppression of salivary antibodies. Oral Microbiol Immunol 1992; 7:137-141.

85. Kroese FG, de Waard R, Bos NA. B-1 cells and their reactivity with the murine intestinal microflora. Semin Immunol 1996; 8:11-18.

86. Kroese FG, Bos NA. Peritoneal B-1 cells switch in vivo to IgA and these IgA antibodies can bind to bacteria of the normal intestinal microflora. Curr Top Microbiol Immunol 1999; 246:343-349.

87. Bos NA, Cebra JJ, Kroese FG. B-1 cells and the intestinal microflora. Curr Top Microbiol Immunol 2000; 252:211-220.

88. Macpherson AJ, Gatto D, Sainsbury E et al. A primitive T cell-independent mechanism of intestinal mucosal IgA responses to commensal bacteria. Science 2000; 288:2222-2226.

89. Hayakawa K, Hardy RR, Parks DR et al. The "Ly-1 B" cell subpopulation in normal immunodefective, and autoimmune mice. J Exp Med 1983; 157:202-218.

90. Hardy RR, Hayakawa K. Development and physiology of Ly-1 B and its human homolog, Leu-1 B. Immunol Rev 1986; 93:53-79.

91. Herzenberg LA, Stall AM, Lalor PA et al. The Ly-1 B cell lineage. Immunol Rev 1986; 93:81-102.

92. Kocks C, Rajewsky K. Stable expression and somatic hypermutation of antibody V regions in B-cell developmental pathways. Annu Rev Immunol 1989; 7:537-559.

93. Vakil M, Kearney JF. Functional characterization of monoclonal auto-anti-idiotype antibodies isolated from the early B cell repertoire of BALB/c mice. Eur J Immunol 1986; 16:1151-1158.

94. Elliott M, Kearney JF. Idiotypic regulation of development of the B-cell repertoire. Ann NY Acad Sci 1992; 651:336-345.

95. Lalor PA, Herzenberg LA, Adams S et al. Feedback regulation of murine Ly-1 B cell development. Eur J Immunol 1989; 19:507-513.

96. Forster I, Rajewsky K. Expansion and functional activity of Ly-1+ B cells upon transfer of peritoneal cells into allotype-congenic, newborn mice. Eur J Immunol 1987; 17:521-528.

97. Karras JG, Wang Z, Huo L et al. Signal transducer and activator of transcription-3 (STAT3) is constitutively activated in normal, self-renewing B-1 cells but only inducibly expressed in conventional B lymphocytes. J Exp Med 1997; 185:1035-1042.

98. Hippen KL, Tze LE, Behrens TW. CD5 maintains tolerance in anergic B cells. J Exp Med 2000; 191:883-890.
99. Gary-Gouy H, Harriague J, Bismuth G et al. Human CD5 promotes B-cell survival through stimulation of autocrine IL-10 production. Blood 2002; 100:4537-4543.
100. Wong SC, Chew WK, Tan JE et al. Peritoneal CD5+ B-1 cells have signaling properties similar to tolerant B cells. J Biol Chem 2002; 277:30707-30715.
101. Cukrowska B, Sinkora J, Mandel L et al. Thymic B cells of pig fetuses and germ-free pigs spontaneously produce IgM, IgG and IgA: detection by ELISPOT method. Immunology 1996; 87:487-492.
102. Klinman DM. Analysis of B lymphocyte cross-reactivity at the single cell level. J Immunol Methods 1992; 152:217-225.
103. Kasaian MT, Casali P. Autoimmunity-prone B-1 (CD5 B) cells, natural antibodies and self recognition. Autoimmunity 1993; 15:315-329.
104. Settmacher U, Delvig A, Jahn S. Anti-bacterial specificities in the human fetal B cell repertoire. Hum Antibodies Hybridomas 1994; 5:91-95.
105. Allison AC, Nawata Y. Cytokines mediating the proliferation and differentiation of B-1 lymphocytes and their role in ontogeny and phylogeny. Ann NY Acad Sci 1992; 651:200-219.
106. Casali P, Schettino EW. Structure and function of natural antibodies. Curr Top Microbiol Immunol 1996; 210:167-179.
107. Wedemayer GJ, Patten PA, Wang LH et al. Structural insights into the evolution of an antibody combining site. Science 1997; 276:1665-1669.
108. Bouvet JP, Dighiero G. Cross-reactivity and polyreactivity: The two sides of a coin. Immunol Today 2000; 21:411-412.
109. Yin J, Mundorff EC, Yang PL et al. A comparative analysis of the immunological evolution of antibody 28B4. Biochemistry 2001; 40:10764-10773.
110. Rothstein TL, Kolber DL. Anti-Ig antibody inhibits the phorbol ester-induced stimulation of peritoneal B cells. J Immunol 1988; 141:4089-4093.
111. Rott O, Charreire J, Mignon-Godefroy K et al. B cell superstimulatory influenza virus activates peritoneal B cells. J Immunol 1995; 155:134-142.
112. Bao S, Beagley KW, Murray AM et al. Intestinal IgA plasma cells of the B1 lineage are IL-5 dependent. Immunology 1998; 94:181-188.
113. Murakami M, Tsubata T, Okamoto M et al. Antigen-induced apoptotic death of Ly-1 B cells responsible for autoimmune disease in transgenic mice. Nature 1992; 357:77-80.
114. Bikah G, Carey J, Ciallella JR et al. CD5-mediated negative regulation of antigen receptor-induced growth signals in B-1 B cells. Science 1996; 274:1906-1909.
115. Nawata Y, Stall AM, Herzenberg LA et al. Surface immunoglobulin ligands and cytokines differentially affect proliferation and antibody production by human CD5+ and CD5- B lymphocytes. Int Immunol 1990; 2:603-614.
116. Murakami M, Honjo T. Involvement of B-1 cells in mucosal immunity and autoimmunity. Immunol Today 1995; 16:534-539.
117. Ray SK, Putterman C, Diamond B. Pathogenic autoantibodies are routinely generated during the response to foreign antigen: A paradigm for autoimmune disease. Proc Natl Acad Sci USA 1996; 93:2019-2024.
118. Adib M, Ragimbeau J, Avrameas S et al. IgG autoantibody activity in normal mouse serum is controlled by IgM. J Immunol 1990; 145:3807-813.
119. Melero J, Tarrago D, Nunez-Roldan A et al. Human polyreactive IgM monoclonal antibodies with blocking activity against self-reactive IgG. Scand J Immunol 1997; 45:393-400.
120. Hayakawa K, Hardy RR, Honda M et al. Ly-1 B cells: functionally distinct lymphocytes that secrete IgM autoantibodies. Proc Natl Acad Sci USA 1984; 81:2494-2498.
121. Tlaskalova-Hogenova H, Mandel L, Stepankova R et al. Autoimmunity: From physiology to pathology. Natural antibodies, mucosal immunity and development of B cell repertoire. Folia Biol.(Praha) 1992; 38:202-215.
122. Murakami M, Tsubata T, Shinkura R et al. Oral administration of lipopolysaccharides activates B-1 cells in the peritoneal cavity and lamina propria of the gut and induces autoimmune symptoms in an autoantibody transgenic mouse. J Exp Med 1994; 180:111-121.
123. Coutinho A, Kazatchkine MD, Avrameas S. Natural autoantibodies. Curr Opin Immunol 1995; 7:812-818.

124. Bendelac A, Bonneville M, Kearney JF. Autoreactivity by design: innate B and T lymphocytes. Nat Rev Immunol 2001; 1:177-186.
125. Bouvet JP,Dighiero G. From natural polyreactive autoantibodies to a la carte monoreactive antibodies to infectious agents: Is it a small world after all? Infect Immun 1998; 66:1-4.
126. Martin F, Oliver AM, Kearney JF. Marginal zone and B1 B cells unite in the early response against T-independent blood-borne particulate antigens. Immunity 2001; 14:617-629.
127. Ochsenbein AF, Fehr T, Lutz C et al. Control of early viral and bacterial distribution and disease by natural antibodies. Science 1999; 286:2156-2159.
128. Carroll MC, Prodeus AP. Linkages of innate and adaptive immunity. Curr Opin Immunol 1998; 10:36-40.
129. Tsuji RF, Szczepanik M, Kawikova I et al. B cell-dependent T cell responses: IgM antibodies are required to elicit contact sensitivity. J Exp Med 2002; 196:1277-1290.
130. Weisz-Carrington P, Schrater AF, Lamm ME et al. Immunoglobulin isotypes in plasma cells of normal and athymic mice. Cell Immunol 1979; 44:343-351.
131. Martin F, Kearney JF. B1 cells: Similarities and differences with other B cell subsets. Curr Opin Immunol 2001; 13:195-201.
132. Fagarasan S, Watanabe N, Honjo T. Generation, expansion, migration and activation of mouse B1 cells. Immunol Rev 2000; 176:205-215.
133. Hayakawa K, Hardy RR, Herzenberg LA et al. Progenitors for Ly-1 B cells are distinct from progenitors for other B cells. J Exp Med 1985; 161:1554-1568.
134. Hiroi T, Yanagita M, Iijima H et al. Deficiency of IL-5 receptor alpha-chain selectively influences the development of the common mucosal immune system independent IgA-producing B-1 cell in mucosa-associated tissues. J Immunol 1999; 162:821-828.
135. Pecquet SS, Ehrat C, Ernst PB. Enhancement of mucosal antibody responses to Salmonella typhimurium and the microbial hapten phosphorylcholine in mice with X-linked immunodeficiency by B-cell precursors from the peritoneal cavity. Infect Immun 1992; 60:503-509.
136. Bos NA, Bun JC, Popma SH et al. Monoclonal immunoglobulin A derived from peritoneal B cells is encoded by both germ line and somatically mutated VH genes and is reactive with commensal bacteria. Infect Immun 1996; 64:616-623.
137. Watanabe N, Ikuta K, Fagarasan S et al. Migration and differentiation of autoreactive B-1 cells induced by activated gamma/delta T cells in antierythrocyte immunoglobulin transgenic mice. J Exp Med 2000; 192:1577-1586.
138. Fujihashi K, McGhee JR, Kweon MN et al. gamma/delta T cell-deficient mice have impaired mucosal immunoglobulin A responses. J Exp Med 1996; 183:1929-1935.
139. Hiroi T, Yanagita M, Ohta N et al. IL-15 and IL-15 receptor selectively regulate differentiation of common mucosal immune system-independent B-1 cells for IgA responses. J Immunol 2000; 165:4329-4337.
140. Fagarasan S, Kinoshita K, Muramatsu M et al. In situ class switching and differentiation to IgA-producing cells in the gut lamina propria. Nature 2001; 413:639-643.
141. Litinskiy MB, Nardelli B, Hilbert DM et al. DCs induce CD40-independent immunoglobulin class switching through BLyS and APRIL. Nat Immunol 2002; 3:822-829.
142. Brandtzaeg P, Baekkevold ES, Morton HC. From B to A the mucosal way. Nat Immunol 2001; 2:1093-1094.
143. Bos NA, Jiang HQ, Cebra JJ. T cell control of the gut IgA response against commensal bacteria. Gut 2001; 48:762-764.
144. Baumgarth N, Herman OC, Jager GC et al. Innate and acquired humoral immunities to influenza virus are mediated by distinct arms of the immune system. Proc Natl Acad Sci USA 1999; 96:2250-2255.
145. Kushnir N, Bos NA, Zuercher AW et al. B2 but not B1 cells can contribute to CD4+ T-cell-mediated clearance of rotavirus in SCID mice. J Virol 2001; 75:5482-5490.
146. Rasooly L, Abouzied MM, Brooks KH et al. Polyspecific and autoreactive IgA secreted by hybridomas derived from Peyer's patches of vomitoxin-fed mice: Characterization and possible pathogenic role in IgA nephropathy. Food Chem Toxicol 1994; 32:337-348.
147. Shimoda M, Inoue Y, Azuma N et al. Natural polyreactive immunoglobulin A antibodies produced in mouse Peyer's patches. Immunology 1999; 97:9-17.

148. Donze HH, Lue C, Julian BA et al. Human peritoneal B-1 cells and the influence of continuous ambulatory peritoneal dialysis on peritoneal and peripheral blood mononuclear cell (PBMC) composition and immunoglobulin levels. Clin Exp Immunol 1997; 109:356-361.
149. Bhat NM, Kantor AB, Bieber MM et al. The ontogeny and functional characteristics of human B-1 (CD5+ B) cells. Int Immunol 1992; 4:243-252.
150. Farstad IN, Carlsen H, Morton HC et al. Immunoglobulin A cell distribution in the human small intestine: phenotypic and functional characteristics. Immunology 2000; 101:354-363.
151. Quan CP, Berneman A, Pires R et al. Natural polyreactive secretory immunoglobulin A autoantibodies as a possible barrier to infection in humans. Infect Immun 1997; 65:3997-4004.
152. McGhee JR, Mestecky J, Dertzbaugh MT et al. The mucosal immune system: From fundamental concepts to vaccine development. Vaccine 1992; 10:75-88.
153. Mestecky J, Bienenstock J, McGhee JR et al. Historical aspects of mucosal immunology. In: Ogra PL et al, eds. Mucosal Immunology. Academic Press, 1999:xxiii-xliii.
154. Winner L, Mack J et al. New model for analysis of mucosal immunity: Intestinal secretion of specific monoclonal immunoglobulin A from hybridoma tumors protects against Vibrio cholerae infection. Infect Immun 1991; 59:977-982.
155. Macpherson AJ, Hunziker L, McCoy K et al. IgA responses in the intestinal mucosa against pathogenic and non-pathogenic microorganisms. Microbes Infect 2001; 3:1021-1035.
156. Williams RC, Gibbons RJ. Inhibition of bacterial adherence by secretory immunoglobulin A: A mechanism of antigen disposal. Science 1972; 177:697-699.
157. Reinholdt J, Kilian M. Interference of IgA protease with the effect of secretory IgA on adherence of oral streptococci to saliva-coated hydroxyapatite. J Dent Res 1987; 66:492-497.
158. Hajishengallis G, Nikolova E, Russell MW. Inhibition of Streptococcus mutans adherence to saliva-coated hydroxyapatite by human secretory immunoglobulin A (S-IgA) antibodies to cell surface protein antigen I/II: Reversal by IgA1 protease cleavage. Infect Immun 1992; 60:5057-5064.
159. Liljemark WF, Bloomquist CG, Germaine GR. Effect of bacterial aggregation on the adherence of oral streptococci to hydroxyapatite. Infect Immun 1981; 31:935-941.
160. Edebo L, Lindstrom F, Skoldstom L et al. On the physical-chemical effect of colostral antibody binding to Escherichia coli O 86. Immunol Commun 1975; 4:587-601.
161. Lindh E. Increased risistance of immunoglobulin A dimers to proteolytic degradation after binding of secretory component. J Immunol 1975; 114:284-286.
162. Crottet P, Corthesy B. Secretory component delays the conversion of secretory IgA into antigen-binding competent F(ab')2: A possible implication for mucosal defense. J Immunol 1998; 161:5445-5453.
163. Bronson RA, Cooper GW, Rosenfeld DL et al. The effect of an IgA1 protease on immunoglobulins bound to the sperm surface and sperm cervical mucus penetrating ability. Fertil Steril 1987; 47:985-991.
164. Phalipon A, Cardona A, Kraehenbuhl JP et al. Secretory component: A new role in secretory IgA-mediated immune exclusion in vivo. Immunity 2002; 17:107-115.
165. Biesbrock AR, Reddy MS, Levine MJ. Interaction of a salivary mucin-secretory immunoglobulin A complex with mucosal pathogens. Infect Immun 1991; 59:3492-3497.
166. Hirano M, Kamada M, Maegawa M et al. Binding of human secretory leukocyte protease inhibitor in uterine cervical mucus to immunoglobulins: Pathophysiology in immunologic infertility and local immune defense. Fertil Steril 1999; 71:1108-1114.
167. Walker WA, Isselbacher KJ, Bloch KJ. Intestinal uptake of macromolecules: Effect of oral immunization. Science 1972; 177:608-610.
168. Stokes CR, Soothill JF, Turner MW. Immune exclusion is a function of IgA. Nature 1975; 255:745-746.
169. Tolo K, Brandtzaeg P, Jonsen J. Mucosal penetration of antigen in the presence or absence of serum-derived antibody. Immunology 1977; 33:733-743.
170. Lim PL, Rowley D. The effect of antibody on the intestinal absorption of macromolecules and on intestinal permeability in adult mice. Int Arch Allergy Appl Immunol 1982; 68:41-46.
171. Johansen FE, Pekna M, Norderhaug IN et al. Absence of epithelial immunoglobulin A transport, with increased mucosal leakiness, in polymeric immunoglobulin receptor/secretory component-deficient mice. J Exp Med 1999; 190:915-922.

172. Stokes CR, Taylor B, Turner MW. Association of house-dust and grass-pollen allergies with specific IgA antibody deficiency. Lancet 1974; 2:485-488.

173. Platts-Mills TA, von Maur RK, Ishizaka K et al. IgA and IgG anti-ragweed antibodies in nasal secretions. Quantitative measurements of antibodies and correlation with inhibition of histamine release. J Clin Invest 1976; 57:1041-1050.

174. Reed CE, Bubak M, Dunnette S et al. Ragweed-specific IgA in nasal lavage fluid of ragweed-sensitive allergic rhinitis patients: Increase during the pollen season. Int Arch Allergy Appl Immunol 1991; 94:275-277.

175. Peebles RS, Jr., Hamilton RG, Lichtenstein LM et al. Antigen-specific IgE and IgA antibodies in bronchoalveolar lavage fluid are associated with stronger antigen-induced late phase reactions. Clin Exp Allergy 2001; 31:239-248.

176. Benson M, Svensson PA, Carlsson B et al. DNA microarrays to study gene expression in allergic airways. Clin Exp Allergy 2002; 32:301-308.

177. Campbell AM, Vignola AM, Chanez P et al. Low-affinity receptor for IgE on human bronchial epithelial cells in asthma. Immunology 1994; 82:506-508.

178. Campbell AM, Vachier I, Chanez P et al. Expression of the high-affinity receptor for IgE on bronchial epithelial cells of asthmatics. Am J Respir Cell Mol Biol 1998; 19:92-97.

179. Yang PC, Berin MC, Perdue MH. Enhanced antigen transport across rat tracheal epithelium induced by sensitization and mast cell activation. J Immunol 1999; 163:2769-2776.

180. Silvey KJ, Hutchings AB, Vajdy M et al. Role of immunoglobulin A in protection against reovirus entry into Murine Peyer's patches. J Virol 2001; 75:10870-10879.

181. Weltzin R, Lucia-Jandris P, Michetti P et al. Binding and transepithelial transport of immunoglobulins by intestinal M cells: demonstration using monoclonal IgA antibodies against enteric viral proteins. J Cell Biol 1989; 108:1673-1685.

182. Mantis NJ, Cheung MC, Chintalacharuvu KR et al. Selective adherence of IgA to murine Peyer's patch M cells: Evidence for a novel IgA receptor. J Immunol 2002; 169:1844-1851.

183. Geissmann F, Launay P, Pasquier B et al. A subset of human dendritic cells expresses IgA Fc receptor (CD89), which mediates internalization and activation upon cross-linking by IgA complexes. J Immunol 2001; 166:346-352.

184. Heystek HC, Moulon C, Woltman AM et al. Human immature dendritic cells efficiently bind and take up secretory IgA without the induction of maturation. J Immunol 2002; 168:102-107.

185. Arulanandam BP, Raeder RH, Nedrud JG et al. IgA immunodeficiency leads to inadequate Th cell priming and increased susceptibility to influenza virus infection. J Immunol 2001; 166:226-231.

186. Kaetzel CS, Robinson JK, Chintalacharuvu KR et al. The polymeric immunoglobulin receptor (secretory component) mediates transport of immune complexes across epithelial cells: A local defense function for IgA. Proc Natl Acad Sci USA 1991; 88:8796-8800.

187. Brown TA, Russell MW, Mestecky J. Hepatobiliary transport of IgA immune complexes: Molecular and cellular aspects. J Immunol 1982; 128:2183-2186.

188. Robinson JK, Blanchard TG, Levine AD et al. A mucosal IgA-mediated excretory immune system in vivo. J Immunol 2001; 166:3688-3692.

189. Mazanec MB, Kaetzel CS, Lamm ME et al. Intracellular neutralization of virus by immunoglobulin A antibodies. Proc Natl Acad Sci USA 1992; 89:6901-6905.

190. Mazanec MB, Nedrud JG, Kaetzel CS et al. A three-tiered view of the role of IgA in mucosal defense. Immunol Today 1993; 14:430-435.

191. Duncan AR, Winter G. The binding site for C1q on IgG. Nature 1988; 332:738-740.

192. Griffiss JM. Bactericidal activity of meningococcal antisera. Blocking by IgA of lytic antibody in human convalescent sera. J Immunol 1975; 114:1779-1784.

193. Russell MW, Reinholdt J, Kilian M. Anti-inflammatory activity of human IgA antibodies and their Fab alpha fragments: inhibition of IgG-mediated complement activation. Eur J Immunol 1989; 19:2243-2249.

194. Nikolova EB, Tomana M, Russell MW. All forms of human IgA antibodies bound to antigen interfere with complement (C3) fixation induced by IgG or by antigen alone. Scand J Immunol 1994; 39:275-280.

195. Nikolova EB, Tomana M, Russell MW. The role of the carbohydrate chains in complement (C3) fixation by solid-phase-bound human IgA. Immunology 1994; 82:321-327.

196. Janoff EN, Fasching C, Orenstein JM et al. Killing of Streptococcus pneumoniae by capsular polysaccharide-specific polymeric IgA, complement, and phagocytes. J Clin Invest 1999; 104:1139-1147.

197. Roos A, Bouwman LH, Gijlswijk-Janssen DJ et al. Human IgA activates the complement system via the mannan-binding lectin pathway. J Immunol 2001; 167:2861-2868.

198. Fanger MW, Goldstine SN, Shen L. Cytofluorographic analysis of receptors for IgA on human polymorphonuclear cells and monocytes and the correlation of receptor expression with phagocytosis. Mol Immunol 1983; 20:1019-1027.

199. Ito S, Mikawa H, Shinomiya K et al. Suppressive effect of IgA soluble immune complexes on neutrophil chemotaxis. Clin Exp Immunol 1979; 37:436-440

200. Kemp AS, Cripps AW, Brown S. Suppression of leucocyte chemokinesis and chemotaxis by human IgA. Clin Exp Immunol 1980; 40:388-395.

201. van Epps DE, Brown SL. Inhibition of formylmethionyl-leucyl-phenylalanine-stimulated neutrophil chemiluminescence by human immunoglobulin A paraproteins. Infect Immun 1981; 34:864-870.

202. Wolf HM, Fischer MB, Puhringer H et al. Human serum IgA downregulates the release of inflammatory cytokines (tumor necrosis factor-alpha, interleukin-6) in human monocytes. Blood 1994; 83:1278-1288.

203. Monteiro RC, Kubagawa H, Cooper MD. Cellular distribution, regulation, and biochemical nature of an Fc alpha receptor in humans. J Exp Med 1990; 171:597-613.

204. Morton HC, van Egmond M, van de Winkel JG. Structure and function of human IgA Fc receptors (Fc alpha R). Crit Rev Immunol 1996; 16:423-440.

205. Weisbart RH, Kacena A, Schuh A et al. GM-CSF induces human neutrophil IgA-mediated phagocytosis by an IgA Fc receptor activation mechanism. Nature 1988; 332:647-648.

206. Hostoffer RW, Krukovets I, Berger M. Enhancement by tumor necrosis factor-alpha of Fc alpha receptor expression and IgA-mediated superoxide generation and killing of Pseudomonas aeruginosa by polymorphonuclear leukocytes. J Infect Dis 1994; 170:82-87.

207. Nikolova EB, Russell MW. Dual function of human IgA antibodies: Inhibition of phagocytosis in circulating neutrophils and enhancement of responses in IL-8-stimulated cells. J Leukoc Biol 1995; 57:875-882.

208. Abu-Ghazaleh RI, Fujisawa T, Mestecky J et al. IgA-induced eosinophil degranulation. J Immunol 1989; 142:2393-2400.

209. Lamkhioued B, Gounni AS, Gruart V et al. Human eosinophils express a receptor for secretory component. Role in secretory IgA-dependent activation. Eur J Immunol 1995; 25:117-125.

210. Motegi Y, Kita H. Interaction with secretory component stimulates effector functions of human eosinophils but not of neutrophils. J Immunol 1998; 161:4340-4346.

211. Ishizaka K, Ishizaka T. Blocking of Prausnitz-Kustner sensitization with reagin by normal human β2A globulin. J Allergy 1963; 34:395-403.

212. Taylor B, Norman AP, Orgel HA et al. Transient IgA deficiency and pathogenesis of infantile atopy. Lancet 1973; 2:111-113.

213. Plebani A, Monafo V, Ugazio AG et al. Comparison of the frequency of atopic diseases in children with severe and partial IgA deficiency. Int Arch Allergy Appl Immunol 1987; 82:485-486.

214. Hanson LA, Bjorkander J, Carlsson B et al. The heterogeneity of IgA deficiency. J Clin Immunol 1988; 8:159-162.

215. Strober W, Sneller MC. IgA deficiency. Ann Allergy 1991; 66:363-375.

216. Steinman RM, Nussenzweig MC. Avoiding horror autotoxicus: the importance of dendritic cells in peripheral T cell tolerance. Proc Natl Acad Sci USA 2002; 99:351-358.

217. Weiner HL. Oral tolerance: Immune mechanisms and the generation of Th3-type TGF-beta-secreting regulatory cells. Microbes Infect 2001; 3:947-954.

218. Kagnoff MF. Oral tolerance: Mechanisms and possible role in inflammatory joint diseases. Baillieres Clin Rheumatol 1996; 10:41-54.

219. Sun J, Dirden-Kramer B, Ito K et al. Antigen-specific T cell activation and proliferation during oral tolerance induction. J Immunol 1999; 162:5868-5875.

220. Meyer AL, Benson J, Song F et al. Rapid depletion of peripheral antigen-specific T cells in TCR-transgenic mice after oral administration of myelin basic protein. J Immunol 2001; 166:5773-5781.

221. Viney JL, Mowat AM, O'Malley JM et al. Expanding dendritic cells in vivo enhances the induction of oral tolerance. J Immunol 1998; 160:5815-5825.
222. Holt PG, Stumbles PA, McWilliam AS. Functional studies on dendritic cells in the respiratory tract and related mucosal tissues. J Leukoc Biol 1999; 66:272-275.
223. Akbari O, DeKruyff RH, Umetsu DT. Pulmonary dendritic cells producing IL-10 mediate tolerance induced by respiratory exposure to antigen. Nat Immunol 2001; 2:725-731.
224. Brandtzaeg P. Nature and function of gastrointestinal antigen-presenting cells. Allergy 2001; 56 Suppl 67:16-20.
225. Iwasaki A, Kelsall BL. Unique functions of CD11b+, CD8 alpha+, and double-negative Peyer's patch dendritic cells. J Immunol 2001; 166:4884-4890.
226. Jonuleit H, Schmitt E, Steinbrink K et al. Dendritic cells as a tool to induce anergic and regulatory T cells. Trends Immunol 2001; 22:394-400.
227. Weiner HL. The mucosal milieu creates tolerogenic dendritic cells and T(R)1 and T(H)3 regulatory cells. Nat Immunol 2001; 2:671-672.
228. Bilsborough J, Viney JL. Getting to the guts of immune regulation. Immunology 2002; 106:139-143.
229. Janeway CA Jr, Medzhitov R. Innate immune recognition. Annu Rev Immunol 2002; 20:197-216.
230. Moreau MC, Corthier G. Effect of the gastrointestinal microflora on induction and maintenance of oral tolerance to ovalbumin in C3H/HeJ mice. Infect Immun 1988; 56:2766-2768.
231. Gaboriau-Routhiau V, Moreau MC. Gut flora allows recovery of oral tolerance to ovalbumin in mice after transient breakdown mediated by cholera toxin or Escherichia coli heat-labile enterotoxin. Pediatr Res 1996; 39:625-629.
232. Wannemuehler MJ, Kiyono H, Babb JL et al. Lipopolysaccharide (LPS) regulation of the immune response: LPS converts germfree mice to sensitivity to oral tolerance induction. J Immunol 1982; 129:959-965.
233. Michalek SM, Kiyono H, Wannemuehler MJ et al. Lipopolysaccharide (LPS) regulation of the immune response: LPS influence on oral tolerance induction. J Immunol 1982; 128:1992-1998.
234. Titus RG, Chiller JM. Orally induced tolerance. Definition at the cellular level. Int Arch Allergy Appl Immunol 1981; 65:323-338.
235. Mowat AM, Thomas MJ, MacKenzie S et al. Divergent effects of bacterial lipopolysaccharide on immunity to orally administered protein and particulate antigens in mice. Immunology 1986; 58:677-683.
236. Sudo N, Sawamura S, Tanaka K et al. The requirement of intestinal bacterial flora for the development of an IgE production system fully susceptible to oral tolerance induction. J Immunol 1997; 159:1739-1745.
237. Kirjavainen PV, Arvola T, Salminen SJ et al. Aberrant composition of gut microbiota of allergic infants: a target of bifidobacterial therapy at weaning? Gut 2002; 51:51-55.
238. Duchmann R, Kaiser I, Hermann E et al. Meyer zum Buschenfelde KH. Tolerance exists towards resident intestinal flora but is broken in active inflammatory bowel disease (IBD). Clin Exp Immunol 1995; 102:448-455.
239. Khoo UY, Proctor IE, Macpherson AJ. CD4+ T cell down-regulation in human intestinal mucosa: evidence for intestinal tolerance to luminal bacterial antigens. J Immunol 1997; 158:3626-3634.
240. Elson CO, Cong Y. Understanding immune-microbial homeostasis in intestine. Immunol Res 2002; 26:87-94.
241. MacDonald TT. Breakdown of tolerance to the intestinal bacterial flora in inflammatory bowel disease (IBD). Clin Exp Immunol 1995; 102:445-447.
242. Shi HN, Ingui CJ, Dodge I et al. A helminth-induced mucosal Th2 response alters nonresponsiveness to oral administration of a soluble antigen. J Immunol 1998; 160:2449-2455.
243. Schwarze J, Gelfand EW. Respiratory viral infections as promoters of allergic sensitization and asthma in animal models. Eur Respir J 2002; 19:341-349.
244. Elson CO, Ealding W. Cholera toxin feeding did not induce oral tolerance in mice and abrogated oral tolerance to an unrelated protein antigen. J Immunol 1984; 133:2892-2897.
245. Rescigno M, Rotta G, Valzasina B et al. Dendritic cells shuttle microbes across gut epithelial monolayers. Immunobiology 2001; 204:572-581.
246. Nagata S, McKenzie C, Pender SL et al. Human Peyer's patch T cells are sensitized to dietary antigen and display a Th cell type 1 cytokine profile. J Immunol 2000; 165:5315-5321.

247. Friedman A, Weiner HL. Induction of anergy or active suppression following oral tolerance is determined by antigen dosage. Proc Natl Acad Sci USA 1994; 91:6688-6692.

248. Whitacre CC, Gienapp IE, Orosz CG et al. Oral tolerance in experimental autoimmune encephalomyelitis. III. Evidence for clonal anergy. J Immunol 1991; 147:2155-2163.

249. Melamed D, Friedman A. Direct evidence for anergy in T lymphocytes tolerized by oral administration of ovalbumin. Eur J Immunol 1993; 23:935-942.

250. Schwartz RH. Models of T cell anergy: Is there a common molecular mechanism? J Exp Med 1996; 184:1-8.

251. Challacombe SJ, Tomasi TB, Jr. Systemic tolerance and secretory immunity after oral immunization. J Exp Med 1980; 152:1459-1472.

252. Melamed D, Friedman A. Modification of the immune response by oral tolerance: Antigen requirements and interaction with immunogenic stimuli. Cell Immunol 1993; 146:412-420.

253. Zivny JH, Moldoveanu Z, Vu HL et al. Mechanisms of immune tolerance to food antigens in humans. ClinImmunol 2001; 101:158-168.

254. Richman LK, Chiller JM, Brown WR et al. Enterically induced immunologic tolerance. I. Induction of suppressor T lymphoyctes by intragastric administration of soluble proteins. J Immunol 1978; 121:2429-2434.

255. Miller SD, Hanson DG. Inhibition of specific immune responses by feeding protein antigens. IV. Evidence for tolerance and specific active suppression of cell-mediated immune responses to ovalbumin. J Immunol 1979; 123:2344-2350.

256. MacDonald TT. Immunosuppression caused by antigen feeding. I. Evidence for the activation of a feedback suppressor pathway in the spleens of antigen-fed mice. Eur J Immunol 1982; 12:767-773.

257. Lider O, Santos LM, Lee CS et al. Suppression of experimental autoimmune encephalomyelitis by oral administration of myelin basic protein. II. Suppression of disease and in vitro immune responses is mediated by antigen-specific CD8+ T lymphocytes. J Immunol 1989; 142:748-752.

258. Miller A, Lider O, Roberts AB et al. Suppressor T cells generated by oral tolerization to myelin basic protein suppress both in vitro and in vivo immune responses by the release of transforming growth factor beta after antigen-specific triggering. Proc Natl Acad Sci USA 1992; 89:421-425.

259. Miller A, Lider O, Weiner HL. Antigen-driven bystander suppression after oral administration of antigens. J Exp Med 1991; 174:791-798.

260. Miller A, al Sabbagh A, Santos LM et al. Epitopes of myelin basic protein that trigger TGF-beta release after oral tolerization are distinct from encephalitogenic epitopes and mediate epitope-driven bystander suppression. J Immunol 1993; 151:7307-7315.

261. Weiner HL. Oral tolerance: Immune mechanisms and treatment of autoimmune diseases. Immunol Today 1997; 18:335-343.

262. Mowat AM, Weiner HL. Oral tolerance, physiological basis and clinical applications. In: Ogra et al, eds. Mucosal Immunology. Academic Press, 1999:587-618.

263. Groux H, O'Garra A, Bigler M et al. A CD4+ T-cell subset inhibits antigen-specific T-cell responses and prevents colitis. Nature 1997; 389:737-742.

264. MacDonald TT. Effector and regulatory lymphoid cells and cytokines in mucosal sites. Curr Top Microbiol Immunol 1999; 236:113-135.

265. Singh B, Read S, Asseman C et al. Control of intestinal inflammation by regulatory T cells. Immunol Rev 2001; 182:190-200.

266. McMenamin C, Pimm C, McKersey M et al. Regulation of IgE responses to inhaled antigen in mice by antigen-specific gamma delta T cells. Science 1994; 265:1869-1871.

267. Yamamoto M, Kiyono H. Immunoregulatory functions of mucosal gammadelta T cells. Microbes Infect 1999; 1:241-246.

268. Yamanaka T, Helgeland L, Farstad IN et al. Microbial colonization drives lymphocyte accumulation and differentiation in the follicle-associated epithelium of Peyer's patches. J Immunol 2003; 170:816-822.

269. Eynon EE, Parker DC. Small B cells as antigen-presenting cells in the induction of tolerance to soluble protein antigens. J Exp Med 1992; 175:131-138.

270. Fuchs EJ, Matzinger P. B cells turn off virgin but not memory T cells. Science 1992; 258:1156-1159.

271. Vella AT, Scherer MT, Schultz L et al. B cells are not essential for peripheral T-cell tolerance. Proc Natl Acad Sci USA 1996; 93:951-955.

272. Hashimoto A, Yamada H, Matsuzaki G et al. Successful priming and tolerization of T cells to orally administered antigens in B-cell-deficient mice. Cell Immunol 2001; 207:36-40.
273. Gonnella PA, Waldner HP, Weiner HL. B cell-deficient (mu MT) mice have alterations in the cytokine microenvironment of the gut-associated lymphoid tissue (GALT) and a defect in the low dose mechanism of oral tolerance. J Immunol 2001; 166:4456-4464.
274. Fujihashi K, Dohi T, Rennert PD et al. Peyer's patches are required for oral tolerance to proteins. Proc Natl Acad Sci USA 2001; 98:3310-3315.
275. Spahn TW, Fontana A, Faria AM et al. Induction of oral tolerance to cellular immune responses in the absence of Peyer's patches. Eur J Immunol 2001; 31:1278-1287.
276. Spahn TW, Weiner HL, Rennert PD et al. Mesenteric lymph nodes are critical for the induction of high-dose oral tolerance in the absence of Peyer's patches. Eur J Immunol 2002; 32:1109-1113.
277. Andre C, Heremans JF, Vaerman JP et al. A mechanism for the induction of immunological tolerance by antigen feeding: Antigen-antibody complexes. J Exp Med 1975; 142:1509-1519.
278. Kagnoff MF. Effects of antigen-feeding on intestinal and systemic immune responses. III. Antigen-specific serum-mediated suppression of humoral antibody responses after antigen feeding. Cell Immunol 1978; 40:186-203.
279. Kagnoff MF. Effects of antigen-feeding on intestinal and systemic immune responses. II. Suppression of delayed-type hypersensitivity reactions. J Immunol 1978; 120:1509-1513.
280. Kagnoff MF. Effects of antigen-feeding on intestinal and systemic immune responses. IV. Similarity between the suppressor factor in mice after erythrocyte-lysate injection and erythrocyte feeding. Gastroenterology 1980; 79:54-61.
281. Karlsson MR, Kahu H, Hanson LA et al. An established immune response against ovalbumin is suppressed by a transferable serum factor produced after ovalbumin feeding: A role of CD25+ regulatory cells. Scand J Immunol 2002; 55:470-477.
282. Hanson DG, Vaz NM, Maia LC et al. Inhibition of specific immune responses by feeding protein antigens. III. Evidence against maintenance of tolerance to ovalbumin by orally induced antibodies. J Immunol 1979; 123:2337-2343.
283. Jarrett EE, Hall E. The development of IgE-suppressive immunocompetence in young animals: Influence of exposure to antigen in the presence or absence of maternal immunity. Immunology 1984; 53:365-373.
284. Falth-Magnusson K, Kjellman NI, Magnusson KE. Antibodies IgG, IgA, and IgM to food antigens during the first 18 months of life in relation to feeding and development of atopic disease. J Allergy Clin Immunol 1988; 81:743-749.
285. Ogra SS, Weintraub D, Ogra PL. Immunologic aspects of human colostrum and milk. III. Fate and absorption of cellular and soluble components in the gastrointestinal tract of the newborn. J Immunol 1977; 119:245-248.
286. Jarvinen KM, Laine ST, Jarvenpaa AL et al. Does low IgA in human milk predispose the infant to development of cow's milk allergy? Pediatr Res 2000; 48:457-462.
287. Machtinger S, Moss R. Cow's milk allergy in breast-fed infants: The role of allergen and maternal secretory IgA antibody. J Allergy Clin Immunol 1986; 77:341-347.
288. Duchen K, Casas R, Fageras-Bottcher M et al. Human milk polyunsaturated long-chain fatty acids and secretory immunoglobulin A antibodies and early childhood allergy. Pediatr Allergy Immunol 2000; 11:29-39.
289. Saarinen KM, Vaarala O, Klemetti P et al. Transforming growth factor-beta1 in mothers' colostrum and immune responses to cows' milk proteins in infants with cows' milk allergy. J Allergy Clin Immunol 1999; 104:1093-1098.
290. Sly PD, Holt PG. Breast is best for preventing asthma and allergies—Or is it? Lancet 2002; 360:887-888.
291. Sorensen CH, Kilian M. Bacterium-induced cleavage of IgA in nasopharyngeal secretions from atopic children. Acta Pathol Microbiol Immunol Scand [C] 1984; 92:85-87.
292. Kilian M, Husby S, Host A et al. Increased proportions of bacteria capable of cleaving IgA1 in the pharynx of infants with atopic disease. Pediatr Res 1995; 38:182-186.
293. Heppell LM, Kilshaw PJ. Immune responses in guinea pigs to dietary protein. I. Induction of tolerance by feeding with ovalbumin. Int Arch Allergy Appl Immunol 1982; 68:54-59.

294. Mowat AM, Strobel S, Drummond HE et al. Immunological responses to fed protein antigens in mice. I. Reversal of oral tolerance to ovalbumin by cyclophosphamide. Immunology 1982; 45:105-113.

295. Melamed D, Friedman A. In vivo tolerization of Th1 lymphocytes following a single feeding with ovalbumin: Anergy in the absence of suppression. Eur J Immunol 1994; 24:1974-1981.

296. Vives J, Parks DE, Weigle WO. Immunologic unresponsiveness after gastric administration of human gamma-globulin: Antigen requirements and cellular parameters. J Immunol 1980; 125:1811-1816.

297. Husby S, Mestecky J, Moldoveanu Z et al. Oral tolerance in humans. T cell but not B cell tolerance after antigen feeding. J Immunol 1994; 152:4663-4670.

298. Waldo FB, van den Wall Bake AW, Mestecky J et al. Suppression of the immune response by nasal immunization. Clin Immunol Immunopathol 1994; 72:30-34.

299. MacDonald TT. Immunosuppression caused by antigen feeding II. Suppressor T cells mask Peyer's patch B cell priming to orally administered antigen. Eur J Immunol 1983; 13:138-142.

300. Sugita-Konishi Y, Smart CJ, Trejdosiewicz LK. Regulation of intestinal immunoglobulin production in response to dietary ovalbumin. Int Arch Allergy Immunol 1992; 98:64-69.

301. Stok W, Van der Heijden PJ, Bianchi AT. Conversion of orally induced suppression of the mucosal immune response to ovalbumin into stimulation by conjugating ovalbumin to cholera toxin or its B subunit. Vaccine 1994; 12:521-526.

302. Elson CO, Holland SP, Dertzbaugh MT et al. Morphologic and functional alterations of mucosal T cells by cholera toxin and its B subunit. J Immunol 1995; 154:1032-1040.

303. Grdic D, Hornquist E, Kjerrulf M et al. Lack of local suppression in orally tolerant CD8-deficient mice reveals a critical regulatory role of CD8+ T cells in the normal gut mucosa. J Immunol 1998; 160:754-762.

304. Kato H, Fujihashi K, Kato R et al. Oral tolerance revisited: Prior oral tolerization abrogates cholera toxin-induced mucosal IgA responses. J Immunol 2001; 166:3114-3121.

305. Russell MW, Prince SJ, Lidthart GJ et al. Comparison of salivary and serum antibodies to common environmental antigens in elderly, edentulous, and normal adult subjects. AGING: Immunology and infectious disease 1990; 2:275-286.

306. Rumbo M, Chirdo FG, Anon MC et al. Detection and characterization of antibodies specific to food antigens (gliadin, ovalbumin and beta-lactoglobulin) in human serum, saliva, colostrum and milk. Clin Exp Immunol 1998; 112:453-458.

307. Ernst PB, Lee ST, Maeba J et al. A role for isotype-specific binding factors in the regulation of IgA- and IgG-specific responses by the anti/contrasuppressor T cell circuit. J Immunol 1989; 143:1426-1432.

308. Fujihashi K, Taguchi T, Aicher WK et al. Immunoregulatory functions for murine intraepithelial lymphocytes: Gamma/delta T cell receptor-positive (TCR+) T cells abrogate oral tolerance, while alpha/beta TCR+ T cells provide B cell help. J Exp Med 1992; 175:695-707.

309. Iijima H, Takahashi I, Kiyono H. Mucosal immune network in the gut for the control of infectious diseases. Rev Med Virol 2001; 11:117-133

310. Kilian M, Roland K, Mestecky J. Interference of secretory immunoglobulin A with sorption of oral bacteria to hydroxyapatite. Infect Immun 1981; 31:942-951.

311. Ogra PL et al. Mucosal Immunology. Academic Press, 1999:43-64.

312. Pruitt KM, Rahemtulla B, Rahemtulla F et al. Innate humoral factors. In: Ogra PL et al, eds. Mucosal Immunology. Academic Press, 1999:65-88.

313. Brandtzaeg P, Fjellanger I, Gjeruldsen ST. Adsorption of immunolgobulin A onto oral bacteria in vivo. J Bacteriol 1968; 96:242-249.

314. van der Waaij LA, Limburg PC, Mesander G et al. In vivo IgA coating of anaerobic bacteria in human faeces. Gut 1996; 38:348-354.

315. Kilian M, Reinholdt J. A hypothetical model for the development of invasive infection due to IgA1 protease-producing bacteria. Adv Exp Med Biol 1987; 216B:1261-1269.

316. Binscheck T, Bartels F, Bergel H et al. IgA protease from Neisseria gonorrhoeae inhibits exocytosis in bovine chromaffin cells like tetanus toxin. J Biol Chem 1995; 270:1770-1774.

317. Hauck CR, .Meyer TF. The lysosomal/phagosomal membrane protein h-lamp-1 is a target of the IgA1 protease of Neisseria gonorrhoeae. FEBS Lett 1997; 405:86-90.

318. Beck SC, Meyer TF. IgA1 protease from Neisseria gonorrhoeae inhibits TNFalpha-mediated apoptosis of human monocytic cells. FEBS Lett 2000; 472:287-292.
319. Firer MA, Hosking CS, Hill DJ. Cow's milk allergy and eczema: patterns of the antibody response to cow's milk in allergic skin disease. Clin Allergy 1982; 12:385-390.
320. Husby S, Oxelius VA, Teisner B et al. Humoral immunity to dietary antigens in healthy adults. Occurrence, isotype and IgG subclass distribution of serum antibodies to protein antigens. Int Arch Allergy Appl Immunol 1985; 77:416-422.
321. Rothberg RM, Farr RS. Antibodies in rabbits fed milk and their similarities to antibodies in some human sera. J Allergy 1965; 36:450-462.
322. Scott H, Rognum TO, Midtvedt T et al. Age-related changes of human serum antibodies to dietary and colonic bacterial antigens measured by an enzyme-linked immunosorbent assay. Acta Pathol Microbiol Immunol Scand [C] 1985; 93:65-70.
323. Barnes RM. IgG and IgA antibodies to dietary antigens in food allergy and intolerance. Clin Exp Allergy 1995; 25 Suppl 1:7-9.
324. Unsworth DJ, Walker-Smith JA, Holborow EJ. Gliadin and reticulin antibodies in childhood coeliac disease. Lancet 1983; 1:874-875.
325. Kemp M, Husby S, Larsen ML et al. ELISA analysis of IgA subclass antibodies to dietary antigens. Elevated IgA1 antibodies in children with coeliac disease. Int Arch Allergy Appl Immunol 1988; 87:247-253.
326. Hvatum M, Scott H, Brandtzaeg P. Serum IgG subclass antibodies to a variety of food antigens in patients with coeliac disease. Gut 1992; 33:632-638.

CHAPTER 7

Induction of Tolerogenic versus Pathogenic Mucosal Immune Responses by Commensal Enteric Bacteria

Dirk Haller and R. Balfour Sartor

Introduction

Inflammatory bowel diseases (IBD) including ulcerative colitis (UC) and Crohn's disease (CD) are spontaneously relapsing, immunologically-mediated disorders of the gastrointestinal tract. Microbial agents are intimately involved in each of the four major current etiologic theories of these idiopathic disorders (Table 1). Rapidly evolving studies in experimental rodent models of chronic, immune-mediated intestinal inflammation illustrate the critical importance of host genetic susceptibility in determining the aggressiveness and chronicity of inflammation. A characteristic feature of the mucosal immune system in the normal host is that protective cell-mediated and humoral immune responses against invading pathogens are allowed to proceed while pathogenic responses to ubiquitous bacterial antigens of the indigenous intestinal microflora are prevented. Under normal circumstances detrimental inflammatory responses to phlogistic luminal contents are prevented by several mechanisms including exclusion of bacterial antigens or macromolecules by a viscous mucus layer, an intact epithelial barrier, secreted antibodies, regulatory T lymphocytes which mediate tolerance, immunosuppressive mediators, as well as intestinal epithelial cells and lamina propria macrophages which are relatively refractory to luminal stimulants. Episodic breaks in the mucosal barrier due to transient infections or luminal toxins occur frequently, challenging the mucosal immune system with bacterial components. Homeostasis (tolerance) versus chronic intestinal inflammation is determined by either a regulated or an uncontrolled response of the host, respectively, to the constant antigenic drive of its resident flora. These responses are genetically determined. In genetically susceptible hosts, the lack of appropriate mechanisms to downregulate mucosal immune responses (loss of immunologic tolerance) and an ineffective mucosal barrier function results in continuous stimulation of the mucosal immune system with chronic inflammation as a the consequence. In this Chapter, we will discuss immunological and bacterial mechanisms which mediate tolerance and inflammation in response to resident enteric bacteria in experimental animals, with selected clinical examples documenting relevance to IBD.

Oral Tolerance: The Response of the Intestinal Mucosa to Dietary Antigens,
edited by Olivier Morteau. ©2004 Eurekah.com and Kluwer Academic / Plenum Publishers.

Table 1. Current etiologic theories of inflammatory bowel disease

1. Persistent infection with a pathogen
   Crohn's disease: Mycobacterium tuberculosis, Listeria monocytogenes
                      paramyxovirus (measles)
   Ulcerative colitis: Pathogenic E.coli
2. Microbial dysbiosis: subtle alterations in bacterial function and composition
3. Deranged mucosal barrier: defective mucus, tight junctions, epithelial restitution
4. Defective regulation of mucosal immune response: deficient downregulation, overly
   aggressive induction (dysregulation of antigen presentation, Th1 lymphocyte activation,
   or cytokine and soluble mediator production)

Dysregulated Immune Responses to Resident Enteric Bacteria Induce Chronic Intestinal Inflammation: Lessons from Genetically Engineered Animal Models

In at least 11 separate animal models with induced, spontaneous or genetically engineered disease, chronic intestinal inflammation is initiated and perpetuated in the presence of resident enteric bacteria, whereas germ-free (sterile) conditions prevent or dramatically attenuate the development of disease (Table 2). The proposed mechanisms which lead to an overly aggressive cellular immune response to normal bacteria and the development of experimental colitis in mutant animals include overexpression of proinflammatory mediators,[1] activation of effector T lymphocyte subsets (Th1 or Th2),[2] deficient protective molecules,[3-5] abnormal antigen presentation, aberrant thymic education,[6,7] an imbalance of regulatory T lymphocytes[8] and abnormal signal transduction of regulatory molecules.[9]

The microbial milieu of genetically engineered animals plays an important role in determining their disease. For example, interleukin-10 deficient (IL-10$^{-/-}$) mice raised under conventional conditions develop discontinuous transmural lesions, similar to patients with Crohn's disease and have lethal small intestinal and colonic inflammation.[4] Other pathological changes include epithelial hyperplasia, mucin depletion, crypt abscesses, ulcers and thickening of the bowel wall.[2] In contrast to conventional housing, disease is limited to the colon in specific pathogen free (SPF) IL-10$^{-/-}$ mice. These mice exhibit nonlethal colitis confined to the mucosa, and develop colonic adenocarcinomas during late stages of colitis, but have no small intestinal inflammation. In contrast, IL-10$^{-/-}$ mice raised in a sterile environment have no evidence of clinical disease, histological intestinal inflammation nor immune activation. Colitis and Th1-dominated mucosal immune responses are evident as early as 1 week after colonization of germ-free IL-10$^{-/-}$ mice with SPF colonic bacteria free of *Helicobacter* species. Importantly, wild type animals colonized with the same SPF organisms exhibit no intestinal inflammation or immune activation, demonstrating the nonpathogenic nature of the enteric bacteria causing disease in IL-10$^{-/-}$ mice.[10]

Role of Mucosal Barrier Function in Experimental Colitis

A mechanistic role for loss in barrier function in the pathogenesis of mucosal inflammation is shown in N-cadherin dominant negative mice[11] and mice with disruption of the multidrug resistance gene 1a (mdr1a$^{-/-}$).[12] In the mdr1a$^{-/-}$ mice model chronic experimental inflammation is caused most probably due to defective intestinal epithelial cells rather than defective lymphocyte function, since irradiated bone-marrow chimeras of mutant mice that are repleted with lymphocytes still develop disease whereas normal mice repleted with mutant mdr$^{-/-}$

Table 2. Rodent models of inflammatory bowel disease

A. Enhanced Mucosal Permeability	
Genetically Engineered	**Chemical Triggers**
N-cadherin dominant negative transgene	Dextran sodium sulphate
Gai2-/-(?)	TNBS/ETOH
Intestinal trefoil factors-/-*	Carrageenan
mdra-/-	Indomethacin
	Acetic Acid

B. Immunoregulatory Abnormalities	
Altered Balance of Immunoregulatory Molecules	**Defective T-Lymphocyte Regulation/Education**
IL-2-/-, IL-2R-/-	TCRα-/-
IL-7 transgene	IL-2-/-
IL-10-/-, IL-10R-/-	HLA-B$_{27}$/β$_2$μ transgene
TGF-β-/-	CD4$^+$CD45RB^{high} into SCID
TNFΔARE	BM transplant into CD3e26 transgene
IL-1RA-/-*	MHC class I -/-
Cox-2-/-*	
Indomethacin	
A20-/-	
STAT4 transgene	

* Potentiates induced colitis, but no spontaneous colitis

lymphocytes do not. In recombination activating gene (Rag$^{-/-}$) deficient mice, the development of colitis associated with *H. hepaticus* required the presence of IL-7 and was downregulated by IL-10.[13] IL-7 production by intestinal epithelial cells, which are an important source of this cytokine, has been shown as the cause of experimental colitis when overexpressed in epithelial cells as a transgene.[14] Finally, deficiency of intestinal trefoil factor, a substance which enhances mucus viscosity and potentiates epithelial restitution, results in increased mortality from dextran sodium sulphate (DSS)-induced colitis.[15] Presumably increased mucosal permeability leads to enhanced uptake of bacteria, bacterial polymers and antigens which overwhelm the normal protective forces of the mucosal immune system.

Immunological Effector Mechanisms of Mucosal Inflammation

In rodent models of experimental intestinal inflammation, infiltration of the lamina propria by CD4$^+$ T cells plays a key role in the pathogenesis of chronic mucosal inflammation. These models include the SCID and CDεTg26 transfer models, several knockout mice (IL-10$^{-/-}$, IL-2$^{-/-}$, T cell receptor (TCR) α$^{-/-}$) and the murine model of induced inflammation with 2,4,6-trinitrobenzene sulphonic acid (TNBs) administration. Most of these models are characterized by dominant Th1 cytokine profiles (interferon (IFN) γ and IL-12) but only a few models develop transmural lesions resembling Crohn's disease (e.g., peptidoglycan-polysaccharide polymer-induced enterocolitis, IL-10$^{-/-}$, SAMP-1/Yit spontaneous colitis, TNBS-induced colitis and TNFΔARE models).[16,17] Additionally, another class of CD4$^+$ T cells producing Th2 cytokines (IL-4) has been shown to induce experimental colitis in TCRα[-/-] mice and oxazolone-induced colitis.[18,19] These animals developed superficial ulcerations of the epithelium characteristic for ulcerative colitis, demonstrating that different engineered animal mutants exhibit distinct pathological changes and cytokine profiles that have been associated with Crohn's disease or ulcerative colitis in humans. However, rodent models with Th1 cytokine profiles have inflammation confined to the colonic mucosa (e.g., HLA-B27 transgenic rats, IL-2[-/-] mice, CDεTG26 mice and SPF IL-10[-/-] mice) demonstrating the complexity of clinical phenotypes and immune responses in these models.

Identifying the immune abnormalities which play a causal role in the development of chronic colitis in IL-10[-/-] mice has been the focus of many studies.[20] Davidson et al[21] showed that T cell deficient IL-10[-/-] mice failed to develop disease and CD4[+] T cells isolated from the colons of IL-10[-/-] mice transferred colitis to immunodeficient Rag 2[-/-] recipients. It was concluded that colitis in IL-10[-/-] mice was mediated by activated CD4[+] Th1 cells producing predominantly IFNγ. Infusing neonatal IL-10[-/-] mice with anti-IFNγ monoclonal antibodies (mAbs) significantly diminished the onset and severity of disease, whereas the treatment with anti-IL-12 mAbs completely prevented colitis in these animals. Cong et al[22] showed that IFNγ producing C3H/HeJBir CD4[+] cells were strongly reactive to cecal lysates antigens but not epithelial or food antigens, strongly implicating antigens of the enteric flora. Adoptive transfer of cecal-antigen-activated CD4[+] T cells from colitic C3H/HeJBir mice but not control C3H/HeJ mice into C3H/HeSnJ *scid/scid* recipients induced colitis. Of importance, cecal-antigen mediated activation of pathogenic C3H/HeJBir CD4[+] T cells required a CD40-CD40 ligand interaction for a sustained IL-12 production in mucosal lesions.[23] IL-12 plays a pivotal role in initiating Th1 cytokine pathways by stimulating T cells to induce the production of tumour necrosis factor (TNF) and IFNγ, and both of these cytokines induce positive feedback for further IL-12 production as well as proinflammatory macrophage-derived cytokines including IL-1β, IL-6 and TNF.[24] The key role of IL-12 in Th1/TNF-mediated pathways of inflammation was demonstrated in the SCID[25] and CDεTg26 transfer models[7] as well as the TNBS-induced colitis model.[26] In each of these models, either inter-crossing with IL-12[-/-] mice or administration of anti-IL-12 mAbs prevented the development of colitis or treated established disease. Additional support for the role of Th1/TNF mediated pathways in the development of chronic inflammation came from TNFΔARE mice.[1,27] These TNF overproducing mice developed Th1-mediated disease primarily in the small intestine rather than the colon and displayed a granulomatous histology that is similar to that of human Crohn's disease, consistent with the dramatic ability of anti-TNF antibodies to treat Crohn's disease.[28]

The importance of the constant antigenic drive of luminal bacteria in inducing and maintaining immune-mediated colitis is illustrated by findings of Veltkamp et al.[29] These authors reported secretion of IFNγ by mesenteric lymph node CD4[+] T cells from bone marrow transplanted CDεTg26 mice with colitis following in vitro incubation with cecal bacterial lysate-pulsed antigen presenting cells (APC), but not colonic epithelial cells or lysates of cecal content from germ-free mice. Activated CD4[+] T cells were present in the mucosa of bone marrow transplanted CDεTg26 mice, but were incapable of inducing disease unless colonic SPF bacteria were present. Activated pathogenic T cells required the continuous presence of bacteria to sustain colitis, indicating a lack of bacterial induction of an autoimmune response to cross reacting host antigens. Taken together, these studies show direct evidence that dysregulated proinflammatory cytokine production in genetically susceptible hosts generate pathogenic T cells reacting to bacterial antigens of the commensal intestinal microflora, which in turn mediate chronic colitis in experimental animals.

Importance of the Host Genetic Background in Experimental Colitis

In each of the genetically engineered rodent models of intestinal inflammation discussed, congenic wild type animals fail to develop disease or immune activation when colonized with identical bacteria,[1,10,22,30,31] demonstrating the nonpathogenic nature of the resident flora and suggesting that normal hosts develop tolerogenic immune responses to commensal bacteria which prevent colitis. In support of this concept, cecal tissue of SPF IL-10[+/+] wild type mice secrete almost undetectable IL-12 levels and cecal bacterial antigen-pulsed APC/CD4[+] T cell cultures from C3H/HeJ or IL-10[+/+] mice produce almost no IFNγ.[10,22,32] Furthermore, different inbred rodent strains exhibit differential susceptibility to immune-mediated colitis. For example, the impact of inheritable factors on disease expression was shown in IL-10[-/-] mice. In IL-10[-/-] mice on three genetic backgrounds with different MHC alleles colitis developed earlier and was more severe in IL-10[-/-] 129/SvEv (H-2b) and BALB/c (H-2d) strains compared with the IL-10[-/-] C57BL/6 (H-2b) strain (JCI 1996).[2] Similarly, C59 BL/6 mice are more resistant to colitis in the T cell receptor knockout and DSS-induced models.[18,33] Moreover, Lewis rats develop chronic, spontaneously relapsing Th1-mediated enterocolitis when injected with sterile bacterial cell wall polymers, while MHC-matched Fischer F_{344} rats exhibit only transient acute inflammation.[34,35,36] These results showed that genetic factors strongly contribute to susceptibility to intestinal inflammation and cellular immune responses to enteric bacteria. Similar differential immune responses may be associated with human genetic susceptibility to Crohn's disease and ulcerative colitis (Fig. 1).

Anti-Inflammatory Mechanisms in Experimental Mucosal Inflammation

The absence of colitis and pathogenic immune responses to commensal bacteria in normal rodents suggests that normal hosts have well developed immunosuppressive mechanisms of their mucosal immune systems. Exposure of the gastrointestinal tract of normal hosts to soluble antigen leads to a state of antigen-specific hyporesponsiveness (oral tolerance) on subsequent antigen challenge. Gonella et al[37] showed that the immunosuppressive cytokines IL-10 and transforming growth factor (TGF) β are secreted in the Peyer's patches and lamina propria shortly after oral administration of antigen, presumably to protect the intestine from pathogenic immune responses to ubiquitous luminal antigens. In a series of elegant studies, Michalek, McGhee and collegues developed the hypothesis that oral tolerance to certain antigens is stimulated by normal bacteria and lipopolysaccharide (LPS). These authors demonstrated that C3H/HeJ LPS-nonresponsive mice lack oral tolerance to sheep red blood cells (SRBC), which is mediated by T lymphocytes.[38,39] Furthermore, germ-free mice have attenuated oral tolerance to SRBC which can be induced by feeding LPS or colonization with normal bacteria.[40] These studies clearly indicate that the luminal microflora in normal hosts are critical stimulants to develop normal mucosal and systemic immune responses.

The ability to induce regulatory cells in response to feeding antigen has been therapeutically used in models of autoimmune diseases.[41] CD4[+] T cells cloned from mesenteric lymph nodes of mice orally tolerized with myelin basic protein (MBP) secreted significant amounts of TGFβ and of importance, these Th3 cells were able to protect susceptible mice from experimental autoimmune encephalomyelitis (EAE) by a TGFβ-mediated immunosuppressive mechanism.[42] The protective role of regulatory cells in experimental colitis was first shown by Powrie and coworkers.[43] Adoptive transfer of CD45RB[high]CD4[+] T cells (naive cells) from normal donors into severe combined immunodeficient (SCID) mice induced a Th1 mediated colitis in the presence of resident enteric bacteria, whereas the reciprocal CD45RB[low]CD4[+] T cell subset (memory cells) did not induce colitis in the recipient host.[44,45] However, when CD45RB[low]CD4[+] T cell were coinjected with pathogenic CD45RB[high] cells disease did not develop. Analysis of the mechanism of immune suppression transferred by CD45RB[low]CD4+ T cells revealed essential roles for both IL-10 and TGFβ. In fact, anti-TGFβ mAbs were able to abrogate

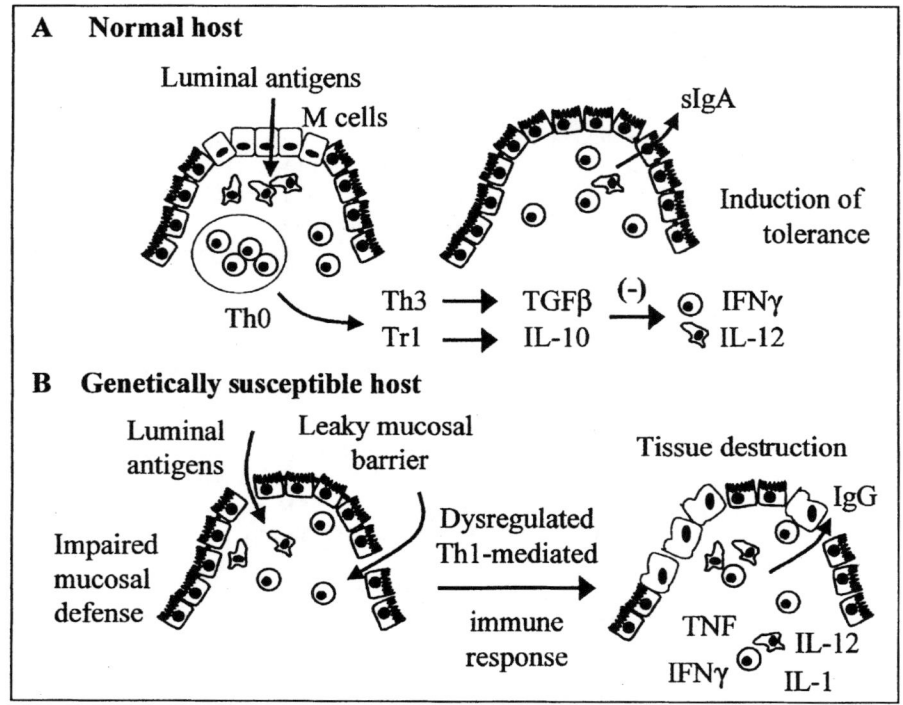

Figure 1. The lumen of the distal ileum and colon contains high concentrations of bacterial products and antigens. A. In the normal host these luminal antigens are preferentially sampled in lymphoid aggregates containing M cells. The induction of regulatory T cells (Th3 and Tr1), which produce immunosuppressive cytokines (TGFβ and IL-10), and of sIgA secreting plasma cells induce tolerance to luminal antigens in the intestinal mucosa. B. In the genetically susceptible host with impaired mucosal defense, luminal antigens can cross a permeable mucosal barrier and induce a dysregulated Th1-mediated immune response. The uncontrolled secretion of proinflammatory cytokines (TNF, IL-1, IL-12, IFNγ) leads to tissue destruction and chronic immune-mediated inflammation.

protection from colitis in CD45RB^{low}CD4^+ T cell cotransferred mice.[46] Moreover, CD45RB^{high}CD4^+ T cells from IL-4^{-/-} mice were equally efficient as wild-type cells in inhibiting colitis, suggesting that this regulatory T cell population is functionally distinct from Th2 cells. These results are consistent with spontaneous development of colitis in IL-10 and TGFβ deficient mice.[4] The immunoregulatory role of TGFβ was further supported by recent findings of Kitani et al[47] showing that intranasal administration of TGFβ1 plasmid prevented experimental TNBS-induced colitis. The authors demonstrated that overexpression of TGFβ in lamina propria tissue and immune cells inhibited Th1-mediated colitis through IL-10-induced suppression of IL-12 production and inhibition of IL-12 signaling via downregulation of the IL-12Rbeta2 chain. It was hypothesized that in hosts with normal immunoregulation enteric antigens induce immunosuppressive IL-10 and TGFβ-secreting T cells (Tr1 and Th3, respectively) that prevent inflammatory responses towards the resident enteric bacteria. Powrie and colleges showed that the administration of murine recombinant IL-10 prevents colitis in SCID mice restored with CD45RB^{high}CD4^+ T cells[25] and CD45RB^{low}CD4^+ T cells from IL-10^{-/-} mice failed to inhibit colitis in the SCID transfer model.[48] In support of these results, administration of anti-IL-10 receptor mAbs completely abrogated protection transferred by

CD45RB^{low}CD4$^+$ T cells from wild-type mice.[49] Taken together, these studies suggest that IL-10 and TGFβ are functional components of regulatory T cell populations important in maintaining the controlled status of physiologic inflammation in the normal intestine (Fig. 2), however the factors that drive the induction of IL-10 and/or TGFβ expressing cells in the gut are not yet well defined. It has been suggested that it is the balance between proinflammatory and anti-inflammatory signals acting on antigen-presenting cells (APC) that direct T cell subset differentiation. A recent preliminary study from Cong et al[50] suggested that enteric bacterial specific regulatory T cells (Tr1) regulate pathogenic Th1 cell activity by inhibiting dendritic cell costimulatory molecule expression and IL-12 production, at least partially through secretion of high amounts of IL-10.

Different Bacterial Species of the Intestinal Microflora Have Variable Abilities to Induce Inflammatory and Protective Intestinal Immune Responses

Selective colonization of germ-free rodents with defined bacterial species show that all enteric bacteria are not equal in their capacities to induce chronic mucosal inflammation. HLA-B27/β$_2$ microglobulin transgenic rats raised under SPF conditions spontaneously develop colitis, gastritis and arthritis but exhibit no inflammation in these organs in a sterile environment.[30,51] Selective bacterial reconstitution studies in gnotobiotic HLA-B27 transgenic rats[30,52] and carrageenan-induced colitis in guinea pigs[53] implicate *Bacteroides vulgatus* as a primary inducer of colitis, with no pathological response to *Escherichia coli*. Gnotobiotic HLA-B27 transgenic rats colonized with a mixture of six different obligate and facultative anaerobic bacteria containing *Streptococcus faecium* (group D), *Streptococcus avium*, *Peptostreptococcus productus*, *E. coli*, *Eubacterium contortum*, and *B. vulgatus* developed much more active colitis and gastritis than did animals colonized with the same mixture without *B. vulgatus*. Of considerable importance, gnotobiotic IL-10$^{-/-}$ mice colonized with either *B. vulgatus* alone or a mixture of 6 different commensal enteric bacteria that caused colitis in HLA B27 transgenic rats developed extremely mild inflammation, whereas *Enterococcus faecalis* monoassociated IL-10$^{-/-}$ mice developed a predominantly distal moderate colitis after 10-12 weeks, with progressive inflammation and dysplasia to at least 35 weeks of age.[32] The concept of specificity of immunologic responses to bacterial stimuli in individual host species was further supported by the finding that IL-10$^{-/-}$ mice with colitis induced by *E. faecalis* monoassociation have selective in vitro mesenteric lymph node T cell secretion of IFNγ in response to *E. faecalis* compared with *E. coli* and *B. vulgatus*. Differences in the kinetics and distribution of colitis between IL-10$^{-/-}$ mice monoassociated with *E. faecalis* and adult germ-free IL-10$^{-/-}$ mice colonized with SPF fecal flora (which develop aggressive cecal inflammation within one week of colonization and show a 50% mortality rate by 5 weeks[10]) indicate that other enteric bacterial species have additive or synergistic activities. Similar results were obtained in SPF HLA B27 transgenic rats which developed a more severe colitis relative to *B. vulgatus* monoassociated animals,[30,52] suggesting synergistic activities of different enteric species in perpetuating intestinal inflammation in genetically susceptible hosts. This concept is independently supported by responses to antibiotics with specific versus broad spectra of activity. Madsen et al[54] demonstrated that the composition of mucosal adherent bacterial species in IL-10$^{-/-}$ mice is altered before the onset of colitis and that broad spectrum antibiotic treatment, which prevented and treated disease, corrected these bacterial changes. Moreover, metronidazole or ciprofloxacin failed to treat established colitis in SPF HLA B27 transgenic rats, whereas inflammation was almost completely resolved following a combination of vancomycin and imipenum.[55] A recent report from Kishi et al[56] showed that colitis in TCRα$^{-/-}$ mice may result from alterations in the microbial homeostasis, emphasizing the pathogenic role of *B. vulgatus*. Together

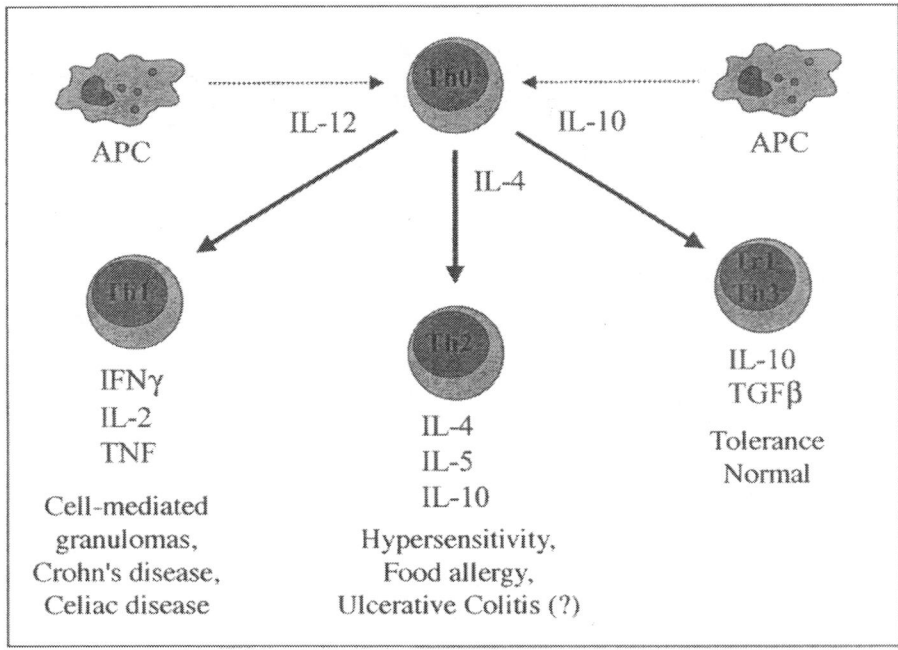

Figure 2. Induction of CD4+ T cell subsets. CD4+ T cells can be subdivided into Th1, Th2 and Tr1/Th3 cells based on their pattern of cytokine secretion. Antigen-presenting cells (APC) which interact first with microbial antigens activate naive T cells and secrete cytokines which affect the differentiation pathway of Th0 cells. IL-12 stimulates Th0 cells to differentiate into the Th1 subset, which produces IFNγ, IL-2 and TNF and mediates cellular immunity. In contrast, if the activated Th0 cells encounters IL-4, it differentiates into the Th2 subset that produces IL-4, IL-5, IL-10, IL-6 and IL-13 and mediates humoral immunity. The presence of IL-10 induces Tr1 and Th3 cells which produce TGFβ and IL-10 and mediate tolerance in the normal intestinal mucosa.

these results demonstrate that all resident bacteria do not have equal capacities to induce intestinal inflammation in genetically susceptible hosts implying that host specific immune responses to dominant commensal enteric bacterial species play an important role in the development of IBD. On the other hand, these results do not exclude a potential role for either microbial dysbiosis in the intestine or enteric pathogens, particularly in the latter case for the induction or reactivation of inflammation which then could be perpetuated by components of the normal intestinal microflora.[57] This possibility is supported by recent observations of chronic, Th1-mediated colitis in IL-10[-/-] mice on the relatively resistant C57/B16 background colonized with *Helicobacter hepaticus*[58] and *Citrobacter rodentium* in immunocompetent normal mice,[59] even though Dieleman et al[60] showed that native *H. hepaticus* strains, either alone in monoassociation studies or combined with SPF bacteria did not induce colitis in more susceptible IL-10[-/-] mouse strains.

Bacteria-Mediated Protection from Intestinal Inflammation

It is now apparent that intestinal bacteria not only have the ability to induce intestinal inflammation, but also mediate beneficial activities. Probiotics are commensal or food-derived micro-organisms with beneficial effects to the host, including stimulation of protective immune responses, enhancement of mucosal barrier function, suppression of pathogenic organisms and treatment of colitis.[61,62] Although the specific properties of probiotic micro-organisms are not yet characterized and validated in well-designed, multicenter clinical trials, studies in several animal models show considerable therapeutic relevance. Madsen et al[63] demonstrated that SPF IL-10[-/-] mice at 2 weeks of age displayed changes in bacterial colonization with increased aerobic adherent and translocated bacteria in conjunction with reduced levels of *Lactobacillus* species. Rectal administration of endogenous *L. reuteri* enhanced mucosal barrier function and attenuated the development of colitis in SPF IL-10[-/-] mice at 4 weeks of age. Similar protective effects of lactobacilli were demonstrated in a rat model of methotrexate-induced enterocolitis showing decreased body weight loss, intestinal permeability and intestinal myeloperoxidase levels after the oral administration of *L. plantarum*.[64] Schultz et al[65] reported that daily administration of *L. plantarum* could reverse established inflammation in SPF IL-10[-/-] mice and prevent the onset of colitis with pretreatment of gnotobiotic mutant mice. Convincing evidence for protective activities of probiotic bacteria in human IBD was provided by Gionchetti et al.[66] The authors reported that VSL-3, a cocktail of 8 different lactic acid bacteria inhibited relapse of chronic pouchitis in a 9 month clinical trial (15% recurrence rate in the VSL-3 treated group versus 100% in the placebo group), with inhibition of mucosal TNF and upregulation of IL-10 in the treated pouches.[67] In vitro studies similarly demonstrated that VSL-3 lysates stimulated IL-10 and inhibited TNF in cecal bacterial lysate-stimulated rat splenocytes (Cender and Sartor, unpublished data). Better understanding of the mechanisms by which normal commensal bacteria induce protective responses in normal hosts and of the bacterial subsets which selectively induce protective versus aggressive immune responses should lead to novel therapeutic approaches to treat diseases. For example, *Bifidobacterium lactis* enhanced neutrophil phagocytosis and natural killer (NK) cell tumoricidal activity[68] and *Lactobacillus casei* strain Shirota induced NK cell cytotoxicity and decreased in vivo tumor incidence.[69] In vitro Gram positive bacteria including lactobacilli revealed selective potential to induce NK cell activation compared to Gram negative *E. coli* through the induction of monocyte-derived IL-12 and costimulatory molecules.[70,71] Importantly, Gram negative bacterial species preferentially induce IL-10 expression while Gram positive bacteria bacteria activate IL-12 in human monocytes.[70,72] Genetically engineered bacteria which secrete immunosuppressive cytokines have already shown the potential of future approaches to immunotherapy of IBD, as validated by the treatment of experimental colitis by *Lactococcus lactis* producing IL-10.[73]

Prebiotics or oral agents such as nonabsorbed carbohydrates which foster the growth of beneficial enteric bacteria, can stimulate protective epithelial cell responses and inhibit intestinal inflammation.[74] Prebiotic substances, including germinated barley extracts, fructo-oligosaccharides and lactulose, stimulate growth of intestinal lactobacilli and bifidobacteria. Production of short chain fatty acids, especially butyrate, can induce protective responses in intestinal epithelial cells, including diminished activation by IL-1β.[75] These agents can prevent experimental colitis[63] and treat active ulcerative colitis.[76]

Bacteria Induced Cross-Talk at the Mucosal Surface: Evidence for Epithelial Cells As a Functional Element in the Initiation and Regulation of Intestinal Immune Responses

Recent observations demonstrate that intestinal epithelial cells, which isolate the host from the gut luminal environment, are an integral and essential component of the host's innate and acquired mucosal immune system. Intestinal epithelial cells constitutively express or can be induced to express costimulatory molecules and MHC molecules, such as class II, classical I and nonclassical class Ib MHC molecules. CD58 (LFA-3) and CD80/CD86 are expressed on normal and inflamed intestinal epithelial cells respectively,[77,78] and can function as costimulatory molecules for T cells in HLA class II-mediated antigen presentation. Mayer et al[79] suggested that there is an intrinsic defect in intestinal epithelial cells from patients with IBD, resulting in their inability to normally stimulate suppressor T cells in an antigen overloaded environment.

Moreover, the stimulation of intestinal epithelial cells by proinflammatory cytokines (e.g., TNF, IL-1) or certain enteric pathogens (e.g., *Salmonella typhimurium, Yersinia enterocolitica* and enteropathogenic *Escherichia coli*) induces the expression and secretion of a wide range of inflammatory and chemoattractive cytokines including TNF, IL-7, IL-8, MCP-1, IP-10 and GROα, of iNOS, prostaglandin (PG) E2 , and the adhesion molecule ICAM-1.[80-82] As shown in multiple cell systems including intestinal epithelial cell lines, most of these proinflammatory molecules are in part regulated at transcriptional level by the transcription factor NF-κB.[83,84] The Gram negative bacterial product LPS, which has emerged as a key bacterial stimulant of innate immune responses, activates the IκB/NF-κB system by using the pattern recognition receptor toll-like receptor (TLR) 4 and down-stream components of the IL-1 signaling cascade.[85] A related receptor, TLR2 transduces parallel signals from the cell wall polymer peptidoglycan found in Gram positive and Gram negative bacteria, and from mycobacterial components.[86] The critical role of LPS-induced signal transduction in intestinal homeostasis is eloquently highlighted by two different observations. First, the mouse strain C3H/HeJ, which harbors a missense mutation in the cytoplasmic domain of TLR4, is more sensitive to DSS-induced colitis.[87-89] Second, point mutations in the intracellular LPS receptor NOD2, which alter LPS-induced NF-κB activation in monocytes, is associated with an increased susceptibility to Crohn's disease in a subset of patients, demonstrating that altered LPS-induced signal transduction might be implicated in the pathogenesis of IBD.[90,91]

Intestinal epithelial cell lines, which express TLR2, TLR3 and TLR4 at variable levels,[92] respond to resident bacteria either directly or through complex interactions with adjacent lamina propria mononuclear cells, which provide regulatory signals in normal hosts as well as inflammatory signals under pathological conditions. For example, we showed that nonpathogenic, noninvasive *B. vulgatus* induce gene expression in intestinal epithelial cell lines through the NF-κB signal transduction pathway by using the TLR-4 signaling cascade.[93a] In addition, we demonstrated the transient induction of phospho-RelA (phospho-p55) followed by persistent activation of phospho-Smad2 in IEC from mucosal tissue sections of *B. vulgatus*-monoassociated rats, indicating that both NF-κB and TGF-β signaling are induced in vivo following bacterial colonization.[93b] Colonic epithelial cells in normal hosts appear to have diminished expression of TLR-4 and the accessory molecule MD-2, which may result in dampened responses to LPS.[94] Similarly, intestinal epithelial cells have delayed, inappropriate degradation of IκBα in response to inflammatory signals, which allows them to exist in the hostile environment of the distal intestine.[95,96] Cario et al[97] showed expression of TLR4 protein in tissue sections from patients with ulcerative colitis and Crohn's disease, suggesting the potential ability of intestinal epithelial cells to respond to luminal Gram negative bacteria or LPS in vivo. The effect of bi-directional cross-talk between intestinal epithelial cells and immuno-competent cells in response to nonpathogenic bacteria was investigated, using enterocyte-like CaCO-2 cells co-cultured with human blood leukocytes in transwell cell cultures.[98] It was demonstrated that commensal bacteria of different origins have the ability to induce a distinct cytokine/chemokine response in leukocyte-sensitized CaCO-2 cells, and to deliver to underlying immuno-competent cells a discriminative signal associated with the production of TNF and IL-10.[98] Additionally, the development of CD14[high] CD16[high] tissue monocytes, observed under certain inflammatory conditions[99,100] was significantly suppressed under the influence of intestinal epithelial cells.[101,102] Hooper et al[103] used elegant microarray and microdissection techniques to identify which genes were modulated when germ-free mice were colonized with a representative anaerobic enteric species. *B. thetaiotaomicron* upregulated a characteristic profile of genes contributing to mucosal barrier function, nutrient absorption, xenobiotic metabolism maturation and angiogenesis. In addition, Lopez-Boado et al[104] showed induction of matrilysin, a matrix metalloprotease which activates prodefensins, in mucosal epithelial cells upon stimulation with *B. thetaiotaomicron.* Taken together these studies support the concept of bacterial-intestinal epithelial cell cross-talk with adjacent mucosal immune cells as a critical determinant in the initiation and regulation of intestinal immune responses, with important immunosuppressive mechanisms in both cell lineages (Fig. 3).

Clinical and Experimental Evidence for Dysregulated Bacteria-Mediated Immune Response in Human IBD

Human Crohn's disease preferentially targets the distal ileum and colon, while ulcerative colitis exclusively involves the colon. These are sites of highest concentrations of commensal luminal bacteria, suggesting that IBD is due to a loss of tolerance to luminal antigens, most likely of bacterial origin. Several groups have reported increased serologic responses to a wide variety of commensal bacteria, including *E. coli, Bacteroides* species, *Pseudomonas fluorescens, Peptostreptococci,* and *Eubacteria.*[57,105-107] Mac Pherson et al[108] demonstrated that the majority of immunoglobulins in Crohn's disease patients recognize luminal bacteria. Moreover, several enteric commensal bacterial species, including *B. caecae* and *E. coli,* cross react with perinuclear antineutrophil cytoplasmic antibodies (pANCA), which are found in approximately sixty percent of ulcerative colitis patients and 15 percent of patients with Crohn's disease.[109] Results in rodent models indicate that chronic intestinal inflammation is mediated by T lymphocyte responses, so it is likely that B cell responses in IBD patients reflect a general loss of immunologic tolerance to commensal bacteria which cross the inflamed mucosal barrier and are not directly involved in disease pathogenesis. However, there is some evidence of complement activation in active Crohn's disease, suggesting a possible mechanism of tissue injury with local bacterial antigen-IgG complexes.[110] Of more obvious pathogenic relevance is the demonstration by Duchmann et al[111-113] of a loss of immunologic tolerance in active IBD with mucosal T lymphocyte proliferation to fecal bacteria, including *B. vulgatus* and *E. coli.* These results are consistent with a lack of inflammation in bypassed distal ileal or colonic segments after proximal diversion of the fecal stream,[114,115] but an immune activation within one week of perfusion of ileal effluent into the bypassed ileum.[116] Clinically Crohn's disease patients with colonic involvement respond to antibiotics with an anaerobic or broad spectrum[117,118] and exhibit a Th1 profile of cytokines with increased IFNγ and IL-12.[119] Cytokine profiles and responses to antibiotics in ulcerative colitis are less consistent but ciprofloxacin may have an adjunctive therapeutic role.[120]

Summary and Clinical Implications

The studies reviewed here suggest that commensal enteric bacteria are key stimulants of mucosal immune responses, with protective versus pathogenic responses determined by both the host genetic background and the composition of the luminal bacterial flora. Normal resistant hosts are genetically programmed to develop immunologic tolerance to commensal bacteria, with tolerogenic responses mediated by regulatory Th3 and Tr1 lymphocytes, which preferentially secrete TGFβ and IL-10 respectively, and perhaps by intestinal epithelial cells. Gram negative bacteria, LPS and lactic acid bacterial species, including lactobacilli and bifidobacteria, appear to be key inducers of protective responses in normal hosts. In contrast, genetically susceptible hosts develop pathogenic Th1 or Th2 immune responses and activation of mucosal macrophages when exposed to commensal bacteria, which leads to chronic, relapsing inflammation in the distal intestine where the contact with commensal bacteria is greatest. Genetic susceptibility is a consequence of either aberrant immunoregulation or defective barrier function, with either abnormality leading to loss of tolerance to ubiquitous luminal antigens (Fig. 4).

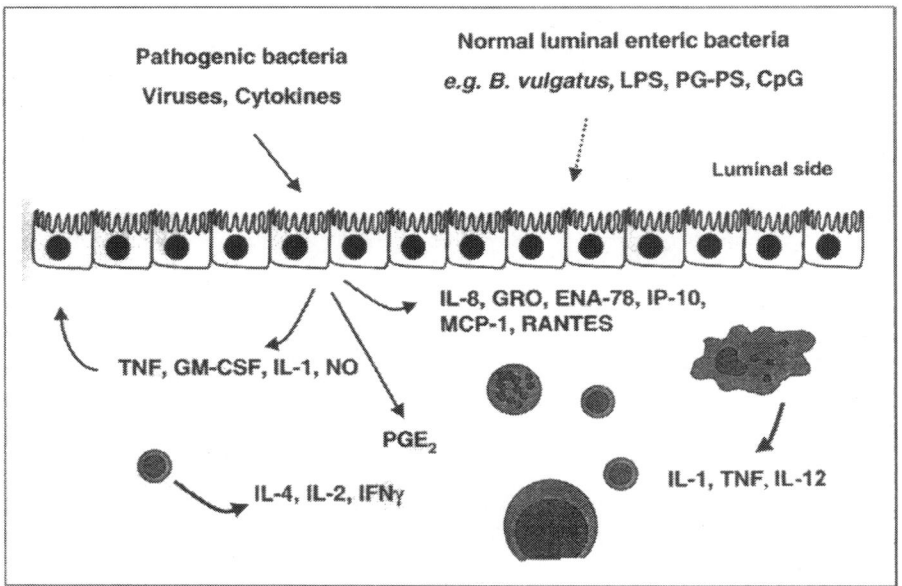

Figure 3. Intestinal epithelial cells are a functional element of the mucosal innate immune system. Cross-talk of bacteria and immune cells with the gut epithelium can influence the phenotype and function of intestinal epithelial cells.

Induction or reactivation of inflammation is triggered by luminal antigens that transiently cross the mucosal barrier and initiate the immune cascade. We hypothesize on the basis of preliminary data that distinct bacterial species preferentially activate pathogenic immune responses in hosts of genetically susceptible backgrounds, which results in a substantial heterogeneity in therapeutic responses from IBD patients to various antibiotic regimens.

These observations provide considerable insights into the pathogenesis of chronic, immune-mediated intestinal inflammation, and an opportunity to develop novel therapeutic approaches for Crohn's disease and ulcerative colitis. Attractive alternatives to the currently used nonspecific immunosuppression include decreasing the load of bacterial antigens which induce pathogenic responses, by selectively altering the composition of enteric bacteria with narrow spectrum antibiotics matched with the patient's genetic background. Another strategy would be to use probiotic bacterial species or prebiotic substances in concert with growth factors and nutritional agents that ensure mucosal healing and barrier function, thereby decreasing bacterial antigen uptake and exposure to underlying lamina propia immune cells. An additional approach, yet underdeveloped, is to upregulate immunosuppressive properties of intestinal epithelial cells perhaps by using probiotic bacteria or prebiotic substances which enhance luminal butyrate concentrations or perhaps by specific pharmacologic stimuli. Finally, genetically engineered bacteria producing immunosuppressive molecules or growth factors which foster epithelial function and mucosal healing offer the potential to reverse the loss of tolerance in genetically susceptible hosts.

Acknowledgement

Original work described in this review was supported by grants from the DFG (HA 3148/ 1-1) and the NIH (DK 40249, DK 53347 and DK 34987).

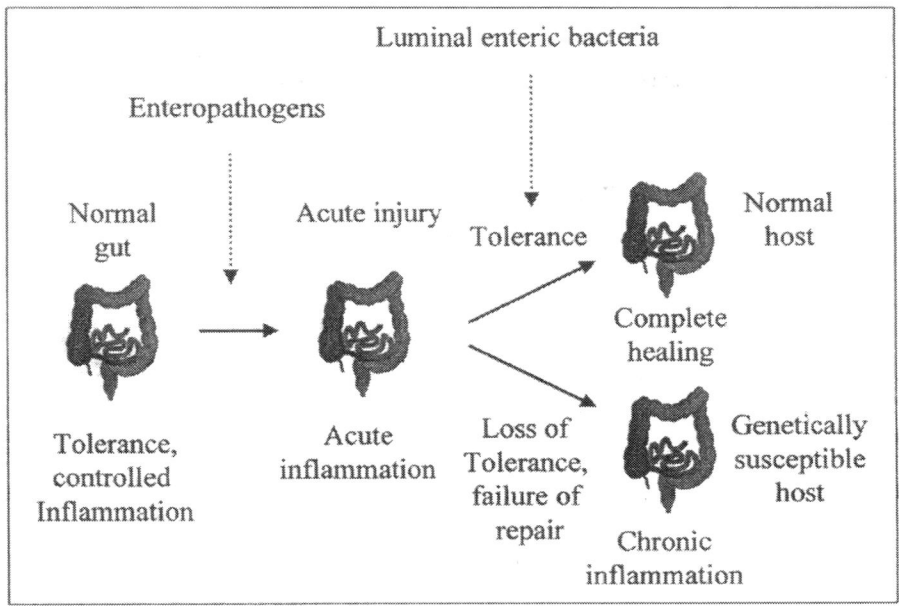

Figure 4. Genetic susceptibility is a consequence of either aberrant immunoregulation or defective barrier function, with either abnormality leading to loss of tolerance to ubiquitous luminal antigens. Induction or reactivation of inflammation are mediated by luminal environmental triggers which initiate chronic immune-mediated inflammation in the genetically susceptible host. Tolerance and complete healing occur in the normal host.

References

1. Kontoyiannis D, Pasparakis M, Pizarro TT et al. Impaired on/off regulation of TNF biosynthesis in mice lacking TNF AU-rich elements: Implications for joint and gut-associated immunopathologies. Immunity 1999; 10:387-398.
2. Berg DJ, Davidson N, Kuhn R et al. Enterocolitis and colon cancer in interleukin-10-deficient mice are associated with aberrant cytokine production and CD4(+) TH1-like responses. J Clin Invest 1996; 98:1010-1020.
3. Morteau O, Morham SG, Sellon R et al. Impaired mucosal defense to acute colonic injury in mice lacking cyclooxygenase-1 or cyclooxygenase-2. J Clin Invest 2000; 105:469-478.
4. Kuhn R, Lohler J, Rennick D et al. Interleukin-10-deficient mice develop chronic enterocolitis. Cell 1993; 75:263-274.
5. Kulkarni AB, Ward JM, Yaswen L et al. Transforming growth factor-beta 1 null mice. An animal model for inflammatory disorders. Am J Pathol 1995; 146:264-275.
6. Sadlack B, Merz H, Schorle H et al. Ulcerative colitis-like disease in mice with a disrupted interleukin-2 gene. Cell 1993; 75:253-261.
7. Hollander GA, Simpson SJ, Mizoguchi E et al. Severe colitis in mice with aberrant thymic selection. Immunity 1995; 3:27-38.
8. Powrie F, Leach MW, Mauze S et al. Phenotypically distinct subsets of CD4+ T cells induce or protect from chronic intestinal inflammation in C. B-17 scid mice. Int Immunol 1993; 5:1461-1471.
9. Monteleone G, Kumberova A, Croft NM et al. Blocking Smad7 restores TGF-beta1 signaling in chronic inflammatory bowel disease. J Clin Invest 2001; 108:601-609.
10. Sellon RK, Tonkonogy S, Schultz M et al. Resident enteric bacteria are necessary for development of spontaneous colitis and immune system activation in interleukin-10-deficient mice. Infect Immun 1998; 66:5224-5231.

11. Hermiston ML, Gordon JI. Inflammatory bowel disease and adenomas in mice expressing a dominant negative N-cadherin. Science 1995; 270:1203-1207.

12. Panwala CM, Jones JC, Viney JL. A novel model of inflammatory bowel disease: mice deficient for the multiple drug resistance gene, mdr1a, spontaneously develop colitis. J Immunol 1998; 161:5733-5744.

13. von Freeden-Jeffry U, Davidson N, Wiler R et al. IL-7 deficiency prevents development of a non-T cell non-B cell-mediated colitis. J Immunol 1998; 161:5673-5680.

14. Watanabe M, Ueno Y, Yajima T et al. Interleukin 7 transgenic mice develop chronic colitis with decreased interleukin 7 protein accumulation in the colonic mucosa. J Exp Med 1998; 187:389-402.

15. Itoh H, Beck PL, Inoue N et al. A paradoxical reduction in susceptibility to colonic injury upon targeted transgenic ablation of goblet cells. J Clin Invest 1999; 104:1539-1547.

16. Elson CO, Sartor RB, Tennyson GS et al. Experimental models of inflammatory bowel disease. Gastroenterology 1995; 109:1344-1367.

17. Blumberg RS, Saubermann LJ, Strober W. Animal models of mucosal inflammation and their relation to human inflammatory bowel disease. Curr Opin Immunol 1999; 11:648-656.

18. Mizoguchi A, Mizoguchi E, Bhan AK. The critical role of interleukin 4 but not interferon gamma in the pathogenesis of colitis in T-cell receptor alpha mutant mice. Gastroenterology 1999; 116:320-326.

19. Boirivant M, Fuss IJ, Chu A et al. Oxazolone colitis: A murine model of T helper cell type 2 colitis treatable with antibodies to interleukin 4. J Exp Med 1998; 188:1929-1939.

20. Rennick DM, Fort MM. Lessons from genetically engineered animal models. XII. IL-10-deficient (IL-10-/-) mice and intestinal inflammation. Am J Physiol Gastrointest Liver Physiol 2000; 278:G829-G833

21. Davidson NJ, Leach MW, Fort MM et al. T helper cell 1-type CD4+ T cells, but not B cells, mediate colitis in interleukin 10-deficient mice. J Exp Med 1996; 184:241-251.

22. Cong Y, Brandwein SL, McCabe RP et al. CD4+ T cells reactive to enteric bacterial antigens in spontaneously colitic C3H/HeJBir mice: increased T helper cell type 1 response and ability to transfer disease. J Exp Med 1998; 187:855-864.

23. Cong Y, Weaver CT, Lazenby A et al. Colitis induced by enteric bacterial antigen-specific CD4+ T cells requires CD40-CD40 ligand interactions for a sustained increase in mucosal IL-12. J Immunol 2000; 165:2173-2182.

24. Hall SS. IL-12 at the crossroads. Science 1995; 268:1432-1434.

25. Powrie F, Leach MW, Mauze S et al. Inhibition of Th1 responses prevents inflammatory bowel disease in scid mice reconstituted with CD45RBhi CD4+ T cells. Immunity 1994; 1:553-562.

26. Neurath MF, Fuss I, Kelsall BL et al. Experimental granulomatous colitis in mice is abrogated by induction of TGF-beta-mediated oral tolerance. J Exp Med 1996; 183:2605-2616.

27. Kosiewicz MM, Nast CC, Krishnan A et al. Th1-type responses mediate spontaneous ileitis in a novel murine model of Crohn's disease. J Clin Invest 2001; 107:695-702.

28. Targan SR, Hanauer SB, van Deventer SJ et al. A short-term study of chimeric monoclonal antibody cA2 to tumor necrosis factor alpha for Crohn's disease. Crohn's Disease cA2 Study Group. N Engl J Med 1997; 337:1029-1035.

29. Veltkamp C, Tonkonogy SL, De Jong YP et al. Continuous stimulation by normal luminal bacteria is essential for the development and perpetuation of colitis in Tg(epsilon26) mice. Gastroenterology 2001; 120:900-913.

30. Rath HC, Herfarth HH, Ikeda JS et al. Normal luminal bacteria, especially Bacteroides species, mediate chronic colitis, gastritis, and arthritis in HLA-B27/human beta2 microglobulin transgenic rats. J Clin Invest 1996; 98:945-953.

31. Schultz M, Tonkonogy SL, Sellon RK et al. IL-2-deficient mice raised under germfree conditions develop delayed mild focal intestinal inflammation. Am J Physiol 1999; 276:G1461-G1472.

32. Kim SC, Tonkonogy SL, Balish E et al. IL-10 deficient mice monoassociated with non-pathogenic Enterococcus faecalis develop chronic colitis. Gastroenterology 2001; A441.

33. Mahler M, Bristol IJ, Leiter EH et al. Differential susceptibility of inbred mouse strains to dextran sulfate sodium-induced colitis. Am J Physiol 1998; 274:G544-G551.

34. McCall RD, Haskill S, Zimmermann EM et al. Tissue interleukin 1 and interleukin-1 receptor antagonist expression in enterocolitis in resistant and susceptible rats. Gastroenterology 1994; 106:960-972.

35. van den Broek MF, van Bruggen MC, Koopman JP et al. Gut flora induces and maintains resistance against streptococcal cell wall-induced arthritis in F344 rats. Clin Exp Immunol 1992; 88:313-317.
36. Sartor RB, DeLa CR, Green KD et al. Selective kallikrein-kinin system activation in inbred rats differentially susceptible to granulomatous enterocolitis. Gastroenterology 1996; 110:1467-1481.
37. Gonnella PA, Chen Y, Inobe J et al. In situ immune response in gut-associated lymphoid tissue (GALT) following oral antigen in TCR-transgenic mice. J Immunol 1998; 160:4708-4718.
38. Kiyono H, McGhee JR, Wannemuehler MJ et al. Lack of oral tolerance in C3H/HeJ mice. J Exp Med 1982; 155:605-610.
39. Michalek SM, Kiyono H, Wannemuehler MJ et al. Lipopolysaccharide (LPS) regulation of the immune response: LPS influence on oral tolerance induction. J Immunol 1982; 128:1992-1998.
40. Wannemuehler MJ, Kiyono H, Babb JL et al. Lipopolysaccharide (LPS) regulation of the immune response:LPS converts germfree mice to sensitivity to oral tolerance induction. J Immunol 1982; 129:959-965.
41. Weiner HL. Oral tolerance: Immune mechanisms and treatment of autoimmune diseases. Immunol Today 1997; 18:335-343.
42. Chen Y, Kuchroo VK, Inobe J et al. Regulatory T cell clones induced by oral tolerance: Suppression of autoimmune encephalomyelitis. Science 1994; 265:1237-1240.
43. Powrie F, Correa-Oliveira R, Mauze S et al. Regulatory interactions between CD45RBhigh and CD45RBlow CD4+ T cells are important for the balance between protective and pathogenic cell-mediated immunity. J Exp Med 1994; 179:589-600.
44. Morrissey PJ, Charrier K, Braddy S et al. CD4+ T cells that express high levels of CD45RB induce wasting disease when transferred into congenic severe combined immunodeficient mice. Disease development is prevented by cotransfer of purified CD4+ T cells. J Exp Med 1993; 178:237-244.
45. Brimnes J, Reimann J, Nissen M et al. Enteric bacterial antigens activate CD4(+)T cells from scid mice with inflammatory bowel disease. Eur J Immunol 2001; 31:23-31.
46. Powrie F, Carlino J, Leach MW et al. A critical role for transforming growth factor-beta but not interleukin 4 in the suppression of T helper type 1-mediated colitis by CD45RB(low) CD4+ T cells. J Exp Med 1996; 183:2669-2674.
47. Kitani A, Fuss IJ, Nakamura K et al. Treatment of experimental (Trinitrobenzene sulfonic acid) colitis by intranasal administration of transforming growth factor (TGF)-beta1 plasmid: TGF-beta1-mediated suppression of T helper cell type 1 response occurs by interleukin (IL)-10 induction and IL-12 receptor beta2 chain downregulation. J Exp Med 2000; 192(1):41-52.
48. Asseman C, Mauze S, Leach MW et al. An essential role for interleukin 10 in the function of regulatory T cells that inhibit intestinal inflammation. J Exp Med 1999; 190:995-1004.
49. Asseman C, Fowler S, Powrie F. Control of experimental inflammatory bowel disease by regulatory T cells. Am J Respir Crit Care Med 2000; 162:S185-S189.
50. Cong Y, Weaver TC, Lazenby A et al. Bacterial-reactive T regulatory cells inhibit pathogenic immune responses to the enteric flora. J Immunol 2002; 169:6112-6119.
51. Khare SD, Luthra HS, David CS. Spontaneous inflammatory arthritis in HLA-B27 transgenic mice lacking beta 2-microglobulin: a model of human spondyloarthropathies. J Exp Med 1995; 182:1153-1158.
52. Rath HC, Wilson KH, Sartor RB. Differential induction of colitis and gastritis in HLA-B27 transgenic rats selectively colonized with Bacteroides vulgatus or Escherichia coli. Infect Immun 1999; 67:2969-2974.
53. Onderdonk AB, Franklin ML, Cisneros RL. Production of experimental ulcerative colitis in gnotobiotic guinea pigs with simplified microflora. Infect Immun 1981; 32:225-231.
54. Madsen KL, Doyle JS, Tavernini MM et al. Antibiotic therapy attenuates colitis in interleukin 10 gene-deficient mice. Gastroenterology 2000; 118:1094-1105.
55. Rath HC, Schultz M, Freitag R et al. Different subsets of enteric bacteria induce and perpetuate experimental colitis in rats and mice. Infect Immun 2001; 69:2277-2285.
56. Kishi D, Takahashi I, Kai Y et al. Alteration of V beta usage and cytokine production of CD4+ TCR beta beta homodimer T cells by elimination of Bacteroides vulgatus prevents colitis in TCR alpha-chain-deficient mice. J Immunol 2000; 165:5891-5899.

57. Sartor RB. Microbial factors in the pathogenesis of Crohn's disease, ulcerative colitis and experimental intestinal inflammation. In: Kirsner JB, ed. 5th Ed. Inflammatory Bowel Disease. W.B. Saunder Co., 2000:153-178.

58. Kullberg MC, Ward JM, Gorelick PL et al. Helicobacter hepaticus triggers colitis in specific-pathogen-free interleukin-10 (IL-10)-deficient mice through an IL-12- and gamma interferon-dependent mechanism. Infect Immun 1998; 66:5157-5166.

59. Higgins LM, Frankel G, Douce G et al. Citrobacter rodentium infection in mice elicits a mucosal Th1 cytokine response and lesions similar to those in murine inflammatory bowel disease. Infect Immun 1999; 67:3031-3039.

60. Dieleman LA, Arends A, Tonkonogy SL et al. Helicobacter hepaticus does not induce or potentiate colitis in interleukin-10-deficient mice. Infect Immun 2000; 68:5107-5113.

61. Shanahan F. Probiotics in inflamatory bowel disease. Gut 2001;4 8(5):609.

62. Schultz M, Sartor RB. Probiotics and inflammatory bowel diseases. Am J Gastroenterol 2000; 95:S19-S21.

63. Madsen KL, Doyle JS, Jewell LD et al. Lactobacillus species prevents colitis in interleukin 10 gene-deficient mice. Gastroenterology 1999; 116:1107-1114.

64. Mao Y, Nobaek S, Kasravi B et al. The effects of Lactobacillus strains and oat fiber on methotrexate-induced enterocolitis in rats. Gastroenterology 1996; 111:334-344.

65. Schultz M, Veltkamp C, Dieleman LA et al. Lactobacillus plantarum 299V in the treatment and prevention of spontaneous colitis in interleukin-10 deficient mice. Inflammat Bowel Dis 2002; 8:71-80.

66. Gionchetti P, Rizzello F, Venturi A et al. Oral bacteriotherapy as maintenance treatment in patients with chronic pouchitis: A double-blind, placebo-controlled trial. Gastroenterology 2000; 119:305-309.

67. Ulisse S, Gionchetti P, D'Alo S et al. Expression of cytokines, inducible nitric oxide synthase, and matrix metalloproteinases in pouchitis: effects of probiotic treatment. Am J Gastroenterol 2001; 96:2691-2699.

68. Chiang BL, Sheih YH, Wang LH et al. Enhancing immunity by dietary consumption of a probiotic lactic acid bacterium (Bifidobacterium lactis HN019): Optimization and definition of cellular immune responses. Eur J Clin Nutr 2000; 54:849-855.

69. Takagi A, Matsuzaki T, Sato M et al. Enhancement of natural killer cytotoxicity delayed murine carcinogenesis by a probiotic microorganism. Carcinogenesis 2001; 22:599-605.

70. Haller D, Blum S, Bode C, Hammes WP, Schiffrin EJ. Activation of human peripheral blood mononuclear cells by nonpathogenic bacteria in vitro: Evidence of NK cells as primary targets. Infect Immun 2000; 68:752-759.

71. Haller D, Serrant P, Granato D et al. Activation of human NK cells by staphylococci and lactobacilli required cell contact-dependent co-stimulation by autologous macrophages. Clin Diag Lab Immunol 2002; 9:649-653.

72. Hessle C, Andersson B, Wold AE. Gram-positive bacteria are potent inducers of monocytic interleukin-12 (IL-12) while gram-negative bacteria preferentially stimulate IL-10 production. Infect Immun 2000; 68:3581-3586.

73. Steidler L, Hans W, Schotte L et al. Treatment of murine colitis by Lactococcus lactis secreting interleukin-10. Science 2000; 289:1352-1355.

74. Roberfroid MB. Prebiotics:preferential substrates for specific germs? Am J Clin Nutr 2001; 73:406S-409S.

75. Böcker U, Nebe T, Herweck F et al. Butyrate modulates intestinal epithelial cell-mediated neutrophil migration. Clin Exp Immunol 2003; 181:53-60.

76. Mitsuyama K, Saiki T, Kanauchi O et al. Treatment of ulcerative colitis with germinated barley foodstuff feeding: A pilot study. Aliment Pharmacol Ther 1998; 12:1225-1230.

77. Framson PE, Cho DH, Lee LY et al. Polarized expression and function of the costimulatory molecule CD58 on human intestinal epithelial cells. Gastroenterology 1999; 116:1054-1062.

78. Nakazawa A, Watanabe M, Kanai T et al. Functional expression of costimulatory molecule CD86 on epithelial cells in the inflamed colonic mucosa. Gastroenterology 1999; 117:536-545.

79. Mayer L, Eisenhardt D. Lack of induction of suppressor T cells by intestinal epithelial cells from patients with inflammatory bowel disease. J Clin Invest 1990; 86:1255-1260.

80. Huang GT, Eckmann L, Savidge TC et al. Infection of human intestinal epithelial cells with invasive bacteria upregulates apical intercellular adhesion molecule-1 (ICAM)-1) expression and neutrophil adhesion. J Clin Invest 1996; 98:572-583.
81. Jung HC, Eckmann L, Yang SK et al. A distinct array of proinflammatory cytokines is expressed in human colon epithelial cells in response to bacterial invasion. J Clin Invest 1995; 95:55-65.
82. Kagnoff MF, Eckmann L. Epithelial cells as sensors for microbial infection. J Clin Invest 1997; 100:6-10.
83. Elewaut D, DiDonato JA, Kim JM et al. NF-kappa B is a central regulator of the intestinal epithelial cell innate immune response induced by infection with enteroinvasive bacteria. J Immunol 1999; 163:1457-1466.
84. Hobbie S, Chen LM, Davis RJ et al. Involvement of mitogen-activated protein kinase pathways in the nuclear responses and cytokine production induced by Salmonella typhimurium in cultured intestinal epithelial cells. J Immunol 1997; 159:5550-5559.
85. Beutler B. Tlr4: Central component of the sole mammalian LPS sensor. Curr Opin Immunol 2000; 12:20-26.
86. Zhang G, Ghosh S. Toll-like receptor-mediated NF-kappaB activation: A phylogenetically conserved paradigm in innate immunity. J Clin Invest 2001; 107:13-19.
87. Hoshino K, Takeuchi O, Kawai T et al. Cutting edge: Toll-like receptor 4 (TLR4)-deficient mice are hyporesponsive to lipopolysaccharide: evidence for TLR4 as the Lps gene product. J Immunol 1999; 162:3749-3752.
88. Qureshi ST, Lariviere L, Leveque G et al. Endotoxin-tolerant mice have mutations in Toll-like receptor 4 (Tlr4). J Exp Med 1999; 189:615-625.
89. Sundberg JP, Elson CO, Bedigian H et al. Spontaneous, heritable colitis in a new substrain of C3H/HeJ mice. Gastroenterology 1994; 107:1726-1735.
90. Hugot JP, Chamaillard M, Zouali H et al. Association of NOD2 leucine-rich repeat variants with susceptibility to Crohn's disease. Nature 2001; 411:599-603.
91. Ogura Y, Bonen DK, Inohara N et al. A frameshift mutation in NOD2 associated with susceptibility to Crohn's disease. Nature 2001; 411:603-606.
92. Cario E, Podolsky DK. Differential alteration in intestinal epithelial cell expression of toll-like receptor 3 (TLR3) and TLR4 in inflammatory bowel disease. Infect Immun 2000; 68:7010-7017.
93a. Haller D, Russo MP, Sartor RB et al. IKKβ and phosphatidyl-inositol 3-kinase/Akt participate in non-pathogenic gram-negative enteric bacteria induced RNA phosphrylations and NFκb activation in both primary and intestinal epithelial cell lines. J Biol Chem 2002; 277:38168-38178.
93b. Haller D, Holt L, Kim SC et al. Transforming growth factor β inhibits non-pathogenic gram negative bacteria-induced NF-κB recruitment to the IL-6 gene promotor in intestinal epithelial cells through modulation of histone acetylation. J Biol Chem 2003; 26:23851-23860.
94. Abreu MT, Vora P, Faure E et al. Decreased expression of Toll-like receptor-4 and MD-2 correlates with intestinal epithelial cell protection against dysregulated proinflammatory gene expression in response to bacterial lipopolysaccharide. J Immunol 2001; 167:1609-1616.
95. Jobin C, Haskill S, Mayer L et al. Evidence for altered regulation of I kappa B alpha degradation in human colonic epithelial cells. J Immunol 1997; 158:226-234.
96. Jobin C, Sartor RB. The I kappa B/NF-kappa B system: A key determinant of mucosalinflammation and protection. Am J Physiol Cell Physiol 2000; 278:C451-C462.
97. Cario E, Podolsky DK. Differential alteration in intestinal epithelial cell expression of toll-like receptor 3 (TLR3) and TLR4 in inflammatory bowel disease. Infect Immun 2000; 68:7010-7017.
98. Haller D, Bode C, Hammes WP et al. Non-pathogenic bacteria elicit a differential cytokine response by intestinal epithelial cell/leucocyte co-cultures. Gut 2000; 47:79-87.
99. Grimm MC, Pavli P, Van de Pol E et al. Evidence for a CD14+ population of monocytes in inflammatory bowel disease mucosa—Implications for pathogenesis. Clin Exp Immunol 1995; 100:291-297.
100. Rugtveit J, Nilsen EM, Bakka A et al. Cytokine profiles differ in newly recruited and resident subsets of mucosal macrophages from inflammatory bowel disease. Gastroenterology 1997; 112:1493-1505.
101. Spottl T, Hausmann M, Kreutz M et al. Monocyte differentiation in intestine-like macrophage phenotype induced by epithelial cells. J Leukoc Biol 2001; 70:241-251.

102. Haller D, Serrant P, Peruisseau G et al. IL-10 producing CD14low monocytes inhibit lymphocyte-dependent activation of intestinal epithetial cells by commensial bacteria. Microbiol Immunol 2002; 46:195-205.
103. Hooper LV, Wong MH, Thelin A et al. Molecular analysis of commensal host-microbial relationships in the intestine. Science 2001; 291:881-884.
104. Lopez-Boado YS, Wilson CL, Hooper LV et al. Bacterial exposure induces and activates matrilysin in mucosal epithelial cells. J Cell Biol 2000; 148:1305-1315.
105. Auer IO, Roder A, Wensinck F et al. Selected bacterial antibodies in Crohn's disease and ulcerative colitis. Scand J Gastroenterol 1983; 18:217-223.
106. Tabaqchali S, O'Donoghue DP, Bettelheim KA. Escherichia coli antibodies in patients with inflammatory bowel disease. Gut 1978; 19:108-113.
107. Sutton CL, Kim J, Yamane A et al. Identification of a novel bacterial sequence associated with Crohn's disease. Gastroenterology 2000; 119:23-31.
108. Macpherson A, Khoo UY, Forgacs I et al. Mucosal antibodies in inflammatory bowel disease are directed against intestinal bacteria. Gut 1996; 38:365-375.
109. Cohavy O, Bruckner D, Gordon LK et al. Colonic bacteria express an ulcerative colitis pANCA-related protein epitope. Infect Immun 2000; 68:1542-1548.
110. Halstensen TS, Mollnes TE, Brandtzaeg P. Persistent complement activation in submucosal blood vessels of active inflammatory bowel disease: immunohistochemical evidence. Gastroenterology 1989; 97:10-19.
111. Duchmann R, Kaiser I, Hermann E et al. Tolerance exists towards resident intestinal flora but is broken in active inflammatory bowel disease (IBD). Clin Exp Immunol 1995; 102:448-455.
112. Duchmann R, Schmitt E, Knolle P et al. Tolerance towards resident intestinal flora in mice is abrogated in experimental colitis and restored by treatment with interleukin-10 or antibodies to interleukin-12. Eur J Immunol 1996; 26:934-938.
113. Duchmann R, May E, Heike M et al. T cell specificity and cross reactivity towards enterobacteria, bacteroides, bifidobacterium, and antigens from resident intestinal flora in humans. Gut 1999; 44:812-818.
114. Harper PH, Lee EC, Kettlewell MG et al. Role of the faecal stream in the maintenance of Crohn's colitis. Gut 1985; 26:279-284.
115. Rutgeerts P, Goboes K, Peeters M et al. Effect of faecal stream diversion on recurrence of Crohn's disease in the neoterminal ileum. Lancet 1991; 338:771-774.
116. D'Haens GR, Geboes K, Peeters M et al. Early lesions of recurrent Crohn's disease caused by infusion of intestinal contents in excluded ileum. Gastroenterology 1998; 114:262-267.
117. Colombel JF, Cortot A, van Kruiningen HJ. Antibiotics in Crohn's disease. Gut 2001; 48:647
118. Sutherland L, Singleton J, Sessions J et al. Double blind, placebo controlled trial of metronidazole in Crohn's disease. Gut 1991; 32:1071-1075.
119. Fuss IJ, Neurath M, Boirivant M et al. Disparate CD4+ lamina propria (LP) lymphokine secretion profiles in inflammatory bowel disease. Crohn's disease LP cells manifest increased secretion of IFN-gamma, whereas ulcerative colitis LP cells manifest increased secretion of IL-5. J Immunol 1996; 157:1261-1270.
120. Turunen U, Farkkila, Valtonen V. Long-term treatment of ulcerative colitis with ciprofloxacin. Gastroenterology 1999; 117:282-300.

CHAPTER 8

Food and Milk Allergies

Mary H. Perdue and Martine Heyman

Introduction

Oral tolerance is the usual response to antigens encountered via the gut mucosal immune system. However in some individuals, ingestion of food antigens does not result in a down-regulated system, but rather an immunologically-mediated allergic reaction. Such reactions occur in ~2-5% of the population and commonly induce gastrointestinal symptoms. Other organ systems, such as the airways and skin, can also be involved. True food allergies/hypersensitivities are caused by antigen cross-linking of IgE antibodies bound to receptors on mucosal mast cells. Mast cell-derived mediators then act on cells in the local environment to alter physiology. A critical step in the reaction is the penetration of antigen through the epithelial lining of the intestine. This Chapter will describe experiments, mainly in animal models, that have contributed to our current understanding of the mechanisms involved in the pathology/pathophysiology of food and milk allergies. We will not provide extensive detail on all studies, but rather will give an overview of the clinical problem and then describe experimental findings with an emphasis on recent novel results related to the role of intestinal epithelial cells in food allergies.

Overview of Food Sensitization

Adverse reactions to foods are relatively common. Symptoms may occur due to the inability to digest or absorb various food constituents, or may be due to chemical sensitivity to certain additives or contaminants. These are food intolerances rather than food allergies and will not be dealt with here. True food allergy is an immunologically-mediated reaction which occurs only in sensitized individuals in response to a specific food antigen. Allergies in general (including asthma) are the largest group of immune disorders affecting 20-30% of the population in North America and Europe. The incidence of food allergy is thought to be ~5% in children under the age of 3 years (with cow's milk allergy being the most significant) and ~2% of adults. However, these figures may not be accurate since food allergies are difficult to diagnose, with symptoms resembling many other enteropathies. In addition, the presenting symptoms may occur in the airways or skin with minimal perturbations of gastrointestinal function. In children, the most common reactions occur to proteins in milk, eggs and nuts, while in adults fish, shellfish and nuts are the major culprits. Celiac disease, which is a specific reaction to the wheat protein, gliadin, involves another category of immune reaction and is the subject of an earlier Chapter.

Exposure to small quantities of antigen intermittently may enhance the allergic reaction. On the other hand, children appear to outgrow some food allergies. However, it is clear that

Oral Tolerance: The Response of the Intestinal Mucosa to Dietary Antigens,
edited by Olivier Morteau. ©2004 Eurekah.com and Kluwer Academic / Plenum Publishers.

intestinal hypersensitivity reactions cause disability for a significant proportion of the population. In addition, peanut allergy can induce systemic anaphylaxis and in some cases be fatal. Hundreds of deaths occur annually due to anaphylactic reactions, with the majority being reactions to food antigens. Currently, the only effective recognized treatment for food allergy is avoidance of offending food(s). In situations where the antigen is unidentified or multiple antigens are involved, diets can become so restrictive that nutrition is compromised. This is true particularly for young children. Therefore, it is important to have a clear understanding of the pathophysiological mechanisms involved in food allergy in order to develop effective therapeutic approaches.

The Clinical Problem of Food and Milk Allergy

Food allergy was first investigated scientifically in 1921, as reported in the classic study by Prausnitz and Kustner.[1] Following injection of serum from Kustner (who reacted to fish) into the skin of Prausnitz, subsequent ingestion of fish by Prausnitz resulted in the development of a wheal-and-flare response at the skin site. We now know that the critical factor in serum responsible for the reaction is IgE immunoglobulin. IgE is the antibody isotype responsible for the rapidly occurring "immediate" hypersensitivity allergic reactions. IgE is normally present in the blood in concentrations which are minimal (1/10,000) compared with IgG. Even in allergic individuals, the level of IgE is well below the mg/ml quantity of IgG in the circulation, and may not be significantly elevated above control values. However, in spite of relatively low circulating levels, IgE can be present in tissues bound to mast cells via its high affinity receptor, FcεRI. Although the half-life of IgE in blood is short, IgE can remain bound to gut mucosal mast cells for a long time. Low affinity IgE receptors, FcεRII, are present on several other cell types. Skin prick tests are often but not always indicative of allergy to a specific food antigen. The only effective and accepted diagnosis of food allergy is a specific response to a double-blind, placebo-controlled oral food challenge.[2]

In most cases of intestinal anaphylaxis, the symptoms include nausea, vomiting, diarrhea and crampy abdominal pain. These may develop as soon as a few minutes after ingesting the food allergen. In controlled trials, local gastrointestinal responses include hyperemia and edema of mucosal tissues, delayed gastric emptying and altered peristalsis of the small intestine associated with mast cell degranulation and histamine release.[3] In oral allergy syndrome, changes in the oropharynx develop rapidly, with symptoms of pruritis and angioedema of the lips, tongue and throat.[4] As indicated above, IgE may not be greatly elevated in the blood of affected individuals. However, high levels of circulating antigen-specific IgE correlate with sensitivity to a wider range of antigens, reactions at extraintestinal sites and longer lasting reactions not outgrown in childhood.[5] In addition, there are several reports of increased concentrations of IgE in duodenal contents of food allergic individuals.[6,7]

Cow's milk allergy in infants and young children is characterized by complex clinical responses. Milk-induced allergic reactions can cause a variety of symptoms involving the gastrointestinal tract, skin and/or respiratory tract. The symptoms are not restricted to anaphylactic IgE-mediated reactions and may develop several hours or days after ingestion of relatively large amount of cow's milk.[2] Although IgE-mediated milk allergy has been most clearly documented, nonIgE-mediated immune reactions, especially of the gastrointestinal tract, are being increasingly recognized. The treatment of cow's milk allergy consists of avoidance of cow's milk protein in the diet and substitution with extensively hydrolyzed casein or whey proteins. In certain circumstances, the maternal diet may also have to involve elimination of dairy products since the child may become allergic to food proteins transferred by breast feeding.[8]

Sensitization to Food Antigens in Humans and Animals

It is not clear how humans become sensitized to food/milk proteins. Increased permeability of the intestinal epithelium during early life when protective immunity is not established may result in an inappropriate immune response to undegraded antigens which gain access to the mucosa. Barrier function can become defective during infectious or inflammatory conditions. Certainly, genetic factors can predispose infants to allergy since it is more common in families with a history of atopy. However, food allergies can also occur without a previous family history.

Some hints on the etiology of food allergy may be gleaned from animal models. Rodents are commonly made sensitive to specific proteins by injection (usually s.c. or i.p.) of the protein together with adjuvants which skew the immune response toward a TH2 response. The most potent adjuvant is pertussis toxin which requires enzymatic activity for its effect.[9] Rats injected with as little as 5-50 ng of pertussis retained sensitivity of the gastrointestinal tract to antigen, in this case ovalbumin (OVA), for at least 8 months, compared with a couple of weeks for rats injected with the protein alone. Pertussis is known to stimulate IL-4 synthesis.[10] In addition, pertussis increases sensitivity to histamine.[11] Other bacterial toxins (e.g., cholera toxin, *E. coli* heat labile toxin) have been used as adjuvants to influence immune responses to antigens delivered via the oral route.[12,13] This suggests that excessive exposure to bacteria or bacterial products/ toxins may be involved in sensitization to foods. However, the oral route of antigen exposure is not commonly used in experimental models of allergy since sensitization is more difficult to achieve, presumably due to limited uptake of intact antigen across the epithelial barrier. Substances which break the epithelial barrier may result in more consistent sensitization to coadministered antigens.[14] In addition, stress has recently been shown to increase gut epithelial permeability for macromolecules in rodents.[15] The role of genetic factors has clearly been established in animal models since certain rat strains are known as high responders (e.g., Brown Norway), and BALB/c mice are much easier to sensitize than C57B6 mice which require several boosts (antigen injections) for a good response. This is due to skewing of the immune response towards TH1 (C57B6) versus TH2 (Brown Norway, BALB/c). In addition, the antigen itself is important since some strains develop sensitivity to one protein, e.g., OVA, but not to another, e.g., horseradish peroxidase (HRP); whereas other strains can be sensitized to almost any protein.

Models of milk allergy have traditionally used guinea pigs since these animals develop milk protein sensitivity after drinking milk for several days.[16] In addition, mice have been sensitized to milk proteins by injection and also by feeding milk or milk proteins with cholera toxin.[17]

Indications of Sensitization in Animal Models

The level of IgE in serum is the most common readout to indicate sensitization in most models of allergy. However, circulating IgE can be low or even below the limit of detection in animals with strong intestinal responses to oral antigen challenge. Receptors on epithelial cells may contribute to removal of IgE from the circulation (to be discussed in a subsequent section). Some subtypes of IgG also have reaginic properties. Other nonfunctional readouts include increased numbers of mast cells (and possibly other inflammatory cells) in the gut mucosa. Histamine release from gut tissues in response to antigen has also been used as well as release of other mast cell mediators, particularly proteases such as rat mast cell protease II (RMCP II).[18,19] With respect to changes in gastrointestinal function, a very sensitive readout is the antigen-induced electrophysiological response of sensitized intestinal tissues in Ussing chambers. The short-circuit current (Isc) is a direct measure of net ion transport and increases within seconds or minutes after addition of specific antigen to either the serosal side or mucosal (luminal) side of the tissue, respectively.[20] The Isc is continuously recorded and provides an instant, consistent and reliable marker of the intestinal anaphylactic reaction. Recently, a more delayed increase in tissue conductance and permeability has been identified to occur, beginning at ~30 minutes post-challenge.[21,22] Generally, in vivo readouts are less sensitive; however, motility changes can also be used if the animal is suitably prepared.[23]

Antigen-Induced Intestinal Pathophysiology in Rodent Models of Food Allergy

Studies conducted over the last 20 years have provided a significant body of information on changes in intestinal function in response to oral antigen in sensitized animals. An early in vivo study[18] reported that perfusion of the jejunum of sensitized rats with antigen (ovalbumin, OVA) containing buffer resulted in decreased absorption of water, Na^+ and K^+, while absorption of Cl^- was reversed to secretion. These transport changes were associated with signs of mast cell activation indicated by fewer stained cells in the perfused tissues and release of histamine into the perfusate. However, when the mast cell stabilizer, doxantrazole, was included in the buffer, the transport defect was prevented.[24] This type of response was more thoroughly investigated by studying tissues from sensitized animals in vitro in Ussing chambers where antigen-induced active secretion of Cl^- was found to be responsible for the Isc increase,[20,25] and in vivo the main driving force for the water secretion.[18] Antagonists or inhibitors added to the bath before the antigen challenge revealed that several mast cell mediators were responsible for the intestinal anaphylactic response. These included histamine, serotonin and prostaglandins, etc.[20] More recently, mast cell proteases acting on protease activated receptors (PARs) have been implicated in secretory responses.[26] Table 1 lists mast cell mediators which can alter gut function. Neural blocking drugs such as tetrodotoxin or capsaicin have been shown to reduce the antigen-induced secretory responses,[20,27] suggesting an amplification step involving mucosal nerves (see below). In addition, exaggerated secretory responses to various agonists were documented in the jejunum of sensitized rats[20] and the colon of milk-sensitized guinea pigs[28] not unlike the hyper-responsiveness in airways of atopic asthmatic patients.

Close anatomical associations between mast cells and nerves were reported in the mucosa of rats, both under baseline conditions and after a nematode infection when mast cell numbers increase dramatically.[29] This intimate relationship was shown statistically to be nonrandom. The types of nerves involved in this study were C-type fibers containing substance P or CGRP. Experiments in mice lacking mast cells confirmed the importance of bidirectional signalling between mast cells and nerves in the gut mucosa.[27] Regardless of which cell type was activated (mast cells by antigen, nerves by transmural field stimulation), the response was greatly diminished without the participation of the other cell type. It is clear that several mast cell mediators act on mucosal nerves to enhance their reactivity and a number of neurotransmitters can activate mast cells.[30]

Another cell type must be included when examining the effects of mast cells/mediators on ion transport. Fibroblasts form a scaffolding supporting the epithelium. These cells synthesize bioactive chemicals, particularly prostaglandins, in response to many inflammatory mediators.[31] The importance of these cells was demonstrated by culturing epithelial cells on a layer of fibroblasts and then comparing responses with those of epithelial cells alone. With epithelial cells alone, only a small response was initiated by several mediators and cytokines; however, larger sustained responses occurred in the presence of fibroblasts.[32] For the most part, inhibition of cyclooxygenase enzymes reversed these effects, suggesting that prostanoids are the final common mediators for changes in immunophysiology.

Thus following oral antigen exposure, the antigen crosses the epithelium and cross-links IgE antibodies on the mast cell surface. A cascade of signals in the mast cell culminates with the release of granular contents from the cells. Mast cell mediators may act directly on epithelial

Table 1. Mast cell mediators

Class of Mediator	Class	Examples
Preformed	Amines	Histamine, serotonin (rodents)
	Proteases	Tryptase, chymase, carboxypeptidase RMCPII, etc (rodents) Metalloprotease
	Proteoglycans	Heparin, chondroitin sulphate
	Cytokines	TNF-α
Rapidly formed	Leukotrienes	LTC$_3$, LTD$_4$, LTE$_4$ PAF
	Prostaglandins	PGD$_2$, PGE$_2$
Newly synthesized	Cytokines	IL-1, IL-3, IL-4, IL-6, IL-9, IL-13, TNF-α
	Chemokines	IL-5, IL-8, IL-16, MIP-1α
	Growth factors	TGF-β, VGF/VEGF, β-FGF GM-CSF, SCF, NGF

Mast cell mediators are either preformed and stored, rapidly synthesized after activation, or slowly generated after IgE cross-linking. Information may be slightly different in different species and different types of mast cells. Abbreviations: βFGF, fibroblast growth factor; GM-CSF, granulocyte-macrophage growth factor; IL, interleukin; LT, leukotriene; MCP, monocyte chemoattractant protein; PAF, platelet-activating factor; PG, prostaglandin; NGF, nerve growth factor; RMCPII, rat mast cell protease II; SCF, stem cell factor; TGF, transforming growth factor; TNF, tumor necrosis factor; VPFF/VEGF, vascular permeability factor/vascular endothelial cell growth factor

cells to induce functional changes, but in most cases the responses are amplified by activation of subepithelial fibroblasts and mucosal nerves. Figure 1 depicts a schema showing the events described. As indicated, mast cell activation leads to ion and water secretion (and ultimately diarrhea). This response occurs within minutes of oral antigen challenge. Epithelial permeability increases, but this appears to be somewhat delayed after mast cell activation, with conductance rising at ~30 minutes,[22] possibly due to RMCP II which has a slower rate of release from mast cells and has been shown to disrupt gut permeability.[33] Lumen to blood transport of both small and large molecules was also enhanced in vivo following intraluminal antigen challenge, and this permeability change was also dependent in part on neural activation.[34] Mucous secretion has also been described following mast cell activation.[35] Motility is also affected with interruption of the migrating motor complex and spike-like contractions developing in association with diarrhea in rats.[23]

The Late Phase Intestinal Anaphylactic Reaction in Rodents

Late phase reactions are well-known in the airways where several hours after an immediate hypersensitivity reaction there is a subsequent phase of release of inflammatory mediators associated with histopathological changes and clinical symptoms.[36] In the gut, functional and structural changes which last for several days after oral antigen challenge have been identified in sensitized rats. Epithelial dysfunction, including ion secretion (elevated Isc) and enhanced permeability, was evident for at least 72 hours associated with intestinal tissue edema and ultrastructural signs of damage.[22] In addition, by 48 hours epithelial mitochondria appeared swollen with loss of cristae, and autophagosomes were present in many mitochondria. The basement

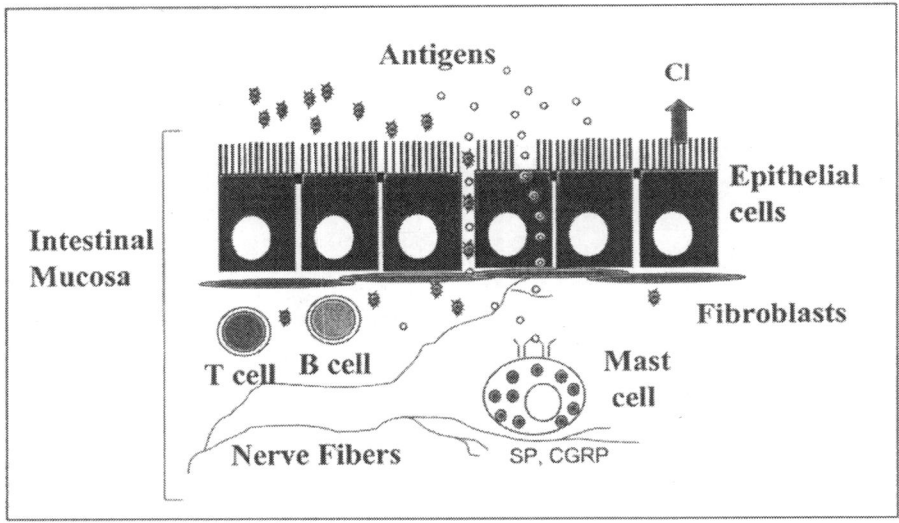

Figure 1. Cross-linking of mast cell-bound IgE by antigen results in release of mediators which stimulate mucosal nerves. In addition, some mediators activate fibroblasts to generate prostaglandins. The overall secretory response is due to both direct effects of the bioactive compounds on the epithelium, as well as indirect effects of nerves and fibroblasts which amplify the response.

membrane was frequently disrupted and eosinophils and lymphocytes were observed penetrating into the epithelial layer. Spaces appeared in these regions with actual sloughing of epithelial cells in some sections.

Infiltration of inflammatory cells into the mucosa was also documented by counting numbers of specific cells within a defined area of the lamina propria. Sensitization alone resulted in greater numbers of mast cells, eosinophils, neutrophils and mononuclear cells in the intestinal mucosa.[22] After antigen challenge, a biphasic pattern of increased mast cells was demonstrated, with peaks at 0.5 and 72 hours, coinciding with release of RMCP II. Neutrophil numbers followed a similar but less obvious pattern to that of mast cells, whereas the number of eosinophils decreased after antigen exposure and then increased again with the greatest number being present at 48 hours. In contrast, mononuclear cells continued to accumulate in the mucosa, reaching a peak at 48 hours when the number was 10 fold greater compared with controls. Studies in mice have also reported gut inflammatory changes in the late phase allergic reaction. For example, several hours after antigen challenge of mice, infiltration into jejunal mucosa of mast cells, eosinophils and intraepithelial lymphocytes was described.[37] Wershil et al[38] reported neutrophil and mononuclear cell infiltration in the stomach of mice after antigen challenge, with neutrophils peaking at 2 hours and mononuclear cells rising several fold at 12-24 hours. In another study,[39] mast cell influx was observed at 1 hour, villus edema at 3 hours, eosinophil infiltration at 6 hours, and villus atrophy associated with increased numbers of lymphocytes at 24 hours, although exact counts were not performed. Increased permeability was documented at 1, 6, and 24 hours with decreases between the peaks. In general, the most severe morphological, ultrastructural and physiological changes appear to coincide in time with the greatest inflammatory cell accumulation within the tissues, suggesting that the additional inflammatory cells contribute to the mucosal damage.

Mast cells appeared to be critical for recruiting (and possibly activating) the other inflammatory cells since no inflammatory cell infiltration occurred in mast cell-deficient rats.[23] Mast cells synthesize and secrete several factors with chemotactic properties, such as TNFα IL-5, leukotriene B4, platelet-activating factor, complement C5a and various other cytokines/chemokines.[40] In addition, cross-linking of the IgE receptor stimulates synthesis of additional mediators and cytokines/chemokines which are likely to be involved in the late phase reaction.[41] Mast cells have been shown to be required for neutrophil accumulation in the stomach after local antigen challenge of sensitized mice, with TNFα playing a major role.[38,42] Thus, there is evidence for mast cell-dependent recruitment of inflammatory cells into the gastrointestinal tract. Data from both in vivo and in vitro systems suggest that mast cells may serve a "gatekeeper" function by regulating leukocyte migration at the level of microvascular endothelium that is a key step in initiating the late phase reaction.[43] In addition, TNFα, RMCP II, histamine and other mast cell mediators have been shown to induce pathophysiological changes in the gastrointestinal tract.[44-46]

Transepithelial Transport of Antigenic Molecules

The pathway/mechanism of transepithelial antigen transport appears to be a critical regulatory step both in the induction of an allergic immune response versus oral tolerance and in the effector reaction occurring in a previously sensitized host. The intestinal epithelium normally acts as a barrier to restrict the uptake of luminal antigens. This barrier is maintained because epithelial cells (mainly absorptive enterocytes) are joined at their apical poles by junctional complexes which prevent the passage of macromolecules between cells. Most ingested protein is digested within the gut lumen by secreted enzymes, by enzymes anchored to the enterocyte microvillus membrane or lysosomal enzymes within the cell. However, a small quantity of intact antigen does escape enzymatic breakdown[47] and therefore has the potential to stimulate the local or systemic immune system. Although tight junctions between intestinal epithelial cells do not allow the diffusion of luminal macromolecules toward the internal milieu by the paracellular route, enterocytes do have the capacity to transport a small proportion of antigenic material from the intestinal lumen to the underlying tissues by transcytosis.

There is evidence that tolerance after feeding is dependent on gut processing of fed antigens, and that "gut processed" antigens may transfer tolerance.[48,49] However, the precise role of the intestinal epithelium in this phenomenon is not clearly understood. Macromolecular transport by the gut epithelium was extensively analyzed in the 1970s by Walker et al.[50] The role of gut epithelium in the processing of food proteins for the mucosal immune system has been evaluated more recently in vitro in human intestinal cell lines or intestinal biopsies mounted in Ussing chambers. Using radiolabelled proteins, it was shown that more than 90% of endocytosed protein is degraded during transepithelial transport, while 10% is transported intact to the serosal compartment[51] (Fig. 2). Both the direct and degradative pathways are transcellular, as shown by the inhibitory effect of metabolic inhibitors and cytoskeleton-disrupting drugs.[51] In the rat, uptake of HRP is greater in the ileum than colon, although only enzymatic activity was measured (MP, unpublished). Paracellular diffusion of antigens through the tight junctions is negligible under physiological conditions, since the integrity of tight junctions is maintained even at sites of desquamation.[52]

Food antigens can be absorbed in the stomach,[53] small intestine[54] and colon.[55] Transcytotic activity increases from the proximal to the distal part of the digestive tract, with the degradative pathway predominating particularly in the distal intestine (MH, unpublished). This might be due to the stimulating role of the intestinal microflora since intestinal antigen transport in germ-free mice is four times less than in conventional mice.[56] The location of antigen sampling is not confined to the absorptive epithelium, but also takes place across M cells in the epithelium overlying Peyer's patches.[54] Peyer's patches are recognized as the inductive site for mucosal immune responses to particulate antigens such as viruses or bacteria, and they may also participate, at least partly, in the acquisition of oral tolerance for soluble antigens.[57]

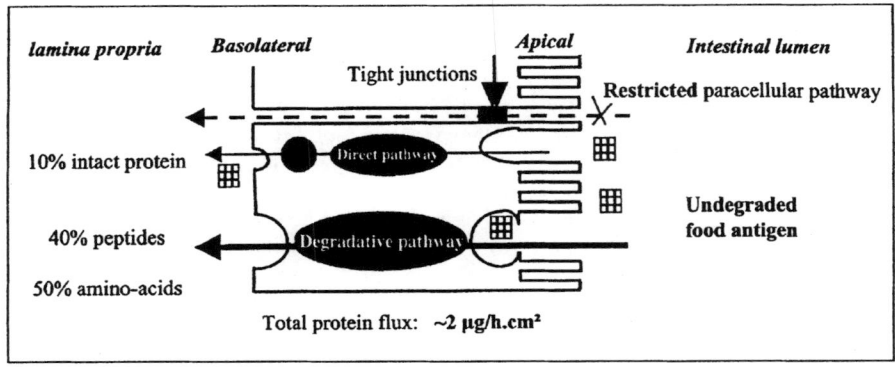

Figure 2. Food antigens that have escaped intraluminal degradation by digestive enzymes reach the intestinal lumen where a small portion is endocytosed and transported toward the lamina propria along two functional pathways, one allowing 10% of the internalized proteins to be transported intact, the other allowing most (90%) of the protein to be processed into peptides or completely hydrolyzed into amino-acids. Peptides formed during transepithelial transport have a molecular mass compatible with the binding to restriction molecules (MHC or MHC-like molecules). In normal conditions, the paracellular (between intestinal epithelial cells) pathway is impermeant to macomolecules. Although the amount of antigenic material absorbed remains very small (less than 2 µg per hour and cm^2 of surface area, it plays an important role in directing the mucosal immune response (from refs 22 and 41).

Intestinal epithelial cells have been described as nonprofessional antigen presenting cells,[58-61] at least in vitro. The studies on epithelial antigen processing and presentation were stimulated by the discovery of MHC molecule expression by absorptive enterocytes.[61] Therefore, one might postulate that MHC class II molecules (HLA-DR), which are moderately expressed in basal conditions in vivo, and highly up-regulated in inflammatory conditions, may interfere with the nature and/or the quantity of antigen-derived peptides formed during transepithelial transport. Indeed, a recent study has shown that the processing of HRP by HT29-19A intestinal monolayers led to the transport of 10% intact protein, 40% peptides and 50% aminoacids,[62] indicating that half of the protein endocytosed by these cells may still retain the potential to react with immune cells. Interestingly, the peptides formed during the transepithelial transport had a molecular mass (~1100 daltons) compatible with their binding to restriction molecules. In addition, IFNγ stimulated not only a paracellular leakage of the protein but also transcellular transport, enhancing the quantity of peptides penetrating the mucosa. It is possible that binding to restriction molecules protects peptides/proteins from further degradation.

Recent studies have identified that intestinal epithelial cells secrete exosome-like vesicles which express MHC class II/peptide complexes, at least in inflammatory conditions.[63] These exosomes may act as messengers to transmit peptidic information to nonadjacent T cells. Indeed, exosomes are small membrane vesicles secreted by multiple cell types. Professional antigen presenting cells such as dendritic cells or B lymphocytes secrete class-I and class-II carrying exosomes that stimulate T cell proliferation in vitro.[64] The role of epithelial-derived exosomes in the induction of oral tolerance or hypersensitivity is currently a matter of investigation. On the other hand, it is noteworthy that either differential induction of immediate-type hypersensitivity or T cell proliferation may occur, depending on whether there are changes in peptide structure or in MHC haplotype, at least when conventional antigen presenting cells are concerned.[65] This possibility might explain why an association between HLA haplotypes and susceptibility to various diseases such as celiac disease is often reported.

The Potential Role of Epithelial Cells in the Development of Food Allergies

Both the quantity of antigen absorbed together with the effect of enteric infections and inflammation are thought to influence the outcome of antigen presentation to underlying T cells and to direct the immune response toward tolerance or allergy. During viral or bacterial infections of the digestive tract, intestinal permeability to food antigens generally increases, due to epithelial damage induced by the infectious agents and to the inflammatory reaction. In the context of such an inflammatory environment, the local antigen presenting cells (mainly dendritic cells) are switched from a tolerogenic to an immunogenic state.[66] Indeed, in a model of sulfonic acid-induced colitis in guinea-pigs, it was shown that the rate and intensity of sensitization to cow's milk proteins was increased compared to nontreated animals.[14]

Few studies have reported a clear link between increased uptake of food antigens and the development of food allergy (or the breakdown of oral tolerance). It has often been suggested that infections, by disrupting the epithelial barrier and increasing antigen absorption, would lead to intestinal dysfunction and persistent diarrhea. Rotavirus infection, which is the most frequent cause of diarrhea in childhood, has been shown to disturb antigen handling by the gut.[67] The frequency of persistent diarrhea following viral enteritis suggests that sensitization to food antigens may occur during the infection[68] and certain viruses may contribute to the allergic sensitization process.[69] Bacterial enteric infections also lead to intestinal lesions, such as the effacement of microvilli or damage to the intercellular junctions by cytotoxins.[70] These lesions may interfere with the barrier function of the epithelium or with the endocytic capacity of enterocytes.[55,71] In weanling rabbits, enteroadherent *E. coli* infection (RDEC1) increased the rate of transcytosis and delayed the gut closure to food protein antigens.[72] However, this increased intestinal transport did not lead to increased allergic sensitization.[73] It was recently reported that the gastric pathogen *H. pylori* induces altered protein processing by the digestive epithelium, leading to increased transepithelial transport of intact proteins.[74] This result may be linked to the observation that persistent gastric inflammation is often observed, even after eradication of the bacteria, suggesting that sensitization to bystander food antigens may have occurred. This hypothesis is strengthened by the observation that *H. pylori* infection is often associated with the development of allergic disorders.[75,76]

Finally, in guinea pigs, the increased intestinal permeability to milk proteins that was observed in malnourished animals was associated with higher β-lactoglobulin specific IgG and IgE titers and with an enhanced intestinal anaphylactic response to β-lactoglobulin, compared to the well-nourished animals[77] (Fig. 3). Therefore, not only the genetic susceptibility of the host, but also other factors interfering with antigen presentation (type of antigen, type and status of the antigen presenting cell, presence of bacterial adjuvants, expression of costimulatory molecules at the time of presentation, cytokines present during T cell activation) are likely to play a role in the development of allergic responses to the intestinal absorption of food antigens.

Intestinal Microflora and Allergic Disorders

Among the environmental factors that modulate oral tolerance versus allergy, the bacterial microflora is an important one. There are apparently contradictory findings on the effect of intestinal microorganisms on the immune response to luminal antigens. On the one hand, the commensal microflora are necessary for the full induction and the maintenance of oral tolerance,[78,79] including the IgE production system,[80] but on the other hand, a strong immune response to an orally administered antigen is obtained when the antigen is encountered by the gut associated lymphoid tissue together with microorganisms capable of stimulating antigen presentation.[81] This has recently been explained by the fact that dendritic cells of the intestinal

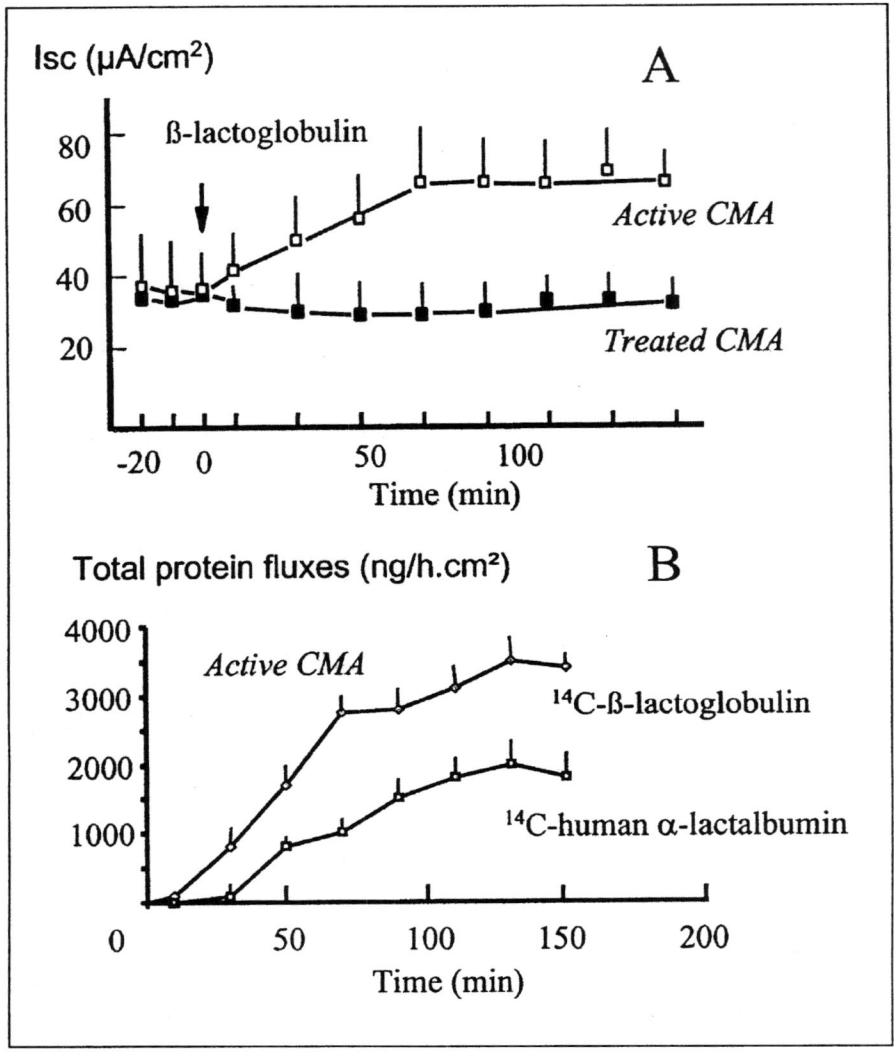

Figure 3. Changes in intestinal function in infants with active cow's milk allergy (CMA, intestinal symptoms) versus treated infants (no symptoms). A) Duodenal biopsies were mounted in Ussing chambers (exposed area 0.1 cm²) and β-lactoglobulin (β-Lg), the antigen) was added to the mucosal compartment. A rise in Isc which was related to an increased chloride secretion (inhibited by bumetanide) was observed in the infants in the active phase of the disease whereas in treated infants (on cow's milk free diet), β-Lg does not trigger any secretion in vitro. B) In Active CMA infants, β-Lg (sensitizing antigen) is transported very rapidly from mucosa to serosa; however, transport is normalized in CMA infants after treatment (from ref 38).

mucosa have an important role to play in the induction of oral tolerance and that the regulation of intestinal responses to soluble antigens via dendritic cell presentation, depends on the presence or the absence of inflammatory signals.[82] In addition, it is interesting to note that nonpathogenic enteric bacteria, interacting directly with a model human epithelium, have recently been shown to attenuate the synthesis of proinflammatory effector molecules (NFkB) elicited by diverse proinflammatory stimuli.[83] The mechanism of such an inhibitory effect consisted in the blockade of IkB-α degradation, preventing subsequent nuclear translocation of active NF-kB dimer and the transcription of genes for inflammatory cytokines. In that context, the use of nonpathogenic enteric organisms such as probiotics are now being explored as therapeutic agents in inflammatory bowel disease.[84] Among their beneficial effects on the intestinal physiology, probiotics have been shown to improve the clinical symptoms of infants with atopic dermatitis. Indeed, an improvement in the clinical score (skin lesions) was observed when the extensively hydrolyzed milk formula used as a treatment, was supplemented with *Lactobacillus rhamnosus GG*.[85] These results suggest that the intestinal microflora are of the utmost importance in maintaining immune homeostasis at the intestinal level. The wide use of antibiotics has been proposed as a contributory factor in the development of atopic diseases,[86] suggesting that frequent unnecessary treatments with antibiotics should be avoided during the first year of life.

Enhanced Transepithelial Antigen Transport in Sensitized Animals

Both in sensitized humans and in animal models of food allergy, it is clear that responses to food antigens can occur very quickly, usually within minutes. Sensitized intestinal tissues in Ussing chambers develop a secretory response, indicated by the rise in Isc, within ~3 minutes after the addition of the sensitizing antigen to the luminal buffer. This is somewhat delayed beyond the beginning of the Isc response to antigen added to the serosal buffer (20 seconds), but much faster than would be expected based on our understanding of transcytosis which normally takes ~20 minutes.[87] It is clear that subepithelial mast cells are the effector cells in both cases. Taken together, these findings suggest that the process for transepithelial antigen transport is altered in food allergy. Rats sensitized to HRP were used to examine the rate and route of antigen transport across the epithelium,[22] since its reaction product can be visualized within tissues by electron microscopy. This study demonstrated that transport was indeed enhanced but only for the sensitizing (but not a bystander) antigen. The specificity implies recognition of antigen at the level of the epithelium, potentially by cell bound immunoglobulin. Further studies[88] identified two phases of antigen transport following sensitization: phase I (described above) is antigen specific but mast cell independent; phase II occurs only after mast cell activation and results in a general increase in permeability of the paracellular pathway (alluded to in an earlier section).

A subsequent paper[89] identified that the specific nature of the enhanced antigen transport is due to expression of CD23/FcεRII, the low affinity IgE receptor, on the apical membrane of epithelial cells following sensitization of rats. CD23 expression has previously been noted on epithelial cells in jejunal biopsies, particularly those from patients with food allergies and inflammatory bowel disease.[90] Following luminal challenge with HRP to the intestine of sensitized rats, the expression of CD23 on the epithelial cell surface decreased and CD23 was subsequently identified on the membrane of endosomes containing HRP antigen.[89] Binding of antigen to the immunoglobulin-receptor complex appeared to reduce degradation since the quantity of intact protein appearing in the serosal buffer was much greater in sensitized rats. Anti-CD23 not only inhibited the enhanced antigen transport, but also reduced the mast cell mediated Isc and permeability responses indicative of the hypersensitivity reaction. These studies suggest that food allergic reactions depend on antigen uptake across the epithelium via this enhanced transport system. This transport system is also likely to serve as a clearance mechanism for circulating IgE into the gut lumen.[91]

Intestinal Function in Cow's Milk Allergy

It is now well recognized that a constitutive abnormality in intestinal antigen handling is not the primary cause for the development of milk allergy. This has been illustrated by studies on macromolecular absorption in jejunal biopsies from infants with cow's milk allergy, during the active symptomatic phase of the disease and after treatment with a cow's milk protein free diet. During active cow's milk allergy, there was an eight-fold increase in the absorption of the bystander protein, HRP, an increase in Cl⁻ secretion and an alteration of the epithelial integrity, as attested by the increased ionic conductance, an index of paracellular permeability.[92] After several months of treatment (cow's milk free diet), i.e., during the symptom-free period, the protein absorption, Cl⁻ secretion and paracellular permeability had returned to normal values, indicating that the increased intestinal permeability to antigens was not the primary cause of the disease. Subsequent experiments analyzing intestinal biopsies from children with cow's milk allergy, clearly confirmed the role of cow's milk antigens in the alteration of antigen handling by the gut.[93] In these studies, bovine β-lactoglobulin (the sensitizing antigen) and human β-lactalbumin (a self antigen) were placed on the luminal surface of the jejunal biopsies from infants with active cow's milk allergy or treated (symptom-free) infants. In infants with active allergy, β-lactoglobulin (but not human-α-lactalbumin) induced an increase in Isc (Fig. 4A), and an increase in conductance, whereas no such effects were observed in treated allergic infants. Moreover, the absorption of the sensitizing antigen, β-lactoglobulin, was faster and higher in active cow's milk allergic infants than in treated infants (Fig. 4B). These results imply that in the sensitized human intestinal mucosa, β-lactoglobulin triggers the release of mast cell mediators which in turn alter intestinal function. Although not examined specifically, these findings also lend support for a potential role for epithelial CD23 in the enhanced transepithelial transport of antigen in allergic humans (as well as in sensitized rodents).

Cow's milk allergy, as previously stated, displays an heterogeneous expression. Children with cow's milk allergy may have a morphologically normal small intestinal mucosa, occasionally with increased IgE plasma cells, and often characterized by enhanced intestinal permeability; whereas cow's milk sensitive enteropathy is characterized by a partially or totally flat intestinal mucosa,[94] such as that observed in gluten-sensitive enteropathy (celiac disease). Abnormal intestinal permeability is a hallmark of an inflamed gut, and it has become clear that the characteristics of intestinal inflammatory response are largely determined by the cytokine responses triggered by the pathological mechanism.[95] Allergic inflammation also leads to the release of T cell cytokines, which are probably involved in the epithelial pathophysiology. In children with cow's milk allergy, oral provocation with milk antigens induces the release of the pro-inflammatory cytokine, TNFα and of eosinophil cationic protein (recovered in feces).[96,97] In parallel, it has been reported that mononuclear cells from infants with active cow's milk allergy and intestinal symptoms, release more TNFα after stimulation than those of children having recovered from the disease.[98] Conditioned media from these mononuclear cells did not directly stimulate electrogenic Cl⁻ secretion by a filter-grown cultured epithelial cells, but reduced epithelial barrier integrity. This effect was inhibited by neutralizing the conditioned media with anti-TNFα antibodies, indicating that TNFα was mostly responsible for the epithelial barrier defect. Moreover, recombinant TNFα was shown to reproduce the increased permeability in HT29-19A cells and to damage tight junctions, as shown by freeze fracture etching.[99] Interestingly, children with cow's milk allergy presenting with cutaneous symptoms, did not display TNFα secretion, suggesting that the mechanism of intestinal alteration may be different according to the symptoms developed. Indeed, children with intestinal symptoms mainly display delayed reactions and do not present with specific IgE antibodies to milk proteins, whereas children with cutaneous symptoms most often present with immediate reactions and greatly elevated levels of milk specific IgE.

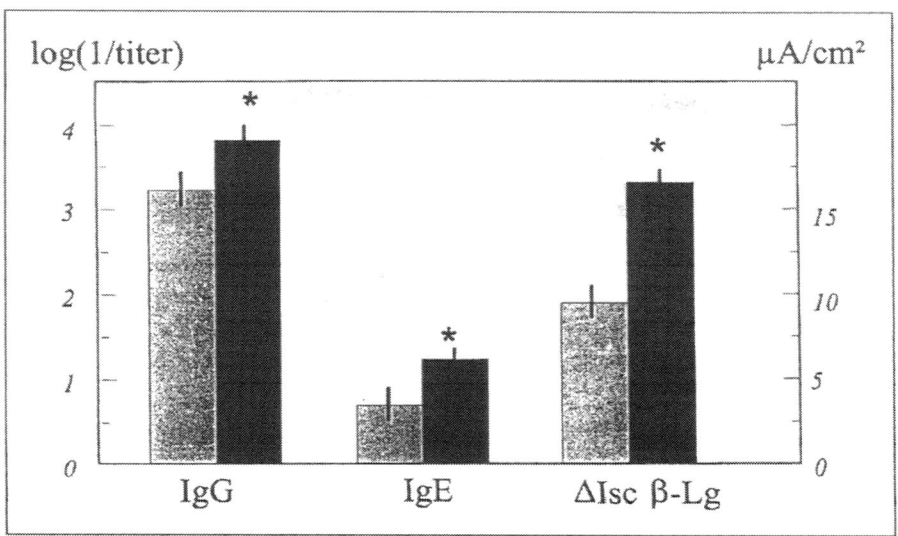

Figure 4. Effect of malnutrition on cow's milk protein sensitization in a guinea-pig model. Anti-β-lactoglobulin IgG1 (the equivalent of IgE in humans) and passive cutaneous anaphylaxis (reaginic antobodies) to β-lactoglobulin, as well as the β-lactoglobulin induced rise in Isc of jejunal segments mounted in Ussing chambers (criteria of milk sensitization) are significantly increased in animals which have been chronically malnourished for 3 weeks (4% protein diet) compared to control well-nourished animals (30% protein diet).

Summary and Conclusions

Several tons of antigens are consumed by each individual over a lifetime. In most instances, no immune reactions takes place, i.e., oral tolerance has been effective. In a minority of the population, ingestion of food results in an adverse reaction. Although the incidence of confirmed food allergy is <5%, up to 25 % of households change their dietary habits due to a perceived food allergy, indicating the level of concern with this problem in the general population.[2] Certainly, individuals affected by food-induced reactions are genuinely disabled and suffer untold stress when eating outside the home. Although much has been learned about the mechanism of food allergic reactions, there still is no effective therapy. Among those being considered, anti-IgE therapy looks promising and is in clinical trials.[100] New emerging information may result in novel therapeutic approaches.

It is clear that the pathway/mechanism of antigen uptake across the gut epithelial barrier is critical in both the inductive phase of food allergy and the effector response to ingested antigen in a previously sensitized host. In the inductive phase, an important factor directing the generation of food allergy versus oral tolerance is the presence of certain microbes (or their secreted products) which act as adjuvants to skew the immune response toward TH2 and the production of reaginic antibodies. In contrast, an inflammatory response to an enteric pathogen results in a barrier break and skews the immune response towards TH1. The balance of TH1, TH2, and regulatory cytokines is obviously pivotal for appropriate mucosal immunity and in part depends on the age of the host, and the maturity of the immune system. A schema depicting our view of the mechanism accounting for the induction of food/milk allergy is shown in Figure 5A.

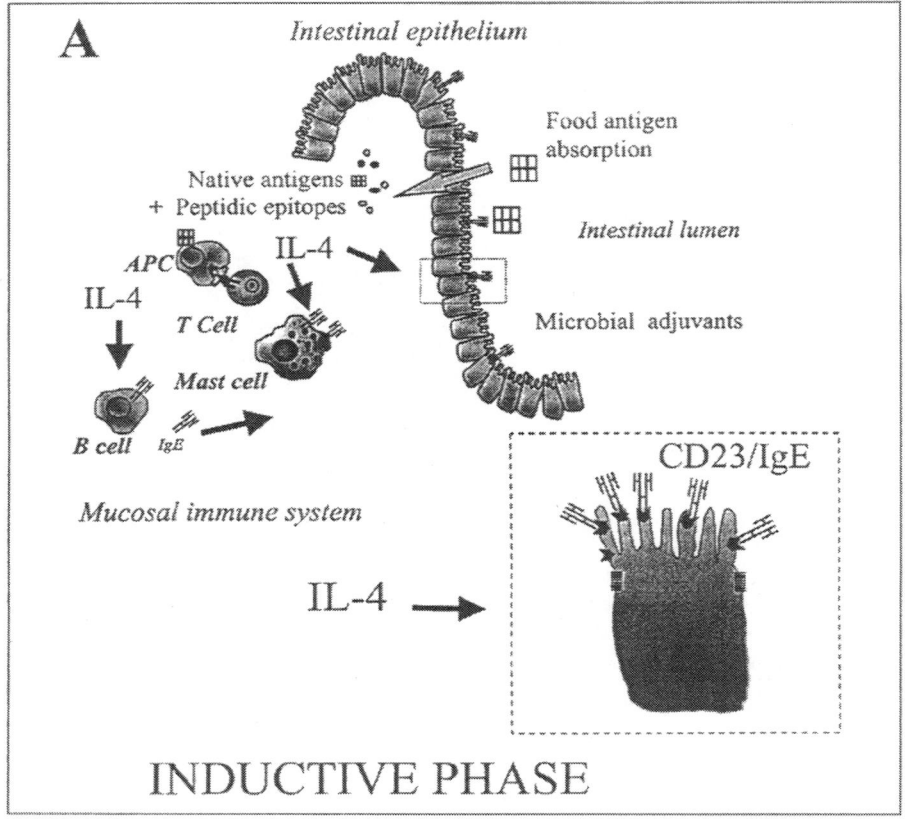

Figure 5A. The pathway/mechanism of the inductive phase and the effector phase of food allergy. A. In the inductive phase, an important factor directing the generation of food allergy versus oral tolerance is the presence of certain microbes (or their secreted products) which act as adjuvants to skew the immune response toward TH2 and the production of reaginic (IgE) antibodies by B cells. Cytokines such as IL-4 upregulate IgE receptor expression, not only FcεRI on mast cells, but also FcεRII/CD23 on epithelial (and some other) cells.

In the effector phase following sensitization, transepithelial antigen transport is dramatically altered such that the speed and quantity of antigenic material taken up is vastly enhanced. The epithelium directs transcellular traffic of both antigens and antibodies into and out of the body by virtue of antibody receptors. It now appears that IgE is not only responsible for binding antigen and activating mast cells, but is also involved in the rapid import of food antigens into the body via binding to CD23 on the enterocyte microvilli. The subsequent activation of mucosal mast cells results in the release of mediators and cytokines, many of which affect the epithelium directly or indirectly via nerves[101,102] to alter its transport and barrier properties. The epithelium not only responds to mast cell and T cell derived compounds, it also produces cytokines, chemokines and other mediators (nitric oxide, lipid mediators, etc) which have the potential for crosstalk with other cells and autocrine action on epithelial cells themselves, all of

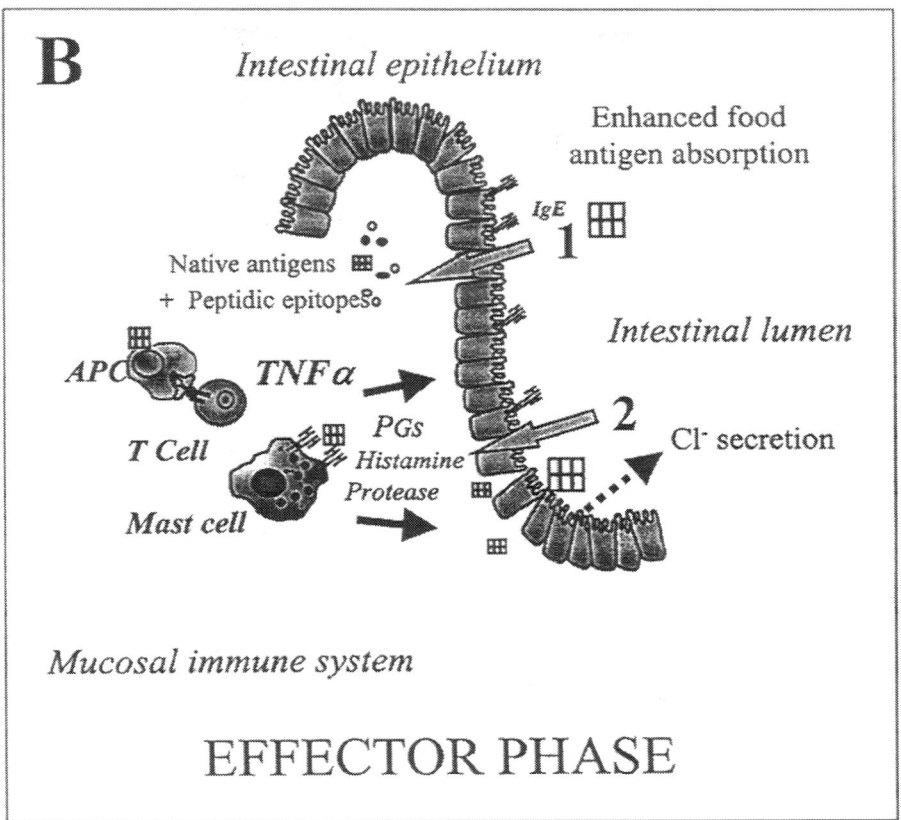

Figure 5B. In the effector phase following sensitization, transepithelial antigen transport is dramatically altered such that the speed and quantity of antigenic material taken up is vastly enhanced. IgE is not only responsible for binding antigen and activating mast cells, but is also involved in the rapid import of food antigens into the body via binding to CD23 on the enterocyte microvilli. The subsequent activation of mucosal mast cells results in the release of mediators and cytokines, many of which affect the epithelium directly or indirectly via nerves to alter its transport and barrier properties. The epithelium not only responds to mast cell and T cell derived compounds, it also produces cytokines, chemokines and other mediators (nitric oxide, lipid mediators, etc.) which have the potential for crosstalk with other cells and autocrine action on epithelial cells themselves, all of which results in amplification of the overall reaction.

which results in amplification of the overall reaction. A schema depicting our view of the mechanism of the effector phase of food allergy is shown in Figure 5B.

In conclusion, food allergy is an example of an immunological mistake, probably similar in nature to an anti-helminthic clearance mechanism evolved to eliminate enteric parasites.[103] Although food allergy has been studied for almost 100 years, new information is still emerging. Hopefully, ongoing experimental and clinical investigations will lead to effective treatments for food and milk allergy within the foreseeable future.

References

1. Prausnitz C, Kustner H. Studien uber die ueberemfindlichkeit (Studies on supersensitivity). Zentralbl Bakteriol Orig 1921; 86:160-169.
2. Sampson HA. Food allergy. Part 2: Diagnosis and management. J Allergy Clin Immunol 1999; 103:981-989.
3. Sampson HA. Food allergy. Part 1: Immunopathogenesis and clinical disorders. J Allergy Clin Immunol 1999; 103:717-728.
4. Ortolani C, Ispano M, Pastorello E et al. The oral allergy syndrome. Ann Allergy 1988; 61:47-52.
5. Yunginger JW, Ahlstedt S, Eggleston PA et al. Quantitative IgE antibody assays in allergic diseases. J Allergy Clin Immunol 2000; 105:1077-1084.
6. Brown WR, Lee EH.. Studies on IgE in human intestinal fluids. Int Arch Allergy Appl Immun 1976; 50:87-94.
7. Belut D, Moneret-Vautrin DA, Nicolas JP et al. IgE levels in intestinal juice. Dig Dis Sci 1980; 25:323-332.
8. De Boissieu D, Matarazzo P, Rocchiccioli F et al. Multiple food allergy: A possible diagnosis in breastfed infants. Acta Paediatr 1997; 86:1042-1046.
9. Kosecka U, Marshall JM, Crowe SE et al. Pertussis toxin stimulates hypersensitivity and enhances nerve-mediated antigen uptake in rat intestine. Am J Physiol 1994; 267:G745-753.
10. Mu HH, Sewell WA. Enhancement of interleukin-4 production by pertussis toxin. Infect Immun 1993; 61:2834-2840.
11. Vleeming W, Hendriksen CF, van de Kuil A et al. Mepyramine but not cimetidine or clobenpropit blocks pertussis toxin-induced histamine sensitization in rats. Br J Pharmacol 2000; 129:1801-1807.
12. Snider DP, Marshall JS, Perdue MH et al. Production of IgE antibody and allergic sensitization of intestinal and peripheral tissues after oral immunization with protein Ag and cholera toxin. J Immunol 1994; 153:647-657.
13. Rappuoli R, Pizza M, Douce G, Dougan G. Structure and mucosal adjuvanticity of cholera and Escherichia coli heat-labile enterotoxins. Immunol Today 1999; 20(11):493-500.
14. Fargeas M J, Theodorou V, More J et al. Boosted systemic immune and local responsiveness after intestinal inflammation in orally sensitized guinea pigs. Gastroenterology 1995; 109:53-62.
15. Kiliaan AJ, Saunders PR, Bijlsma PB et al. Stress stimulates transepithelial macromolecular uptake in rat jejunum. Am J Physiol 1998; 275:G1037-G1044.
16. Baird AW, Coombs RR, McLaughlan P et al. Immediate hypersensitivity reactions to cow milk proteins in isolated epithelium from ileum of milk-drinking guinea-pigs: Comparisons with colonic epithelia. Int Arch Allergy Appl Immunol 1984; 75:255-263.
17. Li XM, Schofield BH, Huang CK et al. A murine model of IgE-mediated cow's milk hypersensitivity. J Allergy Clin Immunol 1999; 103:206-214.
18. Perdue MH, Chung M, Gall DG. The effect of intestinal anaphylaxis on gut function in the rat. Gastroenterology 1984; 86:391-397.
19. Soda S, Kawabori S, Perdue MH et al. Macrophage engulfment of mucosal mast cells treated with dexamethasone. Gastroenterology.1991; 100:929-937.
20. Crowe SE, Sestini P, Perdue MH. Allergic reactions of rat jejunal mucosa. Ion transport responses to luminal antigen and inflammatory mediators. Gastroenterology 1990; 99:74-82.
21. Berin MC, Kiliaan AJ, Groot JA et al. Rapid transepithelial antigen transport in rat jejunum: impact of sensitization and the immediate hypersensitivity reaction. Gastroenterology 1997; 113:856-864.
22. Yang P-C, Berin MC, Yu L, Perdue MH. Mucosal pathophysiology and inflammatory changes in the late phase of the intestinal allergic reaction in the rat. Am J Pathol 2001; 158:681-690.
23. Scott RB, Diamant SC, Gall DG. Motility effects of intestinal anaphylaxis in the rat. Am J Physiol 1988; 255:G505-G511.
24. Perdue MH, Gall DG. Transport abnormalities during intestinal anaphylaxis in the rat. Effect of anti-allergic agents. J Allergy Clin Immunol 1985; 76:498-503.
25. Perdue MH, Gall DG. Intestinal anaphylaxis in the rat: Jejunal response to in vitro antigen exposure. Am J Physiol 1986; 250:G427-G431.

26. Vergnolle N. Review article: Proteinase-activated receptors—Novel signals for gastrointestinal patho-physiology. Aliment Pharmacol Ther 2000; 14:257-266.

27. Perdue MH, Masson S, Wershil B et al. Role of mast cells in ion transport abnormalities associated with intestinal anaphylaxis. Correction of the diminished secretory response in genetically mast cell-deficient W/Wv mice by bone marrow transplantation. J Clin Invest 1991; 87:687-693.

28. Javed NH, Barrett KE, Wang YZ, Bidinger J, Cooke HJ. Enhanced tissue responsiveness in colonic ion transport of cow's milk-sensitized guinea pigs. Agents Actions 1994; 41:25-31.

29. Stead RH, Tomioka M, Quinonez G et al. Intestinal mucosal mast cells in normal and nematode-infected rat intestines are in intimate contact with peptidergic nerves. Proc Natl Acad Sci USA 1987; 84:2975-2979.

30. Yu LCH, Perdue MH. Role of mast cells in intestinal mucosal function: Studies in models of hypersensitivity and stress. Immunol Rev 2001; 179:61-73.

31. Powell DW, Mifflin RC, Valentich JD et al. Myofibroblasts. II. Intestinal subepithelial myofibroblasts. Am J Physiol 1999; 277:C183-C201.

32. Berschneider HM, Powell DW. Fibroblasts modulate intestinal secretory responses to inflammatory mediators. J Clin Invest 1992; 89(2):484-489.

33. Scudamore CL, Thornton EM, McMillan L et al. Release of the mucosal mast cell granule chymase rat mast cell protease II, during anaphylaxis is associated with rapid development of paracellular permeability to macromolecules in rat jejunum. J Exp Med 1995; 182:1871-81.

34. Crowe SE, Perdue MH. Intestinal permeability in allergic rats: Nerve involvement in antigen-induced changes. Am J Physiol 1993; 264:G617-G623.

35. Lake AM, Bloch KJ, Sinclair KJ et al. Anaphylactic release of intestinal goblet cell mucus. Immunology 1980; 39:173-178.

36. Dorsch W. Definitions and clinical symptoms. In: Dorsch W, ed. Late Phase Allergic Reactions. Boca Raton: CRC Press, 1990:9-15.

37. Ohtsuka Y, Yamashiro Y, Maeda M et al. Food antigen activates intraepithelial and lamina propria lymphocytes in food-sensitive enteropathy in mice. Pediatr Res 1996; 39:862-866.

38. Wershil BK, Furuta GT, Wang Z-S et al. Mast cell-dependent neutrophils and mononuclear cell recruitment in immunoglobulin E-induced gastric reactions in mice. Gastroenterology 1996; 110:1482-1490.

39. Sakamoto Y, Ohtsuka T, Yoshida H et al. Time course of changes in the intestinal permeability of food-sensitized rats after oral allergen challenge. Pediatr Allergy Immunol 1998; 9:20-24.

40. Williams CM, Galli SJ. The diverse potential effector and immunoregulatory roles of mast cells in allergic disease. J Allergy Clin Immunol 2000; 105:847-859.

41. Galli SJ, Gordon JR, Wershil BK. Cytokine production by mast cells and basophils. Curr Opin Immunol 1991; 6:865-872.

42. Furuta GT, Schmidt-Choudhury A, Wang MY et al. Mast cell-dependent tumor necrosis factor alpha production participates in allergic gastric inflammation in mice. Gastroenterology 1997; 113:1560-9.

43. Bochner BS, Luscinskas FW, Gimbrone MA Jr et al. Adhesion of human basophils, eosinophils, and neutrophils to interleukin 1-activated human vascular endothelial cells: Contributions of endothelial cell adhesion molecules. J Exp Med 1991; 173:1553-1557.

44. Scott RB, Gall DG, Maric M. Mediation of food protein-induced jejunal smooth muscle contraction in sensitized rats. Am J Physiol 1990; 259:G6-14.

45. Crowe SE, Perdue MH. Gastrointestinal food hypersensitivity: Basic mechanisms of pathophysiology. Gastroenterology 1992; 103:1075-1095.

46. Stenton GR, Vliagoftis H, Befus AD. Role of intestinal mast cells in modulating gastrointestinal pathophysiology. Ann Allergy Asthma Immunol 1998; 81:1-11.

47. Mahe S, Messing B, Thuillier F et al. Digestion of bovine milk proteins in patients with a high jejunostomy. Am J Clin Nutr 1991; 54:534-538.

48. Bruce MG, Ferguson A. Oral tolerance to ovalbumin in mice: studies of chemically modified and 'biologically filtered' antigen. Immunology 1986; 57:627-630.

49. Furrie E, Turner MW, Strobel S. Partial characterization of a circulating tolerogenic moiety which, after a feed of ovalbumin, suppresses delayed-type hypersensitivity in recipient mice. Immunology 1995; 86:480-486.

50. Walker WA, Isselbacher KJ, Bloch KJ. Intestinal uptake of macromolecules: Effect of oral immunization. Science 1972; 177:608-610.

51. Heyman M, Ducroc R, Desjeux JF et al. Horseradish peroxidase transport across adult rabbit jejunum in vitro. Am J Physiol 1982; 242:G558-G564.

52. Madara JL. Maintenance of the macromolecular barrier at cell extrusion sites in intestinal epithelium: Physiological rearrangement of tight junctions. J Membr Biol 1990; 116:177-184.

53. Curtis GH, Gall DG. Macromolecular transport by rat gastric mucosa. Am J Physiol 1992; 262:G1033-G1040.

54. Ducroc R, Heyman M, Beaufrere B et al. Horseradish peroxidase transport across rabbit jejunum and Peyer's patches in vitro. Am J Physiol 1983; 245:G54-G58.

55. Heyman M, Corthier G, Lucas F et al. Evolution of the caecal epithelial barrier during Clostridium difficile infection in the mouse. Gut 1989; 30:1087-1093.

56. Heyman M, Crain-Denoyelle AM, Corthier G et al. Postnatal development of protein absorption in conventional and germ-free mice. Am J Physiol 1986; 251:G326-G331.

57. Gonnella PA, Chen Y, Inobe J et al. In situ immune response in gut-associated lymphoid tissue (GALT) following oral antigen in TCR-transgenic mice. J Immunol 1998; 160:4708-4718.

58. Bland PW, Warren LG. Antigen presentation by epithelial cells of the rat small intestine. I. Kinetics, antigen specificity and blocking by anti-Ia antisera. Immunology 1986; 58:1-7.

59. Hershberg RM, Framson PE, Cho DH et al. Intestinal epithelial cells use two distinct pathways for HLA class II antigen processing. J Clin Invest 1997; 100:204-215.

60. Kaiserlian D, Vidal K, Revillard JP. Murine enterocytes can present soluble antigen to specific class II-restricted CD4+ T cells. Eur J Immunol 1989; 19:1513-1516.

61. Mayer L, Shlien R. Evidence for function of Ia molecules on gut epithelial cells in man. J Exp Med 1987; 166:1471-1483.

62. Terpend K, Boisgerault F, Blaton MA et al. Protein transport and processing by human HT29-19A intestinal cells: Effect of interferon gamma. Gut 1998; 42:538-545.

63. Van Niel G, Raposo G, Hershberg R et al. Intestinal epithelial cells secrete exosome-like vesicles. Gastroenterology 2001; 121:337-349.

64. Denzer K, Kleijmeer MJ, Heijnen HF et al. Exosome: From internal vesicle of the multivesicular body to intercellular signaling device. J Cell Sci 2000; 113:3365-3374.

65. Soloway P, Fish S, Passmore H et al. Regulation of the immune response to peptide antigens: Differential induction of immediate-type hypersensitivity and T cell proliferation due to changes in either peptide structure or major histocompatibility complex haplotype. J Exp Med 1991; 174:847-858.

66. Williamson E, Westrich GM, Viney JL. Modulating dendritic cells to optimize mucosal immunization protocols. J Immunol 1999; 163:3668-3675.

67. Heyman M, Corthier G, Petit A et al. Intestinal absorption of macromolecules during viral enteritis: An experimental study on rotavirus-infected conventional and germ-free mice. Pediatr Res 1987; 22:72-78.

68. Iyngkaran N, Robinson MJ, Sumithran E et al. Cow's milk protein-sensitive enteropathy. An important factor in prolonging diarrhoea of acute infective enteritis in early infancy. Arch Dis Child 1978; 53:150-153.

69. Frick OL, German DF, Mills J. Development of allergy in children. I. Association with virus infections. J Allergy Clin Immunol 1979; 63:228-241.

70. Heyman M, Corthier G, Lucas F et al. Evolution of the caecal epithelial barrier during Clostridium difficile infection in the mouse. Gut 1989; 30:1087-93.

71. Philpott DJ, McKay DM, Mak W et al. Signal transduction pathways involved in enterohemorrhagic Escherichia coli-induced alterations in T84 epithelial permeability. Infect Immun 1998; 66:1680-1687.

72. Gotteland M, Isolauri E, Heyman M et al. Antigen absorption in bacterial diarrhea: In vivo intestinal transport of beta-lactoglobulin in rabbits infected with the entero-adherent Escherichia coli strain RDEC-1. Pediatr Res 1989; 26:237-240.

73. Gotteland M, Crain-Denoyelle AM, Heyman M et al. Effect of cow's milk protein absorption on the anaphylactic and systemic immune responses of young rabbits during bacterial diarrhoea. Int Arch Allergy Immunol 1992; 97:78-82.

74. Matysiak-Budnik T, Terpend K, Alain S et al. Helicobacter pylori alters exogenous antigen absorption and processing in a digestive tract epithelial cell line model. Infect Immun 1998; 66:5785-5791.
75. Corrado G, Luzzi I, Lucarelli S et al. Positive association between Helicobacter pylori infection and food allergy in children. Scand J Gastroenterol 1998; 33:1135-1139.
76. Figura N, Perrone A, Gennari C et al. Food allergy and Helicobacter pylori infection. Ital J Gastroenterol Hepatol 1999; 31:186-191.
77. Darmon N, Heyman M, Candalh C et al. Anaphylactic intestinal response to milk proteins during malnutrition in guinea pigs. Am J Physiol 1996; 270:G442-G448.
78. Gaboriau-Routhiau V, Moreau MC. Gut flora allows recovery of oral tolerance to ovalbumin in mice after transient breakdown mediated by cholera toxin or Escherichia coli heat-labile enterotoxin. Pediatr Res 1996; 39:625-629.
79. Moreau MC, Corthier G. Effect of the gastrointestinal microflora on induction and maintenance of oral tolerance to ovalbumin in C3H/HeJ mice. Infect Immun 1988; 56:2766-2768.
80. Sudo N, Sawamura S, Tanaka K et al. The requirement of intestinal bacterial flora for the development of an IgE production system fully susceptible to oral tolerance induction. J Immunol 1997; 159:1739-1745.
81. Wold AE, Dahlgren UI, Hanson LA et al. Difference between bacterial and food antigens in mucosal immunogenicity. Infect Immun 1989; 57:2666-2673.
82. Viney JL, Mowat AM, O'Malley JM et al. Expanding dendritic cells in vivo enhances the induction of oral tolerance. J Immunol 1998; 160:5815-5825.
83. Neish AS, Gewirtz AT, Zeng H et al. Prokaryotic regulation of epithelial responses by inhibition of IkappaB-alpha ubiquitination. Science 2000; 289:1560-1563.
84. Gupta P, Andrew H, Kirschner BS et al. Is lactobacillus GG helpful in children with Crohn's disease? Results of a preliminary, open-label study. J Pediatr Gastroenterol Nutr 2000; 31:453-457.
85. Majamaa H, Isolauri E. Probiotics: A novel approach in the management of food allergy. J Allergy Clin Immunol 1997; 99:179-185.
86. Wickens K, Pearce N, Crane J et al. Antibiotic use in early childhood and the development of asthma. Clin Exp Allergy 1999; 29:766-771.
87. Bosel M, Prydz K, Parton RG et al. Endocytosis in filter-grown Madin-Darby canine kidney cells. J Cell Biol 1989; 109:3243-3258.
88. Berin MC, Kiliaan AJ, Yang PC et al. The influence of mast cells on pathways of antigen transport in rat intestine. J Immunol 1998; 161:2561-2566.
89. Yang P-C, Berin MC, Yu LCH et al. Enhanced intestinal transepithelial antigen transport in allergic rats is mediated by IgE and CD23 (FceRII). J Clin Invest 2000; 106:879-886.
90. Kaiserlian D, Lachaux A, Grosjean I et al. Intestinal epithelial cells express the CD23/Fc-epsilon-RII molecule—Enhanced expression in enteropathies. Immunology 1993; 80:90-95.
91. Negrao-Correa D, Adams LS, Bell RG. Intestinal transport and catabolism of IgE: A major blood-independent pathway of IgE dissemination during a Trichinella spiralis infection of rats. J Immunol 1996; 157:4037-4044.
92. Heyman M, Grasset E, Ducroc R et al. Antigen absorption by the jejunal epithelium of children with cow's milk allergy. Pediatr Res 1998; 24:197-202.
93. Saidi D, Heyman M, Kheroua O et al. Jejunal response to beta-lactoglobulin in infants with cow's milk allergy. CR Acad Sci III 1995; 318:683-689.
94. Host A. Cow's milk allergy. JR Soc Med 1997; 90 Suppl 30:34-39.
95. Bellanti JA. Cytokines and allergic diseases: Clinical aspects. Allergy Asthma Proc 1998; 19:337-41.
96. Kapel N, Matarazzo P, Haouchine D et al. Fecal tumor necrosis factor alpha, eosinophil cationic protein and IgE levels in infants with cow's milk allergy and gastrointestinal manifestations. Clin Chem Lab Med 1999; 37:29-32.
97. Majamaa H, Miettinen A, Laine S et al. Intestinal inflammation in children with atopic eczema: Faecal eosinophil cationic protein and tumour necrosis factor-alpha as non invasive indicators of food allergy. Clin Exp Allergy 1996; 26:181-187.
98. Heyman M, Darmon N, Dupont C et al. Mononuclear cells from infants allergic to cow's milk secrete tumor necrosis factor alpha, altering intestinal function. Gastroenterology 1994; 106:1514-1523.

99. Rodriguez P, Heyman M, Candalh C et al. Tumour necrosis factor-alpha induces morphological and functional alterations of intestinal HT29 cl.19A cell monolayers. Cytokine 1995; 7:441-448.
100. Sampson HA.. Food allergy: From biology toward therapy. Hospital Practice 2000; May15:67-83.
101. Frieling T, Cooke HJ, Wood JD. Neuroimmune communication in the submucosal plexus of guinea pig colon after sensitization to milk antigen. Am J Physiol 1995; 267:G1087-G1093.
102. Wood JD, Alpers DH, Andrews PLR. Fundamentals of enteric neurogastroenterology. Gut 1999; 45:1-44.
103. Bell RG. IgE, allergies and helminth parasites: A new perspective on an old conundrum. Immunol Cell Biol 1996; 74:337-345.

CHAPTER 9

Physiopathology of Celiac Disease

Katri Kaukinen, Markku Mäki and Pekka Collin

Introduction

In celiac disease, ingestion of gluten results in T-cell-mediated small bowel mucosal damage characterized by subtotal or severe partial villous atrophy with crypt hyperplasia. A life-long gluten-free diet is essential to clinical and small bowel mucosal recovery, and for prevention of complications such as lymphoma and osteoporosis. There is a substantial body of evidence to suggest that celiac disease develops gradually from mucosal inflammation to crypt hyperplasia and finally to overt villous atrophy.[1] Apart from small bowel mucosal villous atrophy and crypt hyperplasia, a prominent feature in untreated celiac disease is an increase in intraepithelial lymphocytes (IELs).

It is nowadays widely accepted that immunological mechanisms are implicated in the development of the mucosal damage in celiac disease, and signs of activation of both mucosal cellular and humoral immune systems have been detected. The risk of developing celiac disease is genetically determined: the disease carries one of the strongest HLA associations, namely HLA DQ2 or DQ8.[2] Moreover, gluten-specific HLA DQ restricted T-cells are present in the small bowel mucosa in untreated disease.[3] IgA-class endomysial antibodies (EmA) are specific markers of the condition and it has recently been found that these antibodies recognize tissue transglutaminase, now considered to be the predominant autoantigen for celiac disease.[4] The actual mechanisms responsible for small bowel mucosal damage remain however so far only partly characterized.

Clinical Features of Celiac Disease

Even though patients affected by celiac disease may suffer from severe malabsorption syndrome with diarrhea and weight loss, abdominal symptoms are nowadays usually mild or absent, and only minor if any hematological or biochemical abnormalities may be evinced.[5,6] Isolated malabsorption of iron, calcium and folic acid are still common, but a deficiency of these nutrients does not invariably lead to clinical consequences.[7-10] Moreover, in many subjects with untreated celiac disease today, the clinical presentation is monosymptomatic or atypical (Table 1). It is often impossible to settle whether these conditions are true immunologically induced, gluten-dependent, extra-intestinal manifestations or complications of malabsorption. Nevertheless, in many cases there is no clear evidence of substantial malabsorption.

An itching and blistering skin disease, dermatitis herpetiformis, is one classical manifestation of celiac disease along with granular IgA deposits in the papillary dermis of unaffected skin.[11] Most patients with dermatitis herpetiformis have small bowel villous atrophy and crypt hyperplasia consistent with celiac disease and, in the remainder, minor mucosal changes with an increased density of IELs can be seen.[12,13] Both cutaneous and small bowel mucosal lesions

Oral Tolerance: The Response of the Intestinal Mucosa to Dietary Antigens, edited by Olivier Morteau. ©2004 Eurekah.com and Kluwer Academic / Plenum Publishers.

Table 1. Atypical symptoms and risk groups in celiac disease

Atypical Symptoms of Celiac Disease

Chronic oral mucosal aphthous ulceration

Dental enamel hypoplasia of permanent teeth

Infertility and unfavorable outcome of pregnancy

Unexplained increase in liver enzymes

Neurological manifestations of unknown origin

(ataxia, polyneuropathy, dementia)

Epilepsy and posterior cerebral calcifications

Non-specific mono- or polyarthritis

Osteopenia or osteporosis

Depression

Small bowel lymphoma or cancer

Risk Groups for Celiac Disease

Insulin dependent diabetes mellitus

Autoimmune thyroid disorders

Alopecia areata

Sjögren's syndrome

First-degree relatives of celiac patients

Selective IgA deficiency

are alleviated during a gluten-free diet.[13,14] Dermatitis herpetiformis may thus be regarded as a celiac disease of the skin.

A typical small bowel mucosal lesion may also be found in apparently asymptomatic subjects, detected by screening in at-risk groups such as first-degree relatives of celiac patients,[15,16] in patients with selective IgA deficiency,[17,18] and in various autoimmune disorders, as shown in Table 1. In the diagnosis of such atypical and asymptomatic cases the determination of circulating antireticulin (ARA) antiendomysial (EmA), antigliadin (AGA) or tissue transglutaminase antibodies (tTG-ab), is helpful.[19-21] Recent studies in the general population suggest that the prevalence of celiac disease may be as high as 1:100.[22]

A gluten-free diet ensures clinical and histological recovery. It is known that patients with untreated celiac disease are at risk of considerable complications such as small bowel lymphoma[23] and osteoporosis,[24] and a long-term gluten-free diet seems to protect from the development of these conditions. Interestingly, in recent observations by Ventura and associates,[25] a prolonged consumption of gluten seemed to predispose celiac patients to the development of other autoimmune diseases such as insulin-dependent diabetes mellitus and autoimmune thyroid disorders. Early detection and treatment of celiac disease is thus clearly warranted.

Role of Cereals

The harmful effect of ingested wheat gluten in celiac disease was first recognized in the 1950s by the Dutch pediatrician W.K. Dicke.[26] A strict life-long gluten-free diet has been since then the cornerstone in celiac disease treatment. Rye (secalins) and barley (hordeins) prolamins bear a close taxonomic relationship to wheat prolamin (gliadin), and are also considered to be toxic in celiac disease.[27] Controversy has prevailed as to the toxicity of oat prolamin (avenin).[28-30] However, recent studies indicate that patients with celiac disease or dermatitis herpetiformis tolerate oats.[31-35] When compared to non-toxic cereals such as rice and maize, a feature common to prolamins of wheat, rye and barley is a high content of glutamine and proline. The oat prolamin has an intermediate amino acid composition and the overall prolamin content of oats is five times less than that in wheat, rye or barley, which may explain the absence of oat toxicity.

The clinical expression of celiac disease may be influenced by the amount and timing of gluten ingestion; early exposure of the immature immune system to gluten seems to be a prominent cofactor for manifestation of clinically overt celiac disease. In the 1980s the incidence of celiac disease in young Swedish children increased fourfold.[36] This was considered to be a result of excessive gluten ingestion related to feeding practices in infants. When infant feeding practices were changed, a rapid decline in celiac incidence rates was observed.[37] Whether feeding practices would affect the overall population prevalence of this condition remains unknown.

Genetics of Celiac Disease

Susceptibility to celiac disease is determined to a significant extent by genetic factors. Liability to the disease runs in families and first-degree relatives of celiac disease patients are known to carry a risk of 10-15%.[38] The concordance between monozygotic twins is reported to be 70%.[39,40] The figure may be even higher: some discordant individuals may later turn out to be concordant, that is, they may have normal biopsy (latent celiac disease) and develop celiac disease during a follow up.

The disease was first described as occurring in patients with human leukocyte antigen (HLA) B8,[41,42] but this HLA association appeared to be secondary and in linkage disequilibrium with alleles in the HLA class II region, namely HLA DR3 and DR5/DR7.[40,43,44] Subsequently, an even stronger association was shown with HLA DQ2 encoded by alleles DQA1*0501 and DQB1*0201 located either in cis (in DR3-DQ2-positive individuals) or in trans position (in DR5/7-DQ2 heterozygous individuals).[2,45] Approximately 90% of celiac disease patients share this HLA DQ2 configuration;[2,46] most of the remainder express the DR4-DQ8 haplotype encoded by DQA1*0301, DQB1*0302 alleles.[47-49] In other words, virtually all Caucasian celiac disease patients share one or other of these HLA DQ2 or DQ8 haplotypes (Table 2). HLA DR3-DQ2 and DR4-DQ8 are also common in many autoimmune diseases such as insulin-dependent diabetes mellitus, autoimmune thyroiditis and Sjögren's syndrome.[50]

The prevalence of HLA DQ2 in the normal population is 20-30%,[2,46] suggesting the involvement of additional non-HLA-linked genes in the pathogenesis of celiac disease.

Table 2. *Frequency of HLA DQ2- or DQ8-positive celiac disease patients in different series*

Authors	Country	No of Patients with Celiac Disease	HLA DQ2- or DQ8-Positive Celiac Disease Patients n	(%)
Sollid et al. 1989 [2]	Norway	94	93*	(99%)
Congia et al. 1994 [130]	Italy (Sardinia)	66	63*	(95%)
Ploski et al. 1996 [131]	Sweden	135	130	(96%)
Michalski et al 1996 [48]	Ireland	90	89	(99%)
Polvi et al 1996 [46]	Finland	45	45	(100%)
Balas et al 1997 [132]	Spain	212	210	(99%)
	Spain	55**	55	(100%)
Polvi et al. 1998 [49]	Finland	84	82	(98%)
	Spain	189	181	(96%)

*only HLA DQ2 studied
**patients with dermatitis herpetiformis

Genome-wide screening studies have resulted in a number of proposals for candidate non-HLA gene regions outside HLA. In Irish celiac disease patients, five other chromosome locations were found: 6p23, 7q31, 11p11, 15q26 and 22cen.[51] In a British study, these findings could not be confirmed, since only one locus in chromosome 15 evinced linkage to celiac disease.[52] Studies elsewhere have pointed to candidate genes in chromosome 5q and possibly in 11q,[53] as well as in the CTLA4/CD28 gene region.[54] In a study by Lie and colleagues,[55] an allele of locus D6S2223 seemed to protect from the development of celiac disease; an allele found in this locus was less frequent among HLA DR3-DQ2 homozygous celiac disease patients than in HLA DR3-DQ2 homozygous non-celiac controls. In summary, no uniform gene or gene region outside HLA DQ has been clearly associated with celiac disease, and any effects of such additional genes are likely to be moderate.

Small Bowel Mucosal Lesion in Celiac Disease

Mucosal Morphological Changes

In untreated celiac disease, the characteristic abnormalities in the small bowel mucosa are villous atrophy, crypt hyperplasia and an increased density of IELs.[56-58] An increased number of chronic inflammatory cells is also found in the lamina propria,[59] and enterocyte height is reduced.[58,60,61] Small bowel mucosal villous atrophy is more prominent in the proximal part of the intestine and the ileal mucosa may even be undamaged.[60,62] It has been suggested that the severity of symptoms correlates with the length of abnormal small bowel mucosa rather than with the degree of villous atrophy. However, this conception was based on data involving only 11 adults.[62]

On a gluten-free diet, histological lesions of the small bowel mucosa are alleviated concomitantly with clinical recovery and reappear when gluten is reintroduced in the diet.[63,64] For the diagnosis of celiac disease, it is crucial to show the gluten dependency of the small bowel mucosal lesion, since villous atrophy and IELs may be seen in other conditions such as cow's

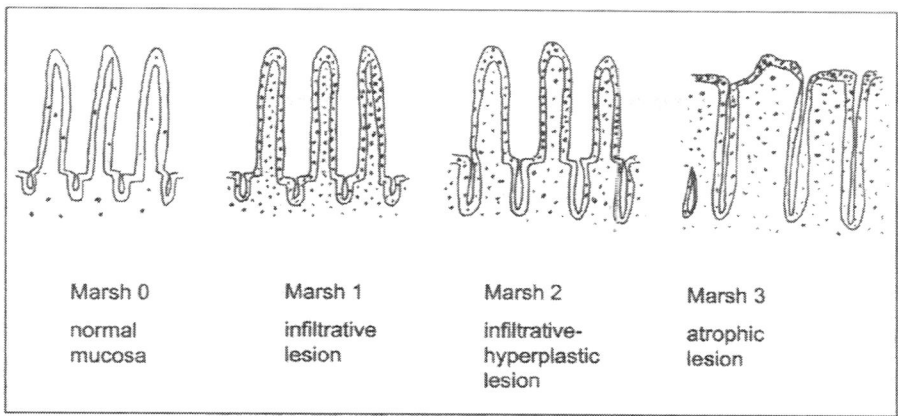

Figure 1. Classification of small bowel mucosal changes according to Marsh.[1]

milk allergy, giardiasis or postenteritis syndrome.[58,65,66] On the other hand, these disorders are rare in adults living in developed countries.

In celiac disease, small bowel mucosal damage develops gradually, as depicted in Figure 1. First, an increased density of IELs is observed in otherwise normal mucosa (infiltrative type); thereafter the crypts become elongated and minor villous shortening ensues (infil-trative-hyperplastic type). The lesion further proceeds to severe partial (PVA) or subtotal villous atrophy (SVA) with crypt hyperplasia (flat destructive type), which finding is today considered diagnostic for celiac disease.[1]

Thus, individuals who consume normal amounts of gluten and have normal small bowel villous architecture may still be gluten-sensitive; they may have latent celiac disease and in the course of time develop typical villous atrophy with crypt hyperplasia.[67] Dermatitis herpetiformis is a good model of celiac disease latency, since the mucosal lesion may be limited to minor villous atrophy or to mucosal inflammation only.[13] In such patients, a typical celiac-like mucosal damage can develop after consumption of extra amounts of gluten.[68,69] Apart from gluten intake,[69,70] the factors responsible for deterioration of the small bowel mucosa remain unclear. In first place, celiac-type genetics, HLA DR3-DQ2 or DR4-DQ8, should be present in patients with latent celiac disease.[71-73] By definition, the diagnosis of latent celiac disease is retrospective, and the concept of potential celiac disease has been applied to patients who are with great likelihood at risk of developing celiac enteropathy later in life.[67] In patients evincing normal villous architecture, an increased density of IELs (especially of $\gamma\delta^+$ cells), a positive serum EmA, or a celiac-like antibody pattern in the jejunal fluid are markers of forthcoming celiac disease.[74-77] The natural history of patients with potential celiac disease is unclear. It is not known if and when an individual patient will develop enteropathy, since only a small number of patients have so far been followed up.[16,74,78-81]

It must be emphasized that, in untreated celiac disease, the small bowel mucosal damage is not characterized simply by atrophy; there is also clear epithelial proliferation in the crypts. An increased mitosis frequency is seen in the crypt epithelium, and the production of these cells is twice that observed in non-celiac control subjects.[82] This enterocyte proliferation appears to be triggered by keratinocyte growth factor (KGF), derived from fibroblasts in the lamina propria.[83] Moss and associates[84] showed that increased enterocyte apoptosis followed crypt cell proliferation, which is in accordance with the occurrence of flat mucosa and hyperproliferation of epithelial cells.

Intraepithelial Lymphocytes

In both celiac disease patients and healthy individuals, most IELs are CD3$^+$ T-cells and B-cells are rarely found in the epithelium.[85,86] The density of CD3$^+$$\alpha\beta^+$ IELs is increased in untreated celiac disease, goes back to normal with a gluten-free diet, and increases again during gluten challenge.[87-89] It has been suggested that $\alpha\beta^+$ IELs are activated by gluten, although there is no evidence that these cells directly recognize gluten peptides. The role of $\alpha\beta^+$ IELs in the pathogenesis of celiac disease is unknown; 80% of $\alpha\beta^+$ IELs are CD8$^+$, suggesting a cytotoxic-suppressor cell function.[90] The cytotoxity of $\alpha\beta^+$ IELs is further suggested by the observation that the density of these cells increases with the density of IELs with cytolytic granules containing granzyme B, a protein characterized in activated lymphocytes.[91]

The increase in $\gamma\delta^+$ IELs density is a typical and constant feature in both untreated celiac disease patients and patients submitted to a gluten-free diet.[87,88,92-94] However, recent studies indicate that the density of $\gamma\delta^+$ IELs decreases on a gluten-free diet, albeit remaining at a high level much longer than other IELs.[95,96] Increased densities of $\gamma\delta^+$ IELs have also been detected in some subjects suspected of having celiac disease but evincing normal small bowel mucosal villous architecture.[79,97] Celiac-type villous atrophy has been reported to develop in some of these patients during follow-up.[74,80,81] A high count of $\gamma\delta^+$ IELs in normal villi can thus be considered indicative of latent celiac disease. However, an increased density of these cells in the small bowel mucosal epithelium was also observed in children with cow's milk allergy or postenteritis syndrome,[93,98,99] and it does not always correlate with celiac-type genetics, HLA DQ2 and DQ8.[81,100]

The role of $\gamma\delta^+$ IELs in the gut epithelium remains unknown. These cells have been thought to be cytotoxic to epithelial cells and to produce proinflammatory mediators.[101-103] However, the slow disappearance of $\gamma\delta^+$ IELs during a gluten-free diet suggests that their role is protective. $\gamma\delta^+$ T-cells express KGF, which may be important in the surveillance and repair of damaged epithelial cells.[104] $\gamma\delta^+$ IELs may also downregulate the inflammatory response of $\alpha\beta^+$ cells.[105] In addition, $\gamma\delta^+$ IELs deficient mice exhibit more severe epithelial damage than wild-type mice in response to intestinal infection by *Eimeria vermiformis*.[106] Recently, a receptor for the HLA class I-like stress-induced protein MICA was identified on $\gamma\delta^+$ T-cells.[107] In this way, activated $\gamma\delta^+$ cells can secrete chemokines, which further influence the antigen-specific immune response towards a Th2 profile by driving $\gamma\delta^+$ cells to secrete IL-4. These various mechanisms may protect the intestinal mucosa from exposure to damaging agents, such as dietary gluten. Animal studies further suggest that $\gamma\delta^+$ cells may play a role in regulating oral tolerance and in mediating autoimmune responses.[108,109]

Lamina Propria Cells

T-lymphocytes constitute 25-40% of total leukocytes in the lamina propria. In addition, large numbers of B-lymphocytes, plasma cells, granulocytes, macrophages and fibroblasts are present. In untreated celiac disease, the density of these cell populations is increased.[110] In contrast to IELs, most lamina propria T-cells are CD4$^+$, and virtually all express the $\alpha\beta^+$ T-cell receptor.[111] Class II HLA-restricted gliadin-specific CD4$^+$ cells are present in the celiac mucosal lesions of the lamina propria. These cells respond to antigen stimulation by secreting cytokines such as interleukin (IL)-2, interferon (IFN)-γ and tumor necrosis factor (TNF) α; this enhanced cytokine production may in turn promote mucosal damage.[3,90,112] Plasma cells, also increased in untreated celiac disease, produce IgA, IgG and IgM in the lamina propria.[113] AGA and EmA can be produced by gluten challenge in small bowel mucosal biopsy samples from celiac patients.[114] Furthermore, IgA- and IgM-class antibodies against gliadin or reticulin have been detected in the jejunal fluid of celiac disease patients.[75,115] These findings suggest that celiac antibodies are of intestinal origin and are produced by lamina propria plasma cells.

Immunological and Pathogenetic Aspects

It is nowadays widely accepted that immunological mechanisms are implicated in the development of the mucosal damage in celiac disease. In untreated celiac patients there are signs of activation of both mucosal cellular and humoral immune systems.[90,116] The major environmental factor is ingested gluten (gliadin), but it has been suggested that enteric adenovirus infection also play a part in the initiation of the disease.[117]

Recently, Dieterich and associates[4] established that serum EmA, a specific indicator of active celiac disease, recognizes tissue transglutaminase. Activated endothelial, fibroblast and mononuclear cells are a rich source of tissue transglutaminase.[118] This enzyme is normally stored intracellularly, where it can be released during cellular wounding brought about by mechanical stress, inflammation, infection, or apoptosis. Tissue transglutaminase is now considered to be the predominant autoantigen for celiac disease, although other autoantigens may also be involved.[119,120] In active celiac disease, the expression of tissue transglutaminase is increased.[121] The enzyme can cross-link with gliadin to generate new antigenic neoepitopes. Gluten-specific HLA DQ2- and DQ8-restricted T-cells are present in the celiac mucosal lesions.[3] Antigen-presenting cells of the lamina propria present digested gluten peptide to CD4⁺ T-cells via their HLA DQ2 molecules. Through deamination of glutamine residues to negatively charged glutamic acid, the enzyme facilitates the binding of gliadin peptides to the peptic groove of HLA DQ2 and DQ8 molecules. This results in better binding affinity and in increased T-cell reactivity.[122] Stimulated T-cells secrete Th2 cytokines such as IL-4, allowing expansion of autoreactive B-cell clones, which induces in turn the formation of autoantibodies. The secretion of IFN-γ, TNFα and other inflammatory cytokines by activated lamina propria T-cells can damage the small bowel mucosa, leading to enteropathy.[116] For example, TNFα triggers intestinal fibroblasts to secrete matrix metalloproteinases (MMPs), which leads to mucosal destruction by dissolution of connective tissue. The inhibition of TNFα and MMP-3, but not of IFN-γ, has been seen to prevent such mucosal damage.[123] In vivo expression of MMP-1 and MMP-3 messenger RNA is increased in fibroblasts of celiac small bowel mucosa.[124]

Antibodies against tissue transglutaminase may play a direct role in the pathogenesis of small bowel mucosal damage in celiac disease. Epithelial differentiation on the crypt-villous axis is inhibited by tTG-ab in vitro.[125] Whether tTG-ab contributes to celiac-type small bowel mucosal damage in vivo has to be confirmed.

Increased Permeability in Celiac Disease

In untreated celiac disease, the epithelial barrier of the small bowel mucosa is deficient, leading to increased molecule permeability.[126] There is some evidence that in active celiac disease, the expression of cell adherence proteins E-cadherin and β-cathenin is decreased and returns to normal after treatment by gluten-free diet. In an in vitro model, pro-inflammatory cytokines such as TNFα, IL-1 and IFN-γ seem to downregulate E-cadherin and β-cathenin expression.[127] According to previous reports, even small changes in cadherin expression have profound effects on cell differentation and epithelial remodelling.[128] Zonulin, a human protein analogue to the *Vibrio cholerae*-derived Zonula occludence toxin, is able to open small bowel mucosal tight junctions. This allows the entry of putative antigens into the intestinal submucosa and can lead to the activation of autoimmune mechanisms. In active celiac disease, zonulin expression is increased.[129] On the whole, defects in the small bowel mucosal barrier may be important in regulating the development of small bowel mucosal lesion in celiac disease and in abrogating oral tolerance.

Table 3. Important steps in the pathogenesis of celiac disease

Factor	Importance
Gluten	Major cause of celiac disease
Other environmental factors, such as adenovirus infection	May be involved in causation of the disease
HLA DQ 2 and DQ8	Found in over 95% of Caucasian celiac disease patients
Non-HLA genes	May be involved, but no uniform gene or gene-region found so far
Tissue transglutaminase	Autoantigen of celiac disease: deamidates gliadin, which results in a better binding affinity of gliadin to HLA-molecule and in an increased T-cell reactivity
Transglutaminase and endomysial antibodies	Specific antibodies for celiac disease; may be involved in the pathogenesis of small bowel mucosal damage
Gluten-specific HLA-DQ restricted T-cells in small bowel mucosa	Activated T-cells secrete pro-inflammatory cytokines, resulting in small bowel mucosal damage

Conclusions

The clinical features of celiac disease are protean and by no means restricted to small bowel mucosa. Gluten, genetic susceptibility to autoimmune disorders, mucosal T-cells, and celiac autoantibodies are all involved in the pathogenesis of the disorder (Table 3). The recognition of tissue transglutaminase as a celiac autoantigen has much advanced the basic research in the field of gluten intolerance. We may soon understand the detailed mechanisms responsible for mucosal damage in celiac disease, leading to therapeutic alternatives to a gluten-free diet.

References

1. Marsh MN. Gluten, major histocompatibility complex, and the small intestine. A molecular and immunobiologic approach to the spectrum of gluten sensitivity ('celiac sprue'). Gastroenterology 1992; 102:330-354.
2. Sollid LM, Markussen G, Ek J et al. Evidence for a primary association of celiac disease to a particular HLA-DQ α/β heterodimer. J Exp Med 1989; 169:345-350.
3. Lundin K, EA, Scott H, Hansen T et al. Gliadin-specific, HLA-DQ(α1*0501, α1*0201) restricted T cells isolated from the small intestinal mucosa of celiac disease patients. J Exp Med 1993; 178:87-96.
4. Dieterich W, Ehnis T, Bauer M et al. Identification of tissue transglutaminase as the autoantigen of celiac disease. Nature Med 1997; 3:797-801.
5. Collin P, Hällström O, Mäki M et al. Atypical coeliac disease found with serologic screening. Scand J Gastroenterol 1990; 25:245-250.
6. Watson RG, McMillan SA, Dickey W et al. Detection of undiagnosed coeliac disease with atypical features using antireticulin and antigliadin antibodies. Q J Med 1992; 84:713-718.
7. Biemond I, Pena AS, Groenland F et al. Coeliac disease in The Netherlands: Demographic data of a patient survey among the members of the Dutch Coeliac Society. Neth J Med 1987; 31:263-268.
8. Ståhlberg MR, Savilahti E, Siimes MA. Iron deficiency in coeliac disease is mild and it is detected and corrected by gluten-free diet. Acta Paediatr Scand 1991; 80:190-193.
9. Bode S, Gudmand-Hoyer E. Symptoms and haematologic features in consecutive adult coeliac patients. Scand J Gastroenterol 1996; 31:54-60.

10. Hin H, Bird G, Fisher P et al. Coeliac disease in primary care, case finding study. BMJ 1999; 318:164-167.
11. van der Meer JB. Granular deposits of immunoglobulins in the skin of patients with dermatitis herpetformis. An immunofluorescent study. Br J Dermatol 1969; 81:493-503.
12. Fry L, Seah PP, McMinn RMH et al. Lymphocytic infiltration of epithelium in diagnosis of gluten-sensitive enteropathy. BMJ 1972; 3:371-374.
13. Reunala T, Kosnai I, Karpati S et al. Dermatitis herpetiformis: Jejunal findings and skin response to gluten-free diet. Arch Dis Child 1984; 59:517-522.
14. Reunala T, Blomqvist K, Tarpila S et al. Gluten-free diet in dermatitis herpetiformis. I. Clinical response of skin lesions in 81 patients. Br J Dermatol 1977; 97:473-480.
15. Auricchio S, Mazzacca G, Tosi R et al. Coeliac disease as a familial condition: Identification of asymptomatic coeliac patients within family groups. Gastroenterol Int 1988; 1:25-31.
16. Mäki M, Holm K, Lipsanen V et al. Serological markers and HLA genes among healthy first-degree relatives of patients with coeliac disease. Lancet 1991; 338:1350-1353.
17. Savilahti E, Pelkonen P, Visakorpi JK. IgA deficiency in children. A clinical study with special reference to intestinal findings. Arch Dis Child 1971; 46:665-670.
18. Meini A, Pillan NM, Villanacci V et al. Prevalence and diagnosis of celiac disease in IgA-deficient children. Ann Allergy Asthma Immunol 1996; 77:33-36.
19. Mäki M. The humoral immune system in coeliac disease. Baillieres Clin Gastroenterol 1995; 9:231-249.
20. Dieterich W, Laag E, Schopper H et al. Autoantibodies to tissue transglutaminase as predictors of celiac disease. Gastroenterology 1998; 115:1317-1321.
21. Sulkanen S, Halttunen T, Laurila K et al. Tissue transglutaminase autoantibody enzyme-linked immunosorbent assay in detecting celiac disease. Gastroenterology 1998; 115:1322-1328.
22. Johnston SD, Watson RGP, McMillan SA et al. Prevalence of coeliac disease in Northern Ireland. Lancet 1997; 350:1370.
23. Holmes GKT, Prior P, Lane MR et al. Malignancy in coeliac disease - effect of a gluten free diet. Gut 1989; 30:333-338.
24. Molteni N, Caraceni MP, Bardella MT et al. Bone mineral density in adult celiac patients and the effect of gluten-free diet from childhood. Am J Gastroenterol 1990; 85:51-53.
25. Ventura A, Magazzu G, Greco L. Duration of exposure to gluten and risk for autoimmune disorders in patients with celiac disease. Gastroenterology 1999; 117:297-303.
26. Dicke WK. Coeliakie, M.D. Thesis, Utrecht 1950.
27. Anand BS, Piris J, Truelove SC. Role of various cereals in coeliac disease. Q J Med 1978; 47:101-110.
28. van de Kamer JH, Weijers HA, Dicke WK. Coeliac disease. IV. An investigation into the injurious constituents of wheat in connection with their action on patients with coeliac disease. Acta Paediatr 1953; 42:223-231.
29. Dissanayake AS, Truelove SC, Whitehead R. Lack of harmful effect of oats on small-intestinal mucosa in coeliac disease. BMJ 1974; 1974:189-191.
30. Baker PG, Read AE. Oats and barley toxicity in coeliac patients. Postgrad Med J 1976; 52:264-268.
31. Janatuinen EK, Pikkarainen PH, Kemppainen TA et al. A comparison of diets with and without oats in adults with celiac disease. N Engl J Med 1995; 333:1033-1037.
32. Srinivasan U, Leonard N, Jones E et al. Absence of oats toxicity in adult coeliac disease. BMJ 1996; 313:1300-1301.
33. Hardman CM, Garioch JJ, Leonard JN et al. Absence of toxicity of oats in patients with dermatitis herpetiformis. N Engl J Med 1997; 337:1884-1887.
34. Reunala T, Collin P, Holm K et al. Tolerance to oats in dermatitis herpetiformis. Gut 1998; 43:490-493.
35. Hoffenberg EJ, Haas J, Drescher A et al. A trial of oats in children with newly diagnosed celiac disease. J Pediatr 2000; 137:361-366.
36. Ascher H, Krantz I, Kristiansson B. Increasing incidence of coeliac disease in Sweden. Arch Dis Child 1991; 66:608-611.
37. Ivarsson A, Persson LA, Nystrom L et al. Epidemic of coeliac disease in Swedish children. Acta Paediatr 2000; 89:165-171.

38. MacDonald WC, Dobbins WO, Rubin CE. Studies on the familial nature of coeliac sprue using biopsy of the small intestine. N Engl J Med 1965; 272:448-456.

39. Polanco I, Biemond I, van Leeuwen A et al. Gluten sensitive enteropathy in Spain: Genetic and environmental factors. In: McConell RB, ed. the genetics of coeliac disease. Lancaster: MTP Press, 1981:211-234.

40. Mearin ML, Biemond I, Pena AS et al. HLA-DR phenotypes in Spanish coeliac children: Their contribution to the understanding of the genetics of the disease. Gut 1983;24:532-537.

41. Falchuk ZM, Rogentine FN, Strober W. Predominance of histocompatibility antigen HLA-A8 in patients with gluten-sensitive enteropathy. J Clin Invest 1972;51:1602-1606.

42. Stokes PL, Asquith P, Holmes GKT et al. Histocompatibility antigens associated with adult coeliac disease. Lancet 1972; 2:162-164.

43. Keuning JJ, Pena AS, van Leeuwen A et al. HLA-DW3 associated with coeliac disease. Lancet 1976; 1:506-508.

44. Verkasalo M, Tiilikainen A, Kuitunen P et al. HLA antigens and atopy in children with coeliac disease. Gut 1983; 24:306-310.

45. Tosi R, Vismara D, Tanigaki N et al. Evidence that celiac disease is primarily associated with a DC locus allelic specificity. Clin Immunol Immunopathol 1983; 28:395-404.

46. Polvi A, Eland C, Koskimies S et al. HLA DQ and DP in Finnish families with coeliac disease. Eur J Immunogen 1996; 23:221-234.

47. Spurkland A, Sollid LM, Polanco I et al. HLA -DR and -DQ genotypes of celiac disease patients serologically typed to be non-DR3 or non-DR 5/7. Human Immunol 1992; 35:188-192.

48. Michalski JP, McCombs CC, Arai T et al. HLA-DR, DQ genotypes of celiac disease patients and healthy subjects from the West of Ireland. Tissue Antigens 1996; 47:127-133.

49. Polvi A, Arranz E, Fernandez-Arquero M et al. HLA-DQ2-negative celiac disease in Finland and Spain. Hum Immunol 1998; 59:169-175.

50. Dalton TA, Bennet JC. Autoimmune disease and major histocompatibility complex: therapeutic implications. Am J Med 1992; 92:183-188.

51. Zhong F, McCombs CC, Olson JM et al. An autosomal screen for genes that predispose to celiac disease in the western counties of Ireland. Nature Genet 1996; 14:329-333.

52. Houlston RS, Tomlinson IP, Ford D et al. Linkage analysis of candidate regions for coeliac disease genes. Hum Mol Genet 1997; 6:1335-1339.

53. Greco L, Corazza G, Babron M-C et al. Genome search in celiac disease. Am J Hum Genet 1998; 62:669-675.

54. Holopainen P, Arvas M, Sistonen P et al. CD28/CTLA4 gene region on chromosome 2q3 confers genetic susceptibility to celiac disease. A linkage and family-based association study. Tissue antigens 1999; 53:470-475.

55. Lie BA, Sollid LM, Ascher H et al. A gene telomeric of the HLA class I region is involved in predisposition to type I diabetes and coeliac disease. Tissue Antigens 1999; 54:162-168.

56. Roy-Choudhury D, Cooke WT, Tan DT et al. Jejunal biopsy: criteria and significance. Scand J Gastroenterol 1966; 1:57-74.

57. Ferguson A, Murray D. Quantitation of intraepithelial lymphocytes in human jejunum. Gut 1971; 12:988-994.

58. Kuitunen P, Kosnai I, Savilahti E. Morphometric study of the jejunal mucosa in various childhood enteropathies with special reference to intraepithelial lymphocytes. J Pediatr Gastroenterol Nutr 1982; 1:525-531.

59. Lancaster-Smith M, Kumar PJ, Dawson AM. The cellular infiltrate of jejunum in adult coeliac disease and dermatitis herpetiformis following the reintroduction of dietary gluten. Gut 1975; 16:683-688.

60. Stewart JS, Pollock DJ, Hoffbrand AV et al. A study of proximal and distal intestinal structure and absorptive function in idiopatic steatorrhoea. Q J Med 1967; 36:425-444.

61. Chapman BL, Henry K, Paice F et al. Measuring the response of the jejunum mucosa in adult coeliac disease to treatment with a gluten-free diet. Gut 1974; 15:870-874.

62. MacDonald WC, Brandborg LL, Flick AL et al. Studies of celiac disease sprue. IV. The response of whole length of the small bowel to a gluten-free diet. Gastroenterology 1964; 47:573-589.

63. McNicholl B, B. E-M, Stevens F et al. Mucosal recovery in treated chilhood celiac disease (gluten-sensitive enteropathy). J Pediatr 1976; 89:418-424.
64. McNicholl B, Egan-Mitchell B, Fottrell PF. Variability of gluten intolerance in treated childhood coeliac disease. Gut 1979; 20:126-132.
65. Kuitunen P, Visakorpi JK, Savilahti E et al. Malabsorption syndrome with cow's milk intolerance. Clinical findings and course in 54 cases. Arch Dis Child 1975; 50:351-356.
66. Katz AJ, Grand RJ. All that flattens is not "sprue". Gastroenterology 1979; 76:375-377.
67. Ferguson A, Arranz E, O'Mahony S. Clinical and pathological spectrum of coeliac disease—Active, silent, latent, potential. Gut 1993; 34:150-151.
68. Weinstein WM. Latent celiac sprue. Gastroenterology 1974; 66:489-493.
69. Ferguson A, Blackwell JN, Barnetson RS. Effects of additional dietary gluten on the small-intestinal mucosa of volunteers and of patients with dermatitis herpetiformis. Scand J Gastroenterol 1987; 22:543-549.
70. Doherty M, Barry RE. Gluten-induced mucosal changes in subjects without overt small-bowel disease. Lancet 1981; 1:517-520.
71. Mäki M, Holm K, Koskimies S et al. Normal small bowel biopsy followed by coeliac disease. Arch Dis Child 1990; 65:1137-1141.
72. Corazza GR, Andreani ML, Biagi F et al. Clinical, pathological, and antibody pattern of latent celiac disease: report of three adult cases. Am J Gastroenterol 1996; 91:2203-2207.
73. Mäki M, Collin P. Coeliac disease. Lancet 1997; 349:1755-1759.
74. Mäki M, Holm K, Collin P et al. Increase in gamma/delta T cell receptor bearing lymphocytes in normal small bowel mucosa in latent coeliac disease. Gut 1991; 32:1412-1414.
75. Arranz E, Ferguson A. Intestinal antibody pattern of celiac disease: Occurrence in patients with normal jejunal biopsy histology. Gastroenterology 1993; 104:1263-1272.
76. Arranz E, Bode J, Kingstone K et al. Intestinal antibody pattern of coeliac disease: Association with gamma/delta T cell receptor expression by intraepithelial lymphocytes, and other indices of potential coeliac disease. Gut 1994; 35:476-482.
77. Troncone R, Greco L, Mayer M et al. Latent and potential coeliac disease. Acta Paediatr Suppl 1996; 412:10-14.
78. Collin P, Helin H, Mäki M et al. Follow-up of patients positive in reticulin and gliadin antibody tests with normal small bowel biopsy findings. Scand J Gastroenterol 1993; 28:595-598.
79. Troncone R. Latent coeliac disease in Italy. Acta Paediatr 1995; 84:1252-1257.
80. Kaukinen K, Collin P, Holm K et al. Small bowel mucosal inflammation in reticulin or gliadin antibody-positive patients without villous atrophy. Scand J Gastroenterol 1998; 33:944-949.
81. Iltanen S, Holm K, Partanen J et al. Increased density of jejunal gamma/delta + T cells in patients having normal mucosa-marker of operative autoimmune mechanisms. Autoimmunity 1999; 29:179-187.
82. Wright N, Watson A, Morley A et al. Cell kinetics in flat (avillous) mucosa of the human small intestine. Gut 1973; 14:701-710.
83. Bajaj-Elliot M, Poulsom R, Pender SL et al. Interactions between stromal cell-derived keratinocyte growth factor and epithelial transforming growth factor in immune-mediated crypt cell hyperplasia. J Clin Invest 1998; 102:1473-1480.
84. Moss SF, Attia L, Scholes JV et al. Increased small intestinal apoptosis in coeliac disease. Gut 1996; 39:811-817.
85. Verkasalo MA, Arato A, Savilahti E et al. Effect of diet and age on jejunal and circulating lymphocyte subsets in children with coeliac disease: persistence of CD4-8-intraepithelial T cells through treatment. Gut 1990; 31:422-425.
86. Selby WS, Janossy G, Bofill M et al. Lymphocyte subpopulations in the human small intestine. The findings in normal mucosa and in the mucosa of patients with adult coeliac disease. Clin Exp Immunol 1983; 52:219-228.
87. Savilahti E, Arato A, Verkasalo M. Intestinal gamma/delta receptor-bearing T lymphocytes in celiac disease and inflammatory bowel diseases in children. Constant increase in celiac disease. Pediatr Res 1990; 28:579-581.
88. Savilahti E, Reunala T, Mäki M. Increase of lymphocytes bearing the gamma/delta T cell receptor in the jejunum of patients with dermatitis herpetiformis. Gut 1992; 33:206-211.

89. Kutlu T, Brousse N, Rambaud C et al. Numbers of T cell receptor (TCR) alpha beta+ but not of TcR gamma delta+ intraepithelial lymphocytes correlate with the grade of villous atrophy in coeliac patients on a long term normal diet. Gut 1993; 34:208-214.

90. Tredjosiewics LK, Howdle PD. T-cell responses and cellular immunity in coeliac disease. Baillieres Clin Gastroenterol 1995; 9:251-272.

91. Oberhuber G, Vogelsang H, Stolte M et al. Evidence that intestinal intraepithelial lymphocytes are activated cytotoxic T cells in celiac disease but not in giardiasis. Am J Pathol 1996; 148:1351-1357.

92. Spencer J, Isaacson PG, Diss TC et al. Expression of disulfide-linked and non-disulfide-linked forms of the T cell receptor gamma/delta heterodimer in human intestinal intraepithelial lymphocytes. Eur J Immunol 1989; 19:1335-1338.

93. Spencer J, Isaacson PG, MacDonald TT et al. Gamma/delta T cells and the diagnosis of coeliac disease. Clin Exp Immunol 1991; 85:109-113.

94. Halstensen TS, Scott H, Brandtzaeg P. Intraepithelial T cells of the TcR gamma/delta+ CD8- and V delta 1/J delta 1+ phenotypes are increased in coeliac disease. Scand J Immunol 1989; 30:665-672.

95. Iltanen S, Holm K, Ashorn M et al. Changing jejunal gamma/delta T cell receptor (TCR)-bearing intraepithelial lymphocyte density in coeliac disease. Clin Exp Immunol 1999; 117:51-55.

96. Kaukinen K, Collin P, Holm K et al. Wheat starch-containing gluten-free flour products in the treatment of coeliac disease and dermatitis herpetiformis. A long-term follow-up study. Scand J Gastroenterol 1999; 34:164-169.

97. Holm K, Mäki M, Savilahti E et al. Intraepithelial gamma/delta T-cell-receptor lymphocytes and genetic susceptibility to coeliac disease. Lancet 1992; 339:1500-1503.

98. Chan KN, Phillips AD, Walker-Smith JA et al. density of gamma/delta T cells in small bowel mucosa realated to HLA-DQ status without coeliac disease. Lancet 1993; 342:492-493.

99. Pesce G, Pesce F, Fiorino N et al. Intraepithelial gamma/delta-positive T lymphocytes and intestinal villous atrophy. Int Arch Allergy Immunol 1996; 110:233-237.

100. Kaukinen K, Turjanmaa K, Mäki M et al. Intolerance to cereals is not specific for coeliac disease. Scand J Gastroenterol 2000; 35:942-946.

101. Brenner MB, McLean J, Scheft H et al. Two forms of the T-cell reseptor gamma protein found on peripherial blood cytotoxic T lymphocytes. Nature 1987; 325:689-694.

102. Viney J, MacDonald TT, Spencer J. Gamma-delta T-cells in gut epithelium. Gut 1990; 31:841-844.

103. McMenamin C, Pimm C, McKersey M et al. Regulation of IgE responses to inhaled antigen in mice by antigen-specific gammadelta T cells. Science 1994; 265:1869-1871.

104. Boismenu R, Havran WL. Modulation of epithelial growth by intraepithelial gamma/delta T cells. Science 1994; 266:1253-1255.

105. Mukasa A, Hiromatsu K, Matsuzaki G et al. Bacterial infection of testis leading to autoaggressive immunity triggers apparently opposed responses of alfa beta and gamma delta T cells. J Immunol 1995; 155:2047-2056.

106. Roberts SJ, Smith AL, West AB et al. T-cell alpha beta+ and gamma delta+ deficient mice display abnormal but distinct phenotypes toward a natural, widespread infection of the intestinal epithelium. Proc Natl Acad Sci USA 1996; 93:11774-11779.

107. Groh V, Steinle A, Bauer S et al. Recognition of stress-induced MHC molecules by intestinal epithelial gamma/delta T cells. Science 1998; 279:1737-1740.

108. Barrett TA, Tatsumi Y, Bluestone JA. Tolerance of T cell reseptor gamma/delta cells in the intestine. J Exp Med 1993; 177:1755-1762.

109. Ke Y, Pearce K, Lake JP et al. Gamma delta T lymphocytes regulate the induction and maintainance of oral tolerance. J Immunol 1997; 158:3610-3618.

110. Dhesi I, Marsh MN, Kelly C et al. Morphometric analysis of small intestinal mucosa. II. Determination of lamina propria volumes; plasma cell and neutrophil populations within control and coeliac disease mucosae. Virchows Arch A Pathol Anat Histopathol 1984; 403:173-180.

111. MacDonald T, Spencer J. T-cell subpopulations in intestinal mucosa. In: Mearin ML, Mulder CJJ, eds. Coeliac Disease. Netherlands: Kluwer Academic Publishers, 1991:51-56.

112. Molberg Ø, Kett K, Scott H et al. Gliadin specific, HLA DQ2-restricted T cells are commonly found in small intestinal biopsies from coeliac disease patients, but not from controls. Scand J Immunol 1997; 46:103-108.

113. Savilahti E. Intestinal immunoglobulins in children with coeliac disease. Gut 1972; 13:958-964.

114. Picarelli A, Maiuri L, Frate A et al. Production of antiendomysial antibodies after in-vitro glaidin challenge af small intestine biopsy samples from patients with coeliac disease. Lancet 1996; 348:1065-1067.

115. O'Mahony S, Arranz E, Barton JR et al. Dissociation between systemic and mucosal humoral immune responses in coeliac disease. Gut 1991; 32:29-35.

116. Sollid LM, Molberg O, McAdam S et al. Autoantibodies in coeliac disease: Tissue transglutaminase— Guilt by association. Gut 1997; 41:851-852.

117. Kagnoff MF, Paterson YJ, Kumar PJ et al. Evidence for the role of a human intestinal adenovirus in the pathogenesis of coeliac disease. Gut 1987; 28:995-1001.

118. Piacentini M, Colizzi V. Tissue transglutamine: apoptosis versus autoimmunity. Immunol Today 1999; 3:130-134.

119. Lock RJ, Gilmour JEM, Unsworth DJ. Anti-transglutaminase, anti-endomysium and anti-R1-reticulin autoantibodies—The antibody trinity of coeliac disease. Clin Exp Immunol 1999; 116:258-262.

120. Brusco G, Muzi P, Ciccocioppo R et al. Transglutaminase and coeliac disease: Endomysial reactivity and small bowel expression. Clin Exp Immunol 1999; 118:371-375.

121. Bruce SE, Bjarnason I, Peters TJ. Human jejunal transglutaminase: Demonstration of activity, enzyme kinetics and substrate specificity with special relation to gliadin and coeliac disease. Clin Sci 1985; 68:573-579.

122. Molberg O, Mcadam SN, Korner R et al. Tissue transglutaminase selectively modifies gliadin peptides that are recognized by gut-derived T cells in celiac disease. Nat Med 1998; 4:713-717.

123. Pender SL, Tickle SP, Docherty AJ et al. A role of matrix metalloproteinases in T cell injury in the gut. J Immunol 1997; 158:1582-1590.

124. Daum S, Bauer U, Foss HD et al. Increased expression of mRNA for matrix metalloproteinase-1 and -3 and tissue inhibitor of metalloproteinases-1 in intestinal biopsy specimens from patients with coeliac disease. Gut 1999; 44:17-25.

125. Halttunen T, Mäki M. Serum immunoglobulin A from patients with celiac disease inhibits human T84 intestinal crypt epithelial cell differentation. Gastroenterology 1999; 116:566-572.

126. Schulzke JD, Schulzke I, Fromm M et al. Epithelial barrier and ion transport in coeliac sprue: Electrical measurements on intestinal aspiration biopsy specimens. Gut 1995; 37:777-782.

127. Perry I, Tselepis C, Hoyland J et al. Reduced cadherin/catenin complex expression in celiac disease can be reproduced in vitro by cytokine stimulation. Lab Invest 1999; 79:1489-1499.

128. Jankowski JA, Bedford FK, Kim YS. Changes in gene structure and regulation of E-cadherin during epithelial development, differentation, and disease. Prog Nucleic Acid Res Mol Biol 1997; 57:187-215.

129. Fasano A, Not T, W. W et al. Zonulin, a newly discovered modulator of intestinal permeability, and its expression in coeliac disease. Lancet 2000; 355:1518-1519.

130. Congia M, Cucca F, Frau F et al. A gene dosage effect of the DQA1*0501/DQ*0201 allelic combination influences the clinical heterogenity of celiac disease. Hum Immunol 1994; 40:138-142.

131. Ploski R, Ascher H, Sollid LM. HLA genotypes and the increased insidence of coeliac disease in Sweden. Scand J Gastroenterol 1996; 31:1092-1097.

132. Balas A, Vicario JL, Zambrano A et al. Absolute linkage of celiac disease and dermatitis herpetiformis to HLA-DQ. Tissue Antigens 1997; 50:52-56.

CHAPTER 10

Clinical Applications of Oral Tolerance

Howard L. Weiner

Introduction

Oral tolerance has classically been defined as the specific suppression of cellular and/or humoral immune responses to an antigen by prior administration of the antigen by the oral route. It presumably evolved to prevent hypersensitivity reactions to food proteins and bacterial antigens present in the mucosal flora. "Immunologic tolerance" has often been defined as a mechanism by which the immune system prevents pathologic autoreactivity against self and thus prevents autoimmune diseases.

The term "tolerance" was first used by Burnet[1] and three assumptions are implicit in Burnet's concept of tolerance: 1) the primary function of the immune system is to defend the organism against pathogens or, in a broader sense, against non-self materials; 2) in order to perform such a function, the major immunologic response is an inflammatory class of response; and 3) since the operation of the immune system is driven by its reactions to foreign pathogens, tolerance is a negative counterpart of the immune system accomplished by neonatal deletion of "forbidden clones".

With a better understanding of the immune system, it is now clear that "tolerance" is a much more complicated and diverse process. Autoreactive cells, such as those reacting with brain antigens, thyroglobulin, serum albumin, collagen and other autoantigens are, in fact, not deleted and are present in all individuals.[2,3] They not only remain harmless under normal conditions, but cells autoreactive with self may have an important function in maintaining tissue homeostasis and may be differentially focused depending on the tissue and the autoantigen.[4] Furthermore, the basis of immunologic tolerance does not appear to simply be distinguishing between self and non-self, but reacting to danger signals that confront the immune system.[5] Thus, immunological tolerance cannot rely solely on neonatal deletional events, but requires an active process that functions during the entire life of the organism.

Tolerance has been defined as a lack of response to self but a more appropriate definition of tolerance is "any mechanism by which a potentially injurious immune response is prevented, suppressed, or shifted to a non-injurious class of immune response". Thus, tolerance is related to productive self-recognition rather than blindness of the immune system to its autocomponents.

Oral tolerance, in this sense, is of unique immunologic importance since it is a continuous natural immunologic event driven by exogenous antigen. Due to their privileged access to the internal milieu, antigens that continuously contact the mucosa represent a frontier between foreign and self components. Thus, oral tolerance is an immunological mechanism that evolved to treat external agents that gain access to the body via a natural route as internal components which then become part of self. Given this, it would seem logical that autoimmune diseases

Oral Tolerance: The Response of the Intestinal Mucosa to Dietary Antigens,
edited by Olivier Morteau. ©2004 Eurekah.com and Kluwer Academic / Plenum Publishers.

caused by an inappropriate response to self antigens might ultimately be treated by presenting such autoantigens to the mucosal surface where they can be dealt with in a non-injurous (non-inflammatory) immunologic environment. Furthermore mucosal tolerance is an attractive treatment for autoimmune diseases as antigen specific therapy is the most physiologic method to manipulate immune responses and mucosal antigen is non-toxic and can be given on a chronic basis (Table 1).

In the eighties, oral tolerance began to attract considerable attention when it was shown to be an effective means of inhibiting immune responses to antigens of immunopathological importance in animals including type II collagen.[6,7] and myelin basic protein.[8,9] In the nineties oral tolerance was then applied for the treatment of human diseases.[10] The potential clinical application of oral or mucosal tolerance has spread beyond autoimmune diseases with positive clinical findings in animal models of transplantation, allergy, asthma and in diseases not classically considered immune mediated in which immune mechanisms play a role such as atherosclerosis, stroke, and Alzheimer's disease.

Because it is known that in autoimmune disease autoreactive T cells are not deleted in the thymus, strategies to deal with these pathogenic cells are required. Oral administration of antigen has the potential to suppress or tolerize these cells through the different mechanisms by which mucosal tolerance operates. In addition to anergy and deletion, one of the most therapeutically attractive approaches involves the generation of regulatory cells, one of the major immunologic mechanisms of oral tolerance.[11] The mucosal milieu creates tolerogenic dendritic cells and Th3 and Tr1 and CD25[+] regulatory cells.[12,13] In addition CD8[+] regulatory cells have been described.[14] The inductive events associated with mucosal tolerance are unique as there are unique dendritic cells in the gastrointestinal and pulmonary compartments.[15] In addition the cytokine environment of the mucosa contains interleukin (IL)-10 and transforming growth factor (TGF)-β which favor the generation of tolerogenic signals. Virtually all immune functions have been reported to be affected by oral tolerance including both Th1 and Th2 responses although larger amounts of antigen are required to suppress Th2 responses. There have been no reports of suppression of TGF-β by oral antigen. The application of mucosal tolerance clinically is complicated by many factors including the age of those being treated and the genetic background. Furthermore oral tolerance is less easily induced in primed immune system although it has been achieved. Thus it is possible that early treatment or treatment following global immunosuppression or removal of primed cells will be required prior to induction of oral tolerance. The intestinal flora may effect oral tolerance and oral tolerance is less easily induced when there is inflammation in the gut associated lymphoid tissue (GALT). Some antigens have better tolerogenic capacities related to both the purity of the antigen and antigen structure. Finally in some instances antigen administered by the nasal route may be preferable to that administered orally. Nasal antigen may require a lower dose and may not be as easily susceptible to degradation in the gut. Furthermore, it may induce responses that are biased more towards IL-10 than TGF-β.[16]

Mechanisms of Oral Tolerance and Immune Functions Affected by Oral Tolerance

It is now clear that oral tolerance is an active immunologic process[11] and is mediated by more than one mechanism (Table 2). Low doses of antigen administration favor the induction of active cellular regulation whereas higher doses favor the induction of anergy or deletion. In many respects the term "oral tolerance" is an inadequate immunologic term as it has primarily been used to define the occurrence of systemic hyporesponsiveness when an animal is immunized after oral antigen administration. We now realize that "oral tolerance" is a complex process that involves suppression of some immune responses and the induction of others. Thus, an understanding of oral tolerance and its use for the treatment of autoimmune or inflammatory

---

Table 1. Therapeutic advantages of mucosal tolerance

---

1. Antigen specific therapy is the most physiologic method to manipulate immune responses
2. Mucosal administration is non-toxic and can be given on a chronic basis
3. Efficacy of mucosal tolerance has been overwhelmingly demonstrated in animals models
4. Tolerance mechanisms better defined

Table 2. Mechanism of oral tolerance

---

1. High doses favor deletion or anergy
2. Low doses favor induction of regulatory cells that secrete Il-4, Il-10 or TGF-β (Th3 type r regulatory cells
3. CD4+CD25+ and Tr1 type regulatory cells are induced by mucosal antigen
4. Intragraft CD8+ regulatory cells are induced by oral alloantigen

---

diseases involves defining the basic immunologic events that occur when antigen encounters the gut associated lymphoid tissue (GALT). Antigen may act directly at the level of the GALT or have an effect following absorption. In this regard, "oral tolerance" and "mucosal immunization" are part of one immunologic continuum and are ultimately explained in the context of how an antigen-presenting cell interacts with a T cell in the GALT and the factors which modulate and regulate this response. Thus in addition to antigen dose, the nature of the antigen, the innate immune system, the genetic background and immunological status of the host, and mucosal adjuvants influence the immunologic outcome following oral antigen administration.

Virtually all manifestations of specific immune responsiveness tested can be suppressed by oral antigen administration (Table 3). This includes in vivo responses such as formation of immunoglobulin of different isotypes,[17,18] delayed hypersensitivity reactions 19, 20, and changes in the rate of antigen clearance from the circulation[21] as well as in vitro assays such as specific plaque forming cells 22, 23, lymphocyte proliferation,[9,23-25] and cytokine production.[10,26] Of note, the suppression of TGF-β response following oral antigen has not been reported for any dose or regimen of orally administered antigen.

Nonetheless, these immunological parameters are differentially affected by oral antigen. Delayed-type hypersensitivity (DTH) is more easily suppressed by oral antigen than is antibody formation in mice,[20,27-29] guinea pigs[30] and humans.[31] Suppression of DTH requires lower doses of oral antigen and tolerance persists longer.[32] Also of note, suppression of DTH induction, but not of antibody responses, may be induced in neonates reconstituted with adult spleen cells.[33,34] On the other hand, oral tolerance to DTH is more readily broken by treatment with cyclophosphamide[20] or stradiol[35] and is more difficult to induce in protein-deprived mice than oral tolerance to humoral responses.[36]

A possible explanation for the in vivo differences in susceptibility to oral tolerance induction may relate to the susceptibility of distinct subsets of CD4+ T cells, namely Th1 and Th2 subpopulations, to oral tolerance induction. Th1- dependent cytokines, such as IL-2 and interferon (IFN)-γ, are readily inhibited by feeding multiple low doses of antigen whereas Th2-dependent cytokines, such as IL-4, IL-5 and IL-10, require high doses of antigen to be suppressed.[10,26,37-39] This would explain also why IL-4-dependent IgG1 responses are more resistant to oral tolerance induction than IFN-γ-dependent IgG2a responses.[37,40]

Table 3. Immune functions affected by oral tolerance

1. DTH responses
2. Lymphocyte proliferation (IL-2;IFNγ)
3. Antibody responses including IgE
4. Th2 responses (Il-4, Il-5, Il-10)
5. Lower doses of antigen required to suppress Th1 than Th2 responses
6. No reports of TFG-β (Th3) suppression

Other studies however argue against such a simple interpretation. It has been known since 1977 that the IL-4-dependent IgE response is highly susceptible to oral tolerance induction.[17,18,41] At the same time, IL-5 and IFN-γ may exhibit similar susceptibilities to feeding over a wide range of single doses of OVA.[40] A number of authors have reported that the development of oral tolerance is preceded by antigen-specific IFN-γ production[40,42-45] raising the theoretical possibility of a role for IFN-γ in oral tolerance. Of note is that nasal tolerance induction to IgE responses seems to be dependent on γδ T cells and IFN-γ production.[46] Investigators working with self antigens and superantigens also suggest that IFN-γ may play a role in tolerance induction.[47] Liu and Janeway[48] reported a reversal of tolerance by depletion of IFN-_ and Cauley and coworkers[47] have shown secretion of IFN-γ by regulatory cells able to transfer suppression to staphylococcal enterotoxin A (SEA) to naive recipients.

Bystander Suppression

Bystander suppression is a concept that regulatory cells induced by a fed antigen can suppress immune responses stimulated by different antigen as long as the fed antigen is present in the anatomic vicinity.[49] Bystander suppression was demonstrated in vitro when it was shown that cells from animals fed low doses of myelin basic protein (MBP) could suppress proliferation of an ovalbumin line across a transwell.[49] The cells from MBP-fed animals suppressed across the transwell only when triggered by the fed antigen. In an analogous fashion, cells from ovalbumin (OVA) fed animals suppressed an MBP line across the transwell when stimulated with OVA. The soluble factor shown to be responsible for the suppression was TGF-β. Bystander suppression was then demonstrated in vivo. Feeding ovalbumin has no effect on MBP-induced experimental allergic encephalomyelitis (EAE) in the Lewis rat. However, if animals are fed ovalbumin and then given aqueous ovalbumin in the footpad following immunization in the footpad with MBP/complete Freund's adjuvant (CFA), EAE is suppressed. Suppression is mediated by OVA-specific regulatory cells which migrate to the draining lymph node and secrete TGF-β upon encountering OVA and thus inhibit the generation of the MBP-specific immune response being generated in the lymph node.[49] Bystander suppression is specific to the fed antigen and is transferable. Further demonstration of bystander or tissue-specific suppression in vivo was obtained using MBP peptides.[50] In the Lewis rat, MBP peptide 21-40 is a non-encephalitogenic epitope whereas 71-90 is the encephalitogenic epitope. Peptide 21-40 triggers TGF-β release following oral tolerization and orally-administered 21-40 suppresses 71-90 induced EAE in the Lewis rat. Furthermore, in 71-90 immunized animals protected by oral administration of peptide 21-40, DTH responses in the ear to peptide 71-90 are not suppressed whereas DTH responses to whole MBP are suppressed and suppression occurs because the 21-40 epitope is present in whole MBP to trigger TGF-β-secreting cells. Another example of tissue-specific bystander suppression is the suppression of proteolipid (PLP)-peptide-induced disease in the SJL mouse by feeding low doses of myelin basic protein or MBP peptides[51]. In addition to its role in EAE,[52] bystander suppression has also been demonstrated in several autoimmune and other models (Table 4).

Bystander suppression solves a major conceptual problem in the design of antigen- or T cell-specific therapy for inflammatory autoimmune diseases such as multiple sclerosis (MS), type 1 diabetes and rheumatoid arthritis (RA), in which the autoantigen is unknown or where there are reactivities to multiple autoantigens in the target tissue. During the course of chronic inflammatory autoimmune processes in animals, there is intra- and interantigenic spread of autoreactivity at the target organ.[53] In human autoimmune diseases, there are reactivities to multiple autoantigens in the target tissue. For example, in MS there is immune reactivity to at least three myelin antigens: MBP, PLP and myelin oligodendrocyte glycoprotein (MOG)·[3,54] In type 1 diabetes, there are multiple islet-cell antigens that could be the target of autoreactivity, including glutamic acid decarboxylase (GAD), insulin and heat shock proteins.[55] Thus for a human organ-specific inflammatory disease, it is not necessary to know the specific antigen that is the target of an autoimmune response, but only to administer orally an antigen capable of inducing regulatory cells, which then migrate to the target tissue and suppress inflammation. Bystander suppression has recently been shown by IL-10 secreting Tr1 cells in which an OVA-specific Tr1 clone could suppress a murine model of inflammatory bowel disease in vivo when fed OVA.[56] In arthritis, bystander suppression was demonstrated by feeding type II collagen (CII) in the antigen arthritis model,[57] the adjuvant arthritis model[58] and the streptococcal cell wall arthritis model.[59] Oral insulin suppresses lymphocytic choriomeningitis virus (LCMV)-induced diabetes.[60] Bystander suppression induced by non-self antigens have been demonstrated by Bloom in the EAE model[61] and by Pullerits[62] in the response to the hapten trimellitic anhydride (TMA), a cause of occupational asthma. In the later model, DTH responses but not antibody levels were suppressed by feeding and co-immunization with ovalbumin.

Bystander suppression may be more difficult to induce in uveitis models[63] where it may occur at the site of induction of autoimmune cells but not in the target organ. A contributing factor could by a difference in the ability of Th1 and Th2 cells to migrate into the target organ. Differential migration has been mentioned by Miossec and van den Berg[64] as a limitation of the oral tolerance approach, specifically in reference to arthritis. Difficulty in recruiting regulatory cells to the target organ could influence the efficacy of the oral tolerance approach to therapy regardless of the antigen. Age may also play a role in bystander suppression. Feeding high doses of OVA has been reported to induce bystander suppression in adult rats but anergy in young animals.[65] In theory, bystander suppression could be applied to the treatment of organ-specific inflammatory conditions that are not classic autoimmune diseases, such as psoriasis, or could be used to target anti-inflammatory cytokines to an organ where inflammation may play a role in disease pathogenesis even if the disease is not primarily autoimmune in nature. For example, oral MBP decreased stroke size in a rat stroke model, presumably by decreasing inflammation associated with ischemic injury.[66] Although bystander suppression was initially described in association with regulatory cells induced by oral antigen, the process could in principal be induced by any immune manipulation that induces Th2- or Th-3-type regulatory cells. Bystander suppression mediated by TGF-β secretion was also reported in a mouse model of transplantation tolerance.[67]

Modulation of Oral Tolerance

A number of factors have been reported to modulate oral tolerance. As oral tolerance has usually been defined in terms of Th1 responses, anything that suppress Th1 and/or enhances Th2 or Th3 cell development would enhance oral tolerance (Table 5). Th3 cells appear to use IL-4 as one of its growth /differentiation factors.[68] Seder have also recently found that IL-4, and TGF-β, may serve to promote growth of TGF-β secreting cells.[69] Thus, IL-4 administra-

Table 4. Models of autoimmune and other diseases that demonstrate bystander suppression

Autoimmune Disease	Immunizing Antigen	Oral Antigen	Target Organ
Arthritis	BSA, mycobacteria	Type II collagen	Joint
EAE	PLP	MBP	Brain
EAE	MBP peptide 71-90	MBP peptide 21-40	Brain
EAE	MBP	OVA	Lymph node, DTH
Diabetes	LCMV	Insulin	Pancreatic islets
IBD	CD4$^+$CD45RBhi T cell transfer	OVA	Intestine
Stroke	None	MBP	Brain

Abbreviation: BSA, bovine serum albumin; DTH, delayed-type hypersensitivity; EAE, experimental allergic encephalomyelitis; LCMV, lymphocytic choriomeningitis virus; MBP, myeline basic protein, OVA, ovalbumin; PLP, proteolipid; IBD, inflammatory bowl disease.

tion i.p. enhances low-dose oral tolerance to MBP in the EAE model and is associated with increased fecal IgA anti-MBP antibodies.[68] Oral IL-10 and IL-4 can also enhance oral tolerance when co-administered with antigen[70] and cytokines have also been administered by the nasal route 71. Large doses of IFN-γ given intraperitoneally abrogate oral tolerance,[72] anti-IL-12 enhances oral tolerance and is associated both with increased TGF-β production and T cell apotosis,[44] and subcutaneous administration of IL-12 reverses mucosal tolerance.[73] In the uveitis model, intraperitoneal IL-2 potentiates oral tolerance and is associated with increased production of TGF-β, IL-10 and IL-4.[74] Oral but not subcutaneous lipopolysaccaride (LPS) enhances oral tolerance to MBP[75] and is associated with increased expression of IL-4 in the brain. Oral IFN-γ synergizes with the induction of oral tolerance in SJL/PLJ mice fed low doses of MBP[76] Cholera toxin (CT) is one of the most potent mucosal adjuvants, and feeding CT abrogates oral tolerance when fed with an unrelated protein antigen.[77] However, when a protein is coupled to recombinant cholera toxin B subunit (CTB) and given orally, there is enhancement of peripheral immune tolerance.[78] Oral administration of corneal epithelial cells markedly enhanced the corneal allograft survival.[79] Antibody to chemokine monocyte chemotactic protein 1 (MCP-1) abrogates oral tolerance.[80] Oral antigen delivery using a multiple emulsion system also enhances oral tolerance.[81] γδ T cells may have important role in oral tolerance induction since it seems more difficult to induce oral tolerance in animals depleted of such cells[82,83] or in delta chain deficient animals.[84] The steroid hormone dehydroepiandrosterone (DHEA) breaks intranasally induced tolerance 85 and diesel exhaust particles block induction of oral tolerance in mice.[86] In the arthritis model, administration of TGF-β or dimaprid (a histamine type 2 receptor agonist) i.p., both of which are believed to promote the development of immunoregulatory cells, enhances the induction of oral tolerance to collagen II even after the onset of arthritis.[87]

Table 5. Modulation of oral tolerance

Augments	Decreases
IL-2	IFN-γ
IL-4	IL-12
IL-10	CT
Anti-IL-12 Ab	Anti-MCP-1
TGF-β	Anti-γδ Ab
IFN-β	GVH
CTB	Anti-B7.2 mAb (low dose tolerance)
F1t-3 ligand	
LPS	
Multiple emulsions	

Abbreviations: Ab, antibody; CT, cholera toxin; CTB, choleran toxin B subunit; GVH, graft-versus-host; IFN, interferon; IL, interleukin; LPS, lipopolysaccharide; MCP, monocyte chemotactic protein 1.

Nasal Tolerance

Similar to the gut mucosa, the respiratory tract is continually exposed to a wide variety of antigens. Moreover, the bronchial-associated lymphoid tissue (BALT) is a well-developed mucosal surface in the respiratory tract. A well-developed lymphoid tissue also surrounds the nasal cavity with its own distinctive environment.[88,89] A network of dendritic antigen-presenting cells exists within the airway epithelium which traps inhaled antigen. γδ T cells are also present in the bronchial epithelium and they express CD8.[90] Presumably some of the antigen that reaches the BALT is processed and presented locally to T cells thus initiating an immune response. Also a small degree of antigen leakage across the intact lung occurs, thus providing a direct route for the penetration of antigen into the peripheral blood.[91,92] This may be particularly relevant in relation to encounters with allergens. These proteins are normally small, highly soluble and have enzymatic activity, and thus may diffuse across the epithelium more readily then larger proteins.[93] Such an event, however, seems to evoke in most circumstances tolerance instead of inflammatory allergic responses. The precise mechanisms by which immunological tolerance to daily sampled antigens in the bronchial epithelia is induced are still unclear although insights are being obtained in this area.

Induction of tolerance to IgE responses to inhaled antigens via the nasal route was first reported in 1981 by Holt and coworkers.[94] This suppression was an active process involving T cells that could transfer suppression. Tolerance developed most rapidly for IgE antibody responses and was followed by suppression of DTH and IgG responses. Suppression was followed by a compensatory rise in IgG2a responses.[95] The regulatory cells that mediated the tolerance described in this system were CD8⁺ γδ T cells and they produced IFN-γ when stimulated in vitro.[46,92,96] In a similar study using nebulised OVA, it was observed that two different populations of CD4+ T cells are activated by inhaled antigen. CD4⁺ T cells expressing a Vβ8.2 TCR appear to be important for the induction of IgE synthesis, whereas CD4+ T cells expressing Vβ2 TCR inhibit the production of IgE in vivo.[97] CD8+ T cells are also activated in this model, which can inhibit IgE synthesis when adoptively transferred into naive animals.[98] Recent studies in which mice were exposed to various concentrations of aerosolized OVA demonstrated prolonged loss of IgE and eosinophil responsiveness which did not require CD8+ cells, γδ T cells or IFN-γ.[99] Other investigators have reported that Th2 responses are not required to suppress Th1 responses by nasal induced tolerance.[100]

Since these first reports on nasal induced tolerance to soluble proteins, a range of self proteins have been tested for the inhibition of experimental autoimmune disease. Daniel and Wegmann[101] demonstrated that intranasal administration of 40 µg of B chain peptide 9-23 during 3 days in pre-diabetic nonobese diabetic (NOD) mice resulted in a marked delay in the onset and a decrease in the incidence of diabetes. The protective effect was associated with a reduced T-cell proliferative response to the peptide and the secretion of Th2 cytokines. Nasal administration of another autoantigen (GAD65) in the NOD mice at the dose of 200 µg reduced insulinitis, long-term insulin-dependent diabetes mellitus (IDDM), inhibited IFN-γ secretion and enhanced the secretion of IL-4 and IL-5.[102] Splenic CD4$^+$ (but not CD8$^+$) T cells from GAD65-treated mice inhibited the adoptive transfer of IDDM to NOD-scid/scid mice. These results suggest immune deviation plays a major role in the tolerance induced. Harrison and coworkers[103] reported similar effects of inhaled aerosol insulin in NOD mice. Insulin-treated mice also showed no proliferative responses to B chain peptide 9-23 and upregulation of IL-4 and IL-10 production by spleen cells. In this model, the cells responsible for adoptive transfer of tolerance were CD8$^+$ γδ T cells. We have also found that nasal administration of insulin B chain peptide 10-24 suppresses diabetes in NOD mice and instillation of 50 µg MBP by nasal route over 3 days prevents EAE induction (Maron and Weiner, unpublished).

Nasal administration of collagen has been shown to suppress arthritis.[104,105] Nasal type II (CII) and type IX (CIX) collagens suppressed pristane-induced arthritis.[106] Interestingly, a single dose of CII given prior to disease suppressed whereas 3 doses given prior exacerbated disease. We also found suppression of collagen arthritis (CIA) by nasal administration of 30 µg CII. T cells from mice treated nasally or orally with CII showed a decrease in IFN-γ production and T cell lines secreted IL-4, IL-10 and TGF-β. Moreover, suppression of CIA by nasal collagen was associated with diminished levels of TNF-β and IL-6 mRNA in the joints of tolerized mice.[107] In the H-2^u mouse model of EAE inhalation but not oral administration of encephalitogenic peptide inhibited disease induction.[108] Oral administration of the encephalitogenic peptide failed to induce oral tolerance to EAE. In contrast, a single intranasal dose of peptide profoundly inhibited EAE induced by subcutaneous injection peptide or a complex mixture of myelin antigens contained in spinal cord homogenate. Inhibition of EAE in rats can also be achieved by nasal administration of a mixture of MBP peptides 68-86 and 87-99,[109] but not of synthetic peptides of AChR.[110] Nasal administration of acetylcholine receptor (AChR) in rats induces effective tolerance to experimental autoimmune myasthenia gravis (EAMG) and the dose required is 1/1000 of the amount of antigen used for oral tolerance induction. Co-administration of minute amounts of IFN-γ nasally blocks tolerance induction.[111] Nasally administered AchR has a protective effect against EAMG even in primed animals.[112] Although the mechanism of nasal tolerance induction in the EAMG model is still unclear, there are data indicating it involves active suppression. Xiao and coworkers[113] showed that tolerance to EAMG by nasal administration of AChR is associated with a decrease in LFA-1 expression on CD4$^+$ T cells and upregulation of TGF-β production. Decreased expression of LFA-1 may contribute to reduction of the infiltration of inflammatory CD4$^+$ T cells, while upregulated TGF-β may inhibit lymphocyte functions. The nasal route is also being explored as a route for immunization against infectious disease such as HIV.[114]

Although most of the work on nasal tolerance indicates a role of immune deviation in this type of mucosal tolerance, Hoyne and coworkers[115-117] demonstrated the presence of anergic cells in mice rendered tolerant by nasal route to Der p1 peptide. Naive mice treated intranasally with the immunodominant peptide p 111-139 could be rendered profoundly unresponsive to an immunogenic challenge with the whole Der p1 protein. The suppression lasts for a period longer than 6 months. Lymph node cells from tolerized mice secreted very low levels of IL-2 and proliferated poorly when restimulated in vitro as compared to the untreated control mice. The authors suggest antigen-specific cells were anergic in this system and they could mediate "linked suppression" to other epitopes in the Der p1 molecule. In summary, nasal administration appears to induce tolerance by many of the same mechanisms as oral antigen although differences exist and remain to be defined.

Of note is that Li and coworkers reported dose-dependent mechanisms related to nasal tolerance induction and protection against EAE in rats. Only low-dose (30 μg) MBP-tolerized rats had high numbers of IL-4 mRNA-expressing lymph node cells and adoptive transfer revealed that only spleen cells from rats pretreated with a low dose, but not from those pretreated with a high (600 μg) dose, of MBP transferred protection against EAE to naive recipients.[111]

Treatment of Autoimmune and Inflammatory Diseases in Animals

Several studies have demonstrated the effectiveness of mucosally (oral, nasal, aerosol) administered autoantigens in animal models of autoimmune and inflammatory diseases.

Experimental Allergic Encephalomyelitis (Table 6)

Lewis Rat (MBP)

The first studies to show that orally administered myelin antigens could suppress EAE were performed in the Lewis rat. EAE was suppressed by low doses of oral MBP and MBP fragments[9] and by high doses of MBP given in bicarbonate.[8] High doses of MBP can suppress EAE via the mechanism of T cell clonal anergy[118] whereas multiple lower doses prevent EAE by transferable active cellular suppression.[119] In the nervous system of low-dose-fed animals, inflammatory cytokines such as TNF and IFN-γ are downregulated and TGF-β is upregulated.[120] Oral MBP partially suppresses serum antibody responses, especially at higher doses. Administration of myelin to sensitized animals in the chronic guinea pig model or larger doses of MBP in the murine EAE model is protective and does not exacerbate disease[121,122] and long term (6 month) administration of myelin in the chronic EAE model was beneficial.[123]

Murine Models (MBP/PLP)

A number of studies have demonstrated suppression of EAE in murine models (see Table 6). Both conventional and T cell receptor transgenic animals have been used and both oral MBP and oral PLP have been administered although the majority of studies have used MBP. In these models, MBP regulatory clones have been described and such cells have also been induced in MBP T cell receptor transgenic mice. Both CD4+ and CD8+ cells have been shown to mediate active suppression and all mechanisms of tolerance including anergy and deletion have also been demonstrated.

Nasal/Aerosol MBP

MBP given by either the nasal or the oral route has been shown to suppress EAE both in mouse and rat models. In some instances, investigators have reported suppression by nasal but not by oral MBP.[108]

Glatiramer Acetate

The latest approach in animal models has been to utilize glatiramer acetate (Cop1, Copaxone), a drug approved for therapy of multiple sclerosis which is given to patients by injection. Teitelbaum et al have found that oral glatiramer acetate suppresses EAE in both the mouse and rat models[124] and we have found that oral glatiramer acetate suppresses EAE in MBP T cell receptor transgenic animals and induces the upregulation of TGF-β when given orally.[125] These effects were not seen in OVA TCR transgenic mice. Our working hypothesis is that glatiramer acetate is acting as an altered peptide ligand and is immunologically active in

Table 6. Mucosal tolerance and experimental autoimmune encephalomyelitis (EAE)

Oral MBP in the Lewis rat
 Suppression by MBP and MBP fragments;[9]
 Suppression by high doses MBP;[8]
 CD8[+] T cells transfer protection;[25]
 Serum IgA/ IgG but not IgM suppressed, increased salivary IgA;[239]
 Suppression enhanced by oral LPS;[75]
 Evidence for clonal anergy;[240]
 Suppression of relapsing EAE;[121]
 Homologous MBP most effective;[241]
 TGF-β upregulated and TNF/IFN-γ downregulated in CNS;[120]
 MBP specific suppressor T cells act via TGF-β;[242]
 Different epitopes of MBP given orally trigger TGF-β;[50]
 Differential effects of oral vs. IV tolerization;[119]
 Oral MBP in neonates enhances EAE in adults;[196]
 Differential effects of GP and rat 68-88;[118]
 Suppression of EAE and EAMG by oral MBP+AchR;[179]
 Reversal of suppressed IgA by IL-4/IL-5;[243]
 Modulation of spinal cord inflammation;[244]
 Effect of oral MBP on Vβ8+ T cells;[245]
 MBP-cholera toxin B conjugates enhance protection;[246,247]
 Nasal MBP plus IL-10 suppresses EAE[248]

Oral MBP in the SJL mouse
 Suppression by recombinant human MBP;[249]
 TGF-β secreting regulatory cells in Peyer's patches;[250]
 Oral MBP suppresses PLP induced EAE;[203]
 MBP regulatory clones suppress EAE;[251]
 CD4[+] and CD8[+] cells mediate active suppression;[252]
 Suppression of chronic relapsing EAE;[198]
 Oral IL-4 enhances protection;[68]
 Oral IL-10 enhances protection;[253]
 Gender differences in oral tolerance to Ac1-11 in B10.PL mice[254]

Oral MBP in TCR transgenic mice
 Suppression of disease and dose-dependent induction of regulatory cells;[255]
 Multiple mechanisms of tolerance following high dose feeding;[122]
 Depletion of antigen specific T cells;[256]

Oral PLP
 Suppression of PLP disease with PLP 140-159;[203]
 Suppression of relapsing-remitting PLP-induced EAE mice with high dose PLP
  139-151;[257]

continued on next page

Table 6. Continued

Nasal/aerosol MBP

 Inhibition of EAE by nasal but not oral MBP peptide;[108]
 Aerosol MBP in the Lewis rat;[131]
 Nasal MBP suppresses relapsing EAE in DA rats;[258]
 Hierarchy in suppressive properties of nasal myelin antigens;[259]
 Synergistic effect of nasal MBP peptides in Lewis rat;[109]
 Nasal MBP in protracted-relapsing EAE;[199]
 Intratracheal MBP peptide suppress EAE[260]

Oral myelin

 Suppression of relapsing EAE;[261]
 Long-term (6month) administration is beneficial;[131]
 Oral MBP is more effective than oral myelin[262]

Oral glatiramer acetate

 Suppression of EAE in both rat and murine models;[124]
 Suppression of EAE in MBP TCR transgenic and SJL mice;[125]

the gut.[126] Trials are currently planned for the oral administration of glatiramer acetate in MS patients (discussed below).

Arthritis Models (Table 7)

There are several animal models of arthritis including collagen induced arthritis (CIA), adjuvant arthritis (AA), pristane induced arthritis (PIA), antigen-induced arthritis (AIA), silicone induced arthritis, and streptococcal cell with arthritis. One of the first studies to demonstrate that an orally administered autoantigen can suppress an autoimmune disease was the use of oral type II collagen in CIA.[6] In addition, oral administration of type II collagen and other antigens have been shown to be effective for suppression of other arthritis models.

Collagen Induced Arthritis (CIA)

Immunization with heterologous or homologous species of type II collagen (CII) produces autoimmune responses to CII that lead to development of arthritis in susceptible mouse strains.[127] CIA has been used as an animal model for RA and is characterized by chronic inflammation within the joints, associated with synovitis and erosion of cartilage and bone.[128] One of the first experiments of oral tolerance using rat CIA was done by Thompson et al.[6] They immunized WA/KIR rat with CII in incomplete Freundís adjuvant (IFA) following oral administration of 2.5 or 25μg CII per gram weight. They found the disease onset was delayed and the severity was reduced at both dosages. At the same time, Nagler-Anderson et al induced CIA in DBA/1 mice by immunizing with CII 300μg in complete Freundís adjuvant (CFA).[7] Oral administration of CII prior to immunization suppressed the incidence of CIA. There was a tendency toward reduced IgG2 responses in the CII fed mice.

Collagen peptides are also capable of inducing CIA. Immunodominant collagen peptides have been used to suppress CIA by oral or nasal administration. Khare et al induced CIA to DBA/1 mice by immunizing with human CII peptide (250-270) in CFA.[129] Human peptide CII (250-270) tolerized mice showed diminished T cell proliferation. Oral tolerance with human peptide CII (250-270) abolished anti-human and anti-mouse CII Ab, and markedly reduced the disease severity both at early and effector phases. Recombinant CII was shown to be

Table 7. Mucosal tolerance and arthritis

Collagen induced arthritis
> Oral CII in rat model;[6]
> Oral CII in DBA mice;[7]
> Oral CII and active peripheral suppression;[264]
> Oral human CII peptide;[129]
> Nasal CII;[105]
> Nasal CII and CII peptide in DBA mice;[104]
> Aerosol CII;[131]
> Anti-IL-4 reverses CII oral tolerance;[133]
> Nasal CII;[106]
> Oral recombinant CII;[130]
> Dose dependent effects of nasal CII[265]

Adjuvant arthritis
> CII suppress at lower not higher doses;[58]
> Oral 65kD HSP;[135]
> Nasal HSP60 peptide;[136]
> Nasal TCR peptide AV11[266]

Pristane induced arthritis
> Oral CII;[137]
> Nasal CIX;[106]

Antigen induced arthritis
> Bystander suppression at lower doses of CII;[141]
> Clonal anergy;[138]
> Anti-IL-4 reverses protection by oral antigen;[133]
> Nasal TCR peptide AVII patients[266]

Streptococcal cell wall (SCW) arthritis
> Oral SCW and CII suppresses;[140]

Silicone induced arthritis
> Oral CII;[267]

Avridine-induced arthritis
> Nasal HSP60 peptide;[136]

effective in CIA.[130] Staines et al showed CIA induced by whole bovine CII was suppressed by nasal administration of bovine CII peptide (184-198).[105] This nasal peptide administration was found to delay the onset of disease, reduce the severity, and shift the anti-CII antibody response from IgG2b to IgG1 isotype.

Other groups have shown that nasally administered CII effectively suppressed CIA in the mouse or rat. Myers et al reported that nasal administration of either intact CII or synthetic peptide reduced the incidence and severity of arthritis.[104] They also showed that lymph node and spleen cells from treated mice secreted more IL-4 or IL-10 in response to CII than non-tolerized mice. Al-Sabbagh et al found that aerosolization of CII suppressed CIA in Wister/Furth rats to a degree similar to that seen with oral administration.[123,131]

Recent analysis of cytokine expression in joint tissue of arthritis showed that proinflammatory cytokines such as TNF-β, IL-1, IL-6, GM-CSF and chemokines such as IL-8 are abundant.[132] We have found that mice treated with CII nasally showed diminished expression of mRNA of TNF-β and IL-6 locally (Garcia et al, unpublished). We also established cell lines producing anti-inflammatory cytokines such as IL-4, IL-10 from mice treated with CII orally or nasally.

Recently it was reported that systemic anti-IL-4 treatment during oral administration of CII blocked the suppression of CIA by oral tolerance.[133] This blockade of suppression of CIA was associated with the blockade of IL-4 secretion, decreases in anti-CII IgG2a Ab, and proliferation of lymphoid cells to CII in CII fed mice.

Adjuvant Arthritis (AA)

Another major model for RA is adjuvant arthritis (AA), which is a well-characterized and fulminant form of experimental arthritis. Oral administration of chicken CII consistently suppressed the development of AA in Lewis rats.[58] A decrease in DTH responses to CII was observed in tolerized animals. Of note is that oral type I collagen was also shown to suppress AA. Suppression of AA could be adoptively transferred by T cells from CII fed animals. Suppression was observed at doses of 3μg and 30μg, but not at 300μg or 1000μg, suggesting that the mechanism involved the generation of suppressive regulatory T cells rather than clonal anergy because active suppression may be lost at higher doses.

Heat shock proteins (HSP) play an important role in the AA model.[134] It was recently reported that oral administration of mycobacterial 65-kDa HSP suppressed the development of AA in rats.[135] Suppression of AA was adoptive transferred by spleen cells from orally tolerized rats. Higher amounts of TGF-β were detected in the culture supernatant of spleen cells from HSP fed rats when cultured with HSP. Prakken et al showed that HSP peptide (176-190) which includes the arthritogenic epitope could induce nasal tolerance for AA.[136] Of note is that this peptide could also inhibit nonmicrobially induced experimental arthritis (avridine-induced arthritis).[136]

Other Arthritis Models

Oral tolerance is also effective in pristane-induced arthritis (PIA).[137] Immunizing mice twice with 2,6,10,14-tetramethylpentadecane (pristane) twice leads to arthritis after 100–200 days. Increasing doses of orally administered CII lowered both the incidence and severity of PIA. Conversely, increasing dose of intraperitoneal administration worsened PIA. Nasal CIX was also effective in PIA.[106]

Yoshino, et al induced antigen-induced arthritis (AIA) in Lewis rats by systemic immunization with methylated bovine serum albumin (mBSA) in CFA, followed by intraarticular injection of mBSA two weeks later.[57] Orally administered CII at lower but not higher doses significantly reduced joint swelling, whereas oral antigen keyhole limpet hemocyanin (KLH) had no effect. These results demonstrate the biologic relevance of bystander suppression associated with oral tolerance. Recently it is reported by the same group that oral tolerance in AIA might also be mediated by clonal anergy.[138] A recent report[139] however showed that suppression of AIA by oral administration of bovine serum albumin was associated with IL-4 secretion and in vivo treatment with monoclonal antibodies to IL-4 abolished the suppression. Other animal models of arthritis that have been successfully treated by mucosal tolerance include streptococcal cell wall arthritis,[140] silicone induced arthritis[141] and avridine induced arthritis.[136]

Methotrexate is a widely used drug in rheumatoid arthritis. Thus we tested the effect of oral collagen on oral tolerance in animals treated with methotrexate. We previously found that there is a synergistic effect between methotrexate and orally administered antigens such as MBP[142] and a synergistic effect with oral methotrexate was also observed in the adjuvant arthritis model.[143]

Diabetes (Table 8)

Oral insulin has been shown to delay and, in some instances, prevent diabetes in the nonobese diabetic (NOD) mouse model. Such suppression is transferable,[144] primarily with CD4+ cells.[145] Immunohistochemistry of pancreatic islets of Langerhans isolated from insulin fed animals demonstrates decreased insulitis associated with decreased IFN-γ, as well as increased expression of tumor necrosis factor (TNF), IL-4, IL-10, TGF-β and prostaglandin (PG)E$_2$.[146] Recently, it was also reported that nasal administration of the insulin B chain or glutamic acid decarboxylase and aerosol insulin suppresses diabetes in the NOD mouse.[101-103] Oral insulin suppressed diabetes in a viral induced model of diabetes in which lymphocytic choriomeningitis virus (LCMV) was expressed under the insulin promoter and animals infected with LCMV to induce diabetes.[60] Protection was associated with protective cytokine shifts (IL-4/IL-10, TGF-β) in the islets. It has also been shown that expression of TGF-β in the pancreatic islets protects the NOD mouse from diabetes and that TGF-β appears to alter the antigen-presenting cell preference, polarizing islet antigen responses towards a Th2 phenotype.[147] Oral administration of B-chain of insulin, a 30-amino-acid peptide slowed the development of diabetes and prevented diabetes in some animals.[148] This effect was associated with a decrease IFN-γ and an increase in IL-4, TGF-β and IL-10 expression. Oral dosing of bacterial stimulants such as LPS and *E. coli* extract OM-89 in NOD mice induces a Th2 shift in the gut cytokine gene expression and, concomitantly, improves diabetes prevention by oral insulin administration.[149] Oral administration of recombinant GAD from plant sources suppressed the development of diabetes in NOD mouse[150] as does oral administration of a plant-based CTB-insulin fusion protein.[151] Of note is that oral insulin is not that effective in the diabetic Biobreeding (BB) rat,[152,153] perhaps due to a defect in regulatory cells in this model. Studies on the pathogenesis of diabetes in NOD mice[154] showed that in prediabetic mice peripheral CD4+ T lymphocytes were highly effective at preventing disease transfer by autoreactive T lymphocytes. These suppressor cells were TCT α/β+ and CD62L+ and they seemed to control peripheral pathogenic autoimmune effectors through an active mechanism. It is possible that oral administration of an autoantigen may potentiate the effect of these cells. Under special experimental conditions, large doses of OVA given to OVA double transgenic mice resulted in diabetes mediated by OVA specific cytotoxic T lymphocytes.[155] These animals expressed OVA on the islets under the rat insulin promoter and were made chimeric to enrich for OVA specific transgenic TCR cytotoxic T lymphocytes.

Uveitis (Table 9)

Oral administration of S antigen (S-Ag), a retinal autoantigen that induces experimental autoimmune uveitis (EAU), or S-Ag peptides prevents or markedly diminishes the clinical appearance of S-Ag-induced disease as measured by ocular inflammation.[156] S-Ag-induced EAU can also be suppressed by feeding an HLA peptide.[157] Feeding interphotoreceptor binding protein (IRBP) suppresses IRBP-induced disease and is potentiated by IL-2.[74] Oral feeding of retinal antigen not only can prevent acute disease but also can effectively suppress second attack in chronic-relapsing EAU, demonstrating that oral tolerance may have practical clinical implications in uveitis, which is predominantly a chronic-relapsing condition in humans.[158-160] Other investigators161 have found that oral administration of bovine S-Ag peptides is very efficient in preventing EAU[162] but could only inhibit mild disease if feeding was delayed until after immunization, and relatively high feeding doses were required.

Myasthenia (Table 10)

Although myasthenia gravis is an antibody-mediated disease, oral and nasal 163 administration of the Torpedo acetylcholine receptor (AchR) to Lewis rats prevented or delayed the

---

Table 8. Mucosal tolerance and diabetes

Oral insulin

      Suppression of diabetes in NOD mouse;[144]
      Induction of regulatory CD4+ T cells;[268]
      Cytokine shifts in pancreatic islets;[269]
      Active suppression is determined by antigen dose;[270]
      Suppression by insulin and adjuvants;[271]
      Suppression of LCMV induced diabetes;[60]
      Insulin B chain suppresses diabetes;[148]
      Enhanced protection by cholera toxin-insulin;[272]
      Enhanced protection by bacterial adjuvant;[273]
      Induction of IL-4 secreting regulatory T cells;[274]
      Protection by a plant-based CTB-insulin fusion protein;[150]
      Neonatal oral insulin suppresses diabetes[197]

Nasal/aerosol insulin

      Nasal insulin peptide suppresses diabetes;[275]
      Aerosol insulin suppresses diabetes and induces CD8 γδ T cells;[103]

Oral glutamic acid decarboxylase (GAD)

      Oral GAD in transgenic plants suppresses diabetes;[150]

Nasal GAD

      Nasal GAD suppresses diabetes;[102]

Transgenic models

      Oral ovalbumin induces diabetes in OVA transgenic model;[155]

BB rat

      Oral insulin is not protective in the BB rat;[152]
      Oral insulin plus adjuvant may exacerbate disease;[153]

---

onset of myasthenia gravis.[164] The levels of anti-AchR antibodies in the serum were lower in orally tolerized animals than in control animals. The effect was dose dependent and large doses of antigen (at least 5mg of AchR) plus soybean tripsin inhibitor (STI)[164] were required, suggesting that anergy may be the primary mechanism. Purified AchR was found more effective than an unpurified mixture.[165] EAMG can also be suppressed by nasally administered AchR[163,166] and AchR peptides.[167]

Autoimmune Diseases and Inflammatory Conditions (Table 11)

Allergy

Both oral and nasal administration of allergens have been shown to be effective ways to suppress both IgE responses and intestinal mast cell responses.[168] The allergens used include the Der P 1 epitope and Dp extract of house mite allergen and pollen extract.[117,169,170] Low and high doses of Dp extract given orally are able to inhibit IgE responses in both naive and sensitized mice.[170] Authors also reported an increase of anti-IgE autoantibodies in orally tolerant mice that may be involved in the modulation of the allergic response. In some instances, linked suppression has been demonstrated in which a single Der P 1 peptide suppresses other epitopes.[171]

Table 9. Mucosal tolerance and uveitis

S-antigen

    Suppression of EAU with oral S-Ag;[156]

    Suppression of EAU by a uveitogenic 20mer peptide;[276]

    Peptide 35 suppresses EAU with suppression of IgA but not IgG;[276]

    Cross reactive homolog of S-Ag can suppress EAU;[277]

    Inhibition of EAU by oral S-Ag and peptides;[278]

    Dose-dependency of mechanism of oral to S-Ag peptides;[39]

    Splenectomy abrogates S-Ag-induced EAU;[279]

    Suppression of EAU by recombinant *E. coli* expressing S-Ag;[280]

    CD8 cells are not essential for "low dose" tolerance to S-Ag;[281]

IRBP

    IL-2 potentiates oral tolerance induction to IRBP;[74]

HLA peptide

    Feeding HLA peptide suppresses S-Ag induced disease;[157,282]

Other

    Bystander suppression in EAU occurs in periphery not in the eye;[63]

    Orally induced peptide specific γδ cells suppress EAU;[283]

    EAU induced by oral or nasal HSP derived peptide;[202]

Antiphospholipid Syndrome

The antiphospholipid syndrome is characterized by the presence of high titers of IgG anticardiolipin antibodies and/or lupus anticoagulant antibodies. Oral administration in Balb/C mice of low doses of β2 glycoprotein prevented the serologic and clinical manifestation of experimental antiphospholipid syndrome upon immunization with the autoantigen.[109] Decreased T cell responses, antibody responses and increased expression of TGF-β which mediated the suppression was demonstrated. Tolerance was transferred by CD8 positive class I restricted TGF-β-secreting cells.[172]

Colitis

TGF-β appears to play a crucial role in the development of animal models of colitis, including 2,4,6-trinitrobenzene sulfonic acid (TNBS)-induced colitis, colitis in the IL-2-deficient animal model following systemic administration of TNP-KLH in adjuvant, and the model of Th1 colitis in SCID mice. It has been shown that TNBS colitis can be prevented by oral administration of TNBS, which acts via the induction of TNBS-specific TGF-β responses.[173] In addition, colitis can be suppressed by orally administered ovalbumin which acts via bystander suppression in an OVA induced colitis model.[56]

Experimental Allergic Neuritis

Experimental allergic neuritis is the counterpart of EAE and can be suppressed both by nasal and oral administration of peripheral nerve proteins.[174,175]

Immune Complex Disease

Immune complex disease can be suppressed both following administration of a single large dose of antigen[176] or by placing antigen in drinking water.[177] These studies were performed before oral tolerance was applied to autoimmune diseases. It has also been raised whether defective oral tolerance may be associated with experimental IgA nephropathy.[178]

Table 10. Mucosal tolerance and myasthenia

Oral acetylcholine receptor (AChR)

Suppression of EAMG with oral AChR in Lewis rats; [164, 284]

Purified AChR is more protective than unpurified AChR; [165]

Induction of IL-4, TGF-β and IFN-γ following oral AChR; [285]

Oral AChR suppresses AChR specific B cell responses; [286]

Oral immunodominant AChR epitope suppresses T cell responses in mice;[287]

Role of tolerogen conformation of AChR fragments [288]

AChR recombinant fragment suppresses ongoing disease [289]

Oral T cell epitope prevents EAMG [290]

Nasal AChR

Suppression of EAMG by nasal AchR; [163]

Upregulation of TGF-β and decreased IFN-γ in tolerized rats; [166]

Nasal AChR peptides can suppress EAMG; [167]

Decreased LFA-1 and increased TGF-β in clones from rats nasally tolerized; [113]

Reversal of nasal tolerance by IFN-γ; [291]

Synthetic peptides failed to suppress EAMG; [110]

Multiple Autoimmune Diseases

Link's group has experimented with administering antigens associated with more than one autoimmune disease and immunizing with a mixture of antigens. They have demonstrated that oral administration of AChR plus MBP suppresses experimental autoimmune myasthenia gravis (EAMG) and EAE, and that nasal administration of three autoantigens suppresses EAMG, EAE and experimental autoimmune neuritis (EAN).[112,179] Thus it appears there is no interference by one autoantigen versus another when they are from different target organs.

Nickel Sensitization

Metals such as nickel and chromium can induce contact sensitivity responses and oral tolerance to nickel has been demonstrated both in the mouse and in the guinea pig.[180,181] Based on these animal findings, oral administration of nickel is being applied to the treatment of allergy in the human condition (discussed below).

Thyroiditis

Thyroiditis has been effectively suppressed following oral administration of either porcine or human thyroglobulin.[182,183] In the murine model, CD8 positive regulatory cells which produce IL-4 and TGF-β mediated the suppression.[184] These cells also appear to induce bystander suppression upon triggering with the fed antigen. Other investigators[185] reported that tolerance induced by IV administration of deaggregated thyroglobulin in experimental autoimmune thyroiditis (EAT) is dependent on CD4+ T cells but independent of IL-4 and IL-10.

Tracheal Eosinophilia

Airway inflammation plays a major role in human asthma and increasing evidence points to a correlation between eosinophilia infiltration and allergic lung disease. In murine models of tracheal eosinophilia, suppression of disease has been achieved by antigen given in high doses[186] or placed in the drinking water.[187] In these instances, both Th1 and Th2 responses were suppressed. The TGF-β induced by oral tolerance appears to be the factor that ameliorates the experimental condition.[188]

Table 11. Mucosal treatment of other autoimmune diseases and inflammatory conditions

1. Allergy

    Sublingual allergen administration suppresses allergen-specific IgE responses;[292]

    Inhibition of T cell and Ab responses to house mite allergen by inhalation of dominant T cell epitope Der p 1;[115]

    Oral tolerance to pollen extract in Balb/c mice suppresses IgE responses;[169]

    Oral Der 1 p cryptic epitopes suppress responses of other epitopes;[293]

    Intranasal Der p 1 peptide transiently activates CD4 cells prior to *in vivo* tolerance;[117]

    Oral and nasal tolerance to ingested allergen suppress IgE and intestinal mast cell responses;[168]

    Intranasal Der p 1 peptides induce T cell tolerance and linked suppression;[171]

    Oral Dp extract inhibits IgE responses;[170]

    Nasal bee venom allergen long peptides suppress Th2 responses;[294]

    Allergen coupled to CTB suppresses IgE responses;[295]

2. Antiphospholipid syndrome

    TGF-β mediated suppression by low-dose oral β2-glycoprotein;[172]

3. Colitis

    TGF-β dependent suppression of TNBS-colitis by oral tolerance;[173]

    Suppression of colitis by orally induced bystander suppression;[56]

    Oral colonic antigens suppress hapten-induced colitis;[296]

4. Experimental allergic neuritis

    Oral bovine peripheral nerve myelin or P2 protein suppresses clinical and histological EAN Gau;[174]

    Nasal administration of P2 57-81 suppresses EAN;[175]

    Adjuvant effects and bystander suppression in P2 peptide induced EAN;[297]

5. Immune complex disease

    Antigen in drinking water modifies antigen-induced immune complex disease;[177]

    Single high dose antigen suppresses immune complex nephritis;[176]

    Defective oral tolerance promotes experimental IgA nephropathy;[178]

6. Multiple autoimmune diseases

    Oral AchR plus oral MBP suppresses EAMG & EAE;[179]

    Nasal administration of multiple autoantigen antigens suppresses EAMG, EAE & EAN;[112]

7. Nickel sensitization

    Oral tolerance to nickel and chromium in guinea pigs;[180]

    Oral tolerance to nickel in mice;[181]

8. Thyroiditis

    Oral porcine thyroglobulin suppression of murine autoimmune thyroiditis;[183]

    Oral human thyroglobulin suppresses autoimmune thyroiditis;[182]

    TGF-β and IL-4 regulatory cells following oral thyroglobulin;[184]

9. Tracheal eosinophilia

    TGF-β induced by oral tolerance ameliorates experimental tracheal eosinophilia;[188]

    High-dose Th1 and Th2 oral tolerance prevents antigen induced eosinophilia recruitment;[186]

    Prevention of Th2 lung eosinophil inflammation by antigen in drinking water;[187]

continued on next page

Table 11. Continued

10. Transplantation

        Allogeneic cells prevent sensitization by skin grafts;[189]

        Oral allopeptides suppress DTH in Lewis rat; [298]

        Oral but not IV alloantigen upregulates intragraft Th2 cells;[190]

        Differential effects of oral vs. intrathymic class II peptide;[269]

        Corneal allograft survival enhanced by oral alloantigen;[299]

        CTB-coupled allogeneic cells enhance survival of corneal grafts;[79,162] and allograft
            rejection[300]

        Oral type V collagen downregulates lung allograft rejection;[301]

        Oral alloantigen generates intragraft CD8+ regulatory cells;[14]

        Non depleting anti-CD4 enhances oral tolerance to allografts[302]

11. Other

        Oral bacterial extract enhances alveolar macrophage activity;[303]

        Oral adenoviral antigen permits long term gene expression;[191]

        Oral casein differentially suppresses certain B and T cell epitopes;[192,193]

        Oral tolerance to milk whey protein;[304]

        Suppression of asthma by oral tolerance;[305]

        Oral tolerance to hepatitis B envelope antigen;[306]

        Amelioration of graft vs. host disease by oral antigen;[307]

        Oral tolerance ameliorates liver disorders in GVH[308]

Transplantation

    Oral administration of allogeneic cells prevents sensitization by skin grafts and changes accelerated rejection of vascularized cardiac allografts to an acute form typical of unsensitized recipients.[189] Orally administered allopeptides in the Lewis rat reduces DTH responses to the peptide.[189] Oral, but not intravenous, alloantigen was accompanied by elevation of intragraft levels of IL-4.[190] Oral alloantigen enhanced corneal allograft survival even in pre-immune hosts.[79] When orally administrered cells are conjugated with cholera toxin B and administered before corneal transplantation, the tolerance effect is optimized.[162]

Other

    Recombinant adenoviruses have been used by many investigators for somatic gene therapy. The duration of transgene expression is limited by the host immune response which precludes gene expression upon readministration of the virus. It has been shown that the immune response can be abrogated by oral tolerization with protein extracts of recombinant adenovirus.[191] Lymphocytes from tolerized rats had increased expression of TGF-β, IL-2 and IL-4 upon exposure to viral antigens whereas IFN-γ expression became undetectable. Thus, oral tolerization of adenoviral antigens has a potential to prevent immune responses associated with repeated injections of recombinant adenoviruses.

    Investigators have studied food allergy using αS1-casein, a major protein in cow's milk. Oral tolerance can be induced by feeding such a protein although antibody responses can occur following immunization. Investigators have found differential suppression in terms of B cell and T cell determinants following oral administration of the casein.[192,193] Thus, orally administered antigen may not induce tolerance to some portions of the repertoire which could lead to food hypersensitivity.

In addition to classic autoimmune diseases it has now become clear that other processes in which inflammation plays a role or a tolerogenic immune response is desired may be helped by oral tolerance. One such example is atherosclerosis in which immune responses against heat shock protein are important. We have demonstrated in our laboratory that nasal administration of heat shock protein can decrease lesions in the aortic arch of low density lipoprotein cholesterol (LDL) deficient animals that develop atherosclerosis.[194] Nasal antigen was more effective than oral antigen. In addition, injury to the nervous system such as that seen with stroke or following crush injury can be ameliorated by administration of oral myelin basic protein.[66] Finally in animal models of Alzheimer's Disease, nasally administered beta amyloid has an ameliorating effect.[195] This effect may be due simply to the generation of antibodies which help clear the beta amyloid from the brain, although cellular immune responses have also been identified and could play an important role in an analogous way that MBP is effective in stroke models.

Worsening of Autoimmune Diseases

Although mucosally administered antigens have been used successfully to treat a wide variety of autoimmune and inflammatory conditions, under certain experimental conditions worsening of autoimmune diseases in animals by oral antigen has been reported.

We have observed that neonatal administration of guinea pig MBP in the Lewis rat does not induce oral tolerance and in fact makes animals more susceptible to EAE induction as adults.[196] This raises the possibility that neonatal exposure to antigen may be a factor in the development of autoimmune disease in adulthood. This indeed has been postulated for diabetes in terms of exposure to cow's milk as a risk factor for development of diabetes. Interestingly, we fed insulin to neonatal NOD mice and did not find an enhancement of diabetes, but better protection against the development of diabetes.[197] We did not observe protection with oral myelin oligodendrocyte glycoprotein (MOG) given to neonates, but it did not exacerbate EAE. Thus worsening of autoimmunity by neonatal exposure may depend on strain of animal and antigen fed.

Meyer et al reported that a single feeding of a small dose of guinea pig MBP exacerbated the clinical course of disease[198] in the B10.PL model of chronic relapsing EAE. Larger single doses suppressed the disease. These investigators also found that multiple oral doses of MBP were required to suppress clinical disease once it was established. We and others have found that there may be initial sensitization of Th1 responses when small doses of antigen are fed, followed by suppression as additional doses are given.[42,45] Thus, in animal models where immunization immediately follows feeding, exacerbation may be observed if only one feeding of a small dose is given. Nasal MBP has been associated with a trend of disease worsening in a protracted relapsing EAE model in DA rats.[199]

In diabetes models, Blanas et al were able to induce diabetes by orally administering large doses of OVA (30mg) to OVA double transgenic mice.[155] The animals expressed OVA on the islets under the rat insulin promoter and were made chimeric to enrich for OVA specific transgenic TCR CTL. Although diabetes was induced, it is not clear the degree to which this transgenic model applies to conventional animals. Nonetheless, these studies demonstrate that orally administered antigen is active immunologically when it encounters the GALT and under special circumstances the immune response generated can have a harmful effect. It has been demonstrated that insulin given with an adjuvant may exacerbate diabetes in the BB rat model.[153] It has been difficult to protect the BB rat from diabetes[152] by oral insulin, which may relate to defects the animals have in regulatory cell populations and could account for the ability to enhance diabetes by coadministered adjuvant. In results reported to date from human trials in which new onset diabetics were fed 1 or 10mg of insulin, there was no evidence of disease worsening.[200]

There have been two instances where investigators have reported the induction of autoimmune disease in animals after oral antigen administration. Terato, et al reported the induction of collagen induced arthritis in animals fed chicken type II collagen for 2-3 week intervals over a 15 week period or fed collagen plus LPS.[201] Hu et al studied HSP peptide 336-351 induced uveitis in the Lewis rat and were unable to protect against disease by mucosal administration of the peptide prior to immunization. They were however, able to induce uveitis with the HSP peptide given orally or nasally in doses ranging from 2.5μg to 250μg.[202] The induction of uveitis could be reversed by treatment with anti-CD4 antibody and suppressed by administration of IL-4 suggesting that CD4+ Th1 type cells were responsible for the uveitis although disease was not transferred from mucosally treated rats. These results suggest that in certain instances, peptides may induce Th1 type autoimmune disease. We have observed that it has been difficult to orally tolerize with the immunodominant PLP peptide 139-151 in SJL mice and in some instances enhancement of disease has been observed when low doses were fed (250μg) (unpublished observations). Protection was observed however with the whole molecule or other peptide fragments of PLP (140-159).[203] Oral tolerance to PLP peptide 139-151 and suppression of EAE in SJL mice was obtained by feeding large doses (2mg).[204] In the Lewis rat we have identified encephalitogenic and tolerogenic epitopes of guinea pig MBP[50] and found that non-encephalitogenic fragments may be more tolerogenic.[9] Careful examination of the work of Metzler and Wraith show a trend toward worsening of EAE relapse in PL/J animals fed the wild type Ac1-11 peptide though the differences were not statistically significant.[108] Taken together, the aforementioned results suggest that there may be peptide fragments of a protein, perhaps the primary immunodominant ones, that have properties resulting in the induction of autoimmunity when given mucosally in appropriate animal strains, something that is not observed when the whole molecule is given. This is not true for all peptides as we have not observed this with the immunodominant peptide of the insulin B chain, MOG, or MBP.

In summary, animal data suggests that worsening of autoimmune disease could theoretically occur in humans treated with oral or mucosal antigen. This was a major concern of our group when we initiated pilot trials of oral myelin and oral type II collagen in MS and RA patients. However no worsening was observed in pilot trials and no worsening has subsequently been observed in 250 MS patients treated with oral bovine myelin or in over 1200 RA patients treated with collagen II, some of whom have been taking these oral preparations for over 3 years. Others have also not reported worsening of RA in patients treated with oral bovine collagen.[205] In a small uveitis trial, however, there was a suggestion (not statistically significant) that oral administration of a retinal mixture appeared to have worsened disease, whereas the purified protein appeared to ameliorate the disease.[206] Thus it is clear that mucosally administered antigens for the treatment of autoimmune or inflammatory conditions must first be tested in dose ranging phase I trials for potential toxic effects and patients must be carefully monitored when larger trials are performed.

Treatment of Autoimmune Diseases in Humans and Human Studies of Mucosal Tolerance (Table 12)

Based on the long history of oral tolerance and the safety of the approach, human trials have been initiated in autoimmune diseases, MS, RA, uveitis and diabetes. These initial trials suggest that there has been no systemic toxicity or exacerbation of disease, although clinical efficacy resulting in an approved drug has not been yet demonstrated. Results in humans however, have paralleled several aspects of what has been observed in animals. In addition, mucosal tolerance has been applied to other conditions.

Allergy

Mucosal tolerance has been used for the treatment of some allergic conditions in humans. In 1987, Taudorf et al demonstrated that capsules of birch pollen extract were effective in decreasing eye symptoms, and allergy scores in conjunctival sensitivity to birch pollen.[207] In 1992, these same investigators treated allergic rhinoconjunctivitis with oral grass pollen and birch pollen.[207] Scadding and Brostoff treated patients with sublingual house dust mite and found a decrease in allergic rhinitis.[208] Litwin et al treated patients with short ragweed extract and found that patients appeared to do better in ragweed season than untreated patients.[209,210] A double-blind study of oral tolerance in pollen respiratory allergy showed statistically significant positive effects in the treated vs. the placebo groups.[211]

Contact Sensitivity

Investigators have shown that exposure of a contact-sensitizing agent via the mucosa prior to subsequent skin challenge led to unresponsiveness in a portion of patients studied.[212]

Diabetes

Six different trials are currently underway or completed in testing mucosally administered recombinant human insulin as a tolerizing agent in type 1 diabetes: (1) A multicenter double-blind study in the U.S. evaluating oral insulin therapy versus placebo in adults and children with new-onset disease. Preliminary analysis suggests preserved beta cell function as measured by endogenous C-peptide insulin responses in patients diagnosed over age 20 years and fed 1 mg. vs. placebo;[213] (2) A double-blind study in France to compare oral insulin therapy and parenteral insulin therapy versus placebo in patients during the remission phase. Evaluation criteria include duration of remission, measures of insulin secretion/sensitivity and immunological parameters; no effect of treatment with 2.5 or 7.5 mg oral insulin was observed.[214] (3) A multicenter double-blind study in Italy to evaluate whether the addition of oral insulin is able to improve the integrated parameters of metabolic control and modify immunological findings compared to placebo in patients with recent onset disease treated with intensive insulin therapy (IMDIAB VI); (4) A multicenter double-blind study in the U.S. to determine if diabetes can be prevented by subcutaneous insulin therapy or oral insulin therapy in subjects at risk for diabetes (DPT-1); (5) A double-blind study in Australia evaluating aerosolized insulin versus placebo in patients with new-onset disease; (6) a double-blind study in Finland evaluating nasally administered insulin versus placebo in patients with new-onset disease.

KLH

KLH administered orally to human subjects has been reported to decrease subsequent cell-mediated immune responses although antibody responses were not affected31 and to decrease KLH-precursor frequency.[215] Nasal KLH has also been reported to induce tolerance in humans.[216]

Maternal Donor Allografts

It is known that a large number of maternal lymphocytes are present in breast milk and investigators asked the question whether exposure of an infant to maternal lymphocytes during breast feeding would have an effect on subsequent reactivity of a patient to a maternal donor related renal transplant. In a study reported in 1984, there was a suggestion that breast fed recipients may have done better than non breast fed recipients.[217] Of note is that it has recently been shown in animal models that transfusion tolerance involving cells may be mediated by TGF-β.[218]

Table 12. Human studies of mucosal tolerance

A. Allergy

Oral immunotherapy for birch pollen hay fever;[207]

Oral encapsulated ragweed extract;[209]

Double-blind study of encapsulated ragweed;[210]

Oral immunotherapy for allergic rhinoconjunctivitis;[309]

HIV patients allergic to sulfonamides desensitized by oral trimethoprim-
sulfamethoxazole;[310]

Double-blind study of oral immunotherapy for respiratory allergy[211]

B. Contact Sensitivity

Oral and mucosal suppression of contact sensitivity to DNCB;[311-314]

C. Diabetes

Preliminary Report: Preserved beta-cell function as measured by endogenous C-peptide
in new onset diabetics over 20 years old fed 1mg;[213]

Oral insulin not beneficial in new onset disease fed 2.5 or 7.5 mg oral insulin for 1
year[214]

D. Keyhole limpet hemocyanin

Oral KLH suppresses T cell but not B cell responses to immunization;[31]

Nasal KLH suppresses antibody and DTH responses to immunization;[216]

Oral KLH decreases KLH-reactive precursor cell frequency;[215]

E. Maternal-Donor renal allografts

Breast-feeding in infancy may benefit maternal-donor renal transplants;[217]

F. Multiple sclerosis

Oral myelin decreased MRI lesions in DR2+ males, no effect on clinical relapse;[10]

Increased TGF-β secreting myelin cells after oral myelin;[219]

G. Nickel

Reduced nickel allergy following oral nickel contact at early age;[315]

Sublingual treatment effective for nickel sulfite dermatitis;[222]

Oral desensitization in nickel allergy decreases nickel-specific T cells;[221]

H. Rheumatoid arthritis

Oral collagen ameliorates rheumatoid arthritis;[226]

Oral collagen benefits juvenile RA in open label trial;[225]

20 μg best in double blind oral dosing trial of type II collagen;[224]

Oral bovine collagen at higher doses without positive effect;[205]

60 μg oral collagen best in composite analysis of dosing trials;[143] no different than
placebo in phase III trial

Bovine collagen (0.5 mg) beneficial in placebo controlled trial[227]

Oral collagen II beneficial in JRA clinically and immunologically in pilot trial[228]

I. Rhinitis

Sublingual therapy with house dust mite benefits patients with perennial rhinitis;[208]

J. Thyroid disease

Decreased cellular immunity to thyroglobulin in patients receiving oral thyroglobulin;[230]

K. Uveitis

Oral S-Ag appeared to allow medication taper, retinal mixture appeared to worsen
uveitis;[206]

Oral HLA peptide allowed steroid taper;[159]

continued on next page

Table 12. Continued

L. Other

Decreased immune responses after oral BSA;[316]

Oral desensitization in Rh disease;[317]

Oral spirochetes suppress lymphocyte responses;[318]

IgA antibody producing cells after oral streptococcus mutans;[319]

Oral bovine type I collagen beneficial in systemic sclerosis in pilot trial[232]

Multiple Sclerosis

In MS patients, MBP- and PLP-specific TGF-β-secreting Th3-type cells have been observed in the peripheral blood of patients treated with an oral bovine myelin preparation and not in patients who were untreated.[219] There was no increase in MBP- or PLP-specific IFN-γ-secreting cells in treated patients. These results demonstrate that it is possible to immunize via the gut for autoantigen-specific TGF-β-secreting cells in a human autoimmune disease by oral administration of the autoantigen. However, a recently completed 515 patient, placebo-controlled, double-blind Phase III trial of single-dose bovine myelin in relapsing-remitting MS did not show differences between placebo and treated groups in the number of relapses; a large placebo effect was observed (AutoImmune Inc., Lexington, MA, USA). The dose of myelin was 300 mg given in capsule form and contained 8 mg MBP and 15 mg PLP. Preliminary analysis of magnetic resonance imaging data showed significant changes favoring oral myelin in certain patient subgroups. Based on the results of oral tolerance in uveitis in humans,[206] and in animal models[165, 220] it appears that protein mixtures may not be as effective oral tolerogens as purified proteins and future trials in MS are being planned with the MBP analogue, glatiramer acetate, which is currently given by injection to MS patients but has been shown to be effective orally in animals and to induce regulatory cells that mediate bystander suppression.[124,126]

Nickel

Oral desensitization to nickel-allergy in humans induces a decrease in nickel-specific T cells and affects cutaneous eczema.[221] Sublingual treatment is effective for nickel sulfite dermatitis[222] and there is reduced nickel allergy in those exposed to nickel at an early age.[223]

Rheumatoid Arthritis

In RA, a 280 patient double-blind phase II dosing trial of type II collagen in liquid doses ranging from 20 µg to 2500 µg per day for six months demonstrated statistically significant positive effects in the group treated with the lowest dose.[224] Oral administration of larger doses of bovine type II collagen (1-10 mg) did not show a significant difference between tested and placebo groups, although a higher prevalence of responders was reported for the groups treated with type II collagen.[223] These results are consistent with animal studies of orally administered type II collagen in which protection against adjuvant- and antigen-induced arthritis and bystander suppression was observed only at the lower doses.[58,141] An open-label pilot study of oral collagen in juvenile RA gave positive results with no toxicity.[225] This lack of systemic toxicity is an important feature for the clinical use of oral tolerance, especially in children for whom the long-term effects of immunosuppressive drugs is unknown.

Five phase II randomized studies of oral type II collagen have been performed, and based on the results obtained, a multi-center double-blind phase III trial study of oral type II collagen (Colloral®) is underway (AutoImmune Inc.). In the five double-blind phase II studies a total of 805 patients were treated with oral type II collagen and 296 treated with placebo. Two of the studies have been published.[224,226] The other three studies were included in a integrated analysis that led to the decision to carry out a phase III trial. A dose refinement study tested doses of 5, 20, and 60µg. Colloral at 60µg was found to be the most significant dose compared to other doses. Weighted averages for the Paulus 20 and Paulus 50 responses were calculated for the 60µg dose and placebo. A significant effect favoring 60µg was observed for both the Paulus 20 and the Paulus 50 response. Integrated efficacy analysis of predictors of response including HLA, phenotype, rheumatoid factor, CII antibodies, duration of disease, and tender and swollen joint count were performed, but no statistically significant predictors were identified. Non steroid antiinflammatory drugs (NSAIDS) did not appear to affect the clinical response of RA patient to oral type II collagen. Safety analysis demonstrated that Colloral was extraordinarily safe with no side effects. The magnitude of the clinical responses of Colloral appear to be on the same level as NSAIDS for the majority of patients. However, there is a sub-group of patients that appear to have a more significant response to the medication. Based on these data, a 760-patient phase III trial was performed comparing 60µg of Colloral to placebo. However, no differences were observed. A large placebo effect (greater than 50%) was observed in the control group. Subsequently a placebo controlled trial of bovine collagen showed significant effects in those receiving 0.5mg, but not in groups receiving 0.05mg or 5mg.[226] Oral CII in juvenile RA was associated with clinical improvement and decreased CII specific IFN-γ and increased TGFβ.[228] Clinical trials are underway to determine whether withholding NSAIDS and prednisone will allow OT to be induced and whether oral CII has meaningful clinical efficacy in RA.[229]

Rhinitis

Low dose sublingual therapy with house dust mite was reported to be effective in relieving symptoms in 72% of a group of patients with perennial rhinitis due to house dust mite in a double-blind placebo-controlled crossover trial.[208]

Thyroid

Thirteen patients receiving thyroid hormone replacement with synthetic thyroxin were randomly assigned to receive oral porcine thyroid or remain on synthetic T4.[230] Humoral and cellular immune responses were measured over the course of a year. A decrease in cellular immunity to thyroid peptides was observed in the fed versus the control group. No changes between groups were observed in autoantibody levels.

Uveitis

In uveitis, a pilot trial of S-Ag and an S-Ag mixture was conducted at the National Eye Institute (Bethesda, MD, USA) and showed positive trends with oral bovine S-Ag but not the retinal mixture.[206] Feeding of peptide derived from patient's own HLA antigen appeared to have effect on uveitis in that patients could discontinue their steroids because of reduced intraocular inflammation mediated by oral tolerance.[160]

Other

Positive effects were reported in an open label pilot study of oral type I collagen in patients with systemic sclerosis.[231,232] A pilot immunological study of oral MHC peptides has been initiated in transplantation patients in our institution. In terms of immune response to food antigens in humans, Husby and coworkers studied humoral immunity to dietary antigens in healthy adults and found 90% of subjects had antibodies to ovalbumin and 24% had antibodies to alpha-lactalbumin.[233] Peripheral and intestinal lymphocyte activation after in vitro exposure to cow's milk antigens was observed in normal subjects and in patients with

Table 13. Application of mucosal tolerance for the treatment of human disease

1. Dose
2. Immune marker of immunologic effect
3. Route (oral vs. Nasal)
4. Mucosal adjuvant
5. Protein preparation
6. Combination therapy
7. Early therapy

Crohn's disease.[234] In another study, humoral response to food antigens were reported to be of the IgG subclass.[235] Immune reactions induced in infants by intestinal absorption of incompletely digested cow's milk protein has also been reported.[236] Recently, Zivny and coworkers reported multiple mechanisms of oral tolerance to food antigens in humans including anergy and active suppression1.[59] Of note, a study reported that grapefruit juice increases felodipine oral availability in humans by decreasing intestinal CYP3A protein expression.[237]

In summary, based on results to date in humans, it appears that the clinical application of oral antigen for the treatment of human conditions will depend on the specific disease, early treatment, the nature and dosages of proteins administered, the use of synergists or mucosal adjuvants to enhance biologic effects, development of immune markers for the biologic effect, and combination therapy (Table 13). Also, recombinant human proteins may be more efficacious than animals proteins.[238]

Future Directions

Although it is clear that oral antigen can suppress autoimmunity and inflammatory diseases in animals, much remains to be learned. Cell surface molecules and cytokines associated with inductive events in the gut that generate and modulate oral tolerance are not completely understood. Important areas of investigation include cytokine milieu, antigen presentation and co-stimulation requirements, routes of antigen processing, form of the antigen, role of the liver, the effect or oral antigens on antibody and IgE responses and on CTLs, and the role of γδ T-cells. As the molecular events associated with the generation and modulation of oral tolerance are better understood, the ability to apply mucosal tolerance successfully for the treatment of human autoimmune and other diseases will be further enhanced.

References

1. Burnet M. The Clonal Selection Theory of Acquired Immunity. Nashville: Vanderbilt University Press, 1959.
2. Avrameas S. Natural autoantibodies: From 'horror autotoxicus' to 'gnothi seauton'. Immunol Today 1991; 12:154-159.
3. Zhang J, Markovic S, Raus J et al. Increased frequency of IL-2 responsive T-cells specific for myelin basic protein and proteolipid protein in peripheral blood and cerebrospinal fluid of patients with multiple sclerosis. J Exp Med 1993; 179:973-984.
4. Cohen I, Young DB. Autoimmunity, microbial immunity and the immunological homunculus. Immunol Today 1991; 12:105-110.
5. Matzinger P. Tolerance, danger, and the extended family. Annu Rev Immunol 1994; 12:991-1045.
6. Thompson HSG, Staines NA. Gastric administration of type II collagen delays the onset and severity of collagen-induced arthritis in rats. Clin Exp Immunol 1986; 64:581-586.

7. Nagler-Anderson C, Bober LA, Robinson ME et al. Suppression of type II collagen-induced arthritis by intragastric administration of soluble type II collagen. Proc Natl Acad Sci USA 1986; 83:7443-7446.

8. Bitar DM, Whitacre CC. Suppression of experimental autoimmune encephalomyelitis by the oral administration of myelin basic protein. Cell Immunol 1988; 112:364-370.

9. Higgins P, Weiner HL. Suppression of experimental autoimmune encephalomyelitis by oral administration of myelin basic protein and its fragments. J Immunol 1988; 140:440-445.

10. Weiner HL. Oral tolerance: Immune mechanisms and treatment of autoimmune diseases. Immunol Today 1997; 18:335-343.

11. Weiner HL. Oral tolerance, an active immunologic process mediated by multiple mechanisms. J Clin Invest 2000; 106:935-937.

12. Weiner HL. The mucosal milieu creates tolerogenic dendritic cells and T(R)1 and T(H)3 regulatory cells. Nat Immunol 2001; 2:671-672.

13. Zhang X, Izikson L, Liu L et al. Activation of cd25(+)cd4(+) regulatory t cells by oral antigen administration. J Immunol 2001; 167:4245-4253.

14. Zhou J, Carr RI, Liwski RS et al. Oral exposure to alloantigen generates intragraft CD8⁺ regulatory cells. J Immunol 2001; 167:107-113.

15. Iwasaki A, Kelsall BL. Freshly isolated Peyer's patch, but not spleen, dendritic cells produce interleukin 10 and induce the differentiation of T helper type 2 cells. J Exp Med 1999; 190:229-239.

16. Akbari O, DeKruyff RH, Umetsu DT. Pulmonary dendritic cells producing IL-10 mediate tolerance induced by respiratory exposure to antigen. Nat Immunol 2001; 2:725-731.

17. Vaz NM, Maia LCS, Hanson DG et al. Inhibition of homocytotropic antibody responses in adult inbred mice by previous feeding of the specific antigen. J Allergy Clin Immunol 1977; 60:110-115.

18. Ngan J, Kind LS. Suppressor T-cells for IgE and IgG in Peyer's patches of mice made tolerant by the oral administration of ovalbumin. J Immunol 1978; 120:861-865.

19. Miller S, Hanson D. Inhibition of specific immune responses by feeding protein antigens. IV. Evidence for tolerance and specific active suppression of cell-mediated immune responses to ovalbumin. J Immunol 1979; 123:2344-2350.

20. Mowat AM, Strobel S, Drummond HE et al. Immunological response to fed protein antigens in mice: I. Reversal of oral tolerance to ovalbumin by cyclophosphamide. Immunology 1982; 45:105-113.

21. Hanson DG, Vaz NM, Maia LCS et al. Inhibition of specific immune responses by feeding protein antigens. III. Evidence against maintenance of tolerance to ovalbumin by orally-induced antibodies. J Immunol 1979; 123:2337-2344.

22. Richman LK, Chiller JM, Brown WR et al. Enterically induced immunological tolerance. I. Induction of suppressor T lymphocytes by intragastric administration of soluble proteins. J Immunol 1978; 121:2429-2433.

23. Titus RG, Chiller JM. Orally induced tolerance. Definition at the cellular level. Int Arch Allergy Appl Immunol 1981; 65:323-338.

24. Hanson DG, Miller SD. Inhibition of specific immune responses by feeding protein antigens. V. Induction of the tolerant state in the absence of specific suppressor T-cells. J Immunol 1982; 128:2378-2381.

25. Lider O, Santos LM, Lee CS et al. Suppression of experimental autoimmune encephalomyelitis by oral administration of myelin basic protein. II. Suppression of disease and in vitro immune responses is mediated by antigen-specific CD8+ T lymphocytes. J Immunol 1989; 142:748-752.

26. Fishman-Lobell J, Friedman A, Weiner HL. Different kinetic patterns of cytokine gene expression in vivo in orally tolerant mice. Eur J Immunol 1994; 24:2720-2724.

27. Mowat AM, Thomas MJ, MacKenzie S et al. Divergent effects of bacterial lipopolysaccharide on immunity to orally administered protein and particulate antigens in mice. Immunology 1986; 58:677-683.

28. Kay RA, Ferguson A. The immunological consequences of feeding cholera toxin. II Mechanisms responsible for the induction of oral tolerance for DTH. Immunology 1989; 66:416-421.

29. Ke Y, Kapp JA. Oral antigen inhibits priming of CD8+ CTL, CD4+ T-cells, and antibody responses while activating CD8⁺ suppressor T-cells. J Immunol 1996; 156:916-921.

30. Heppell LMJ, Kilshaw PJ. Immune responses in guinea pigs to dietary protein. Int Arch Allergy Appl Immunol 1982; 68:54-59.

31. Husby S, Mestecky J, Moldoveanu Z et al. Oral tolerance in humans. T-cell but not B cell tolerance after antigen feeding. J Immunol 1994; 152:4663-4670.

32. Strobel S, Ferguson A. Persistence of oral tolerance in mice fed ovalbumin is different for humoral and cell-mediated immune responses. Immunology 1987; 60:317-318.

33. Hanson DG, Morimoto T. Delayed recovery of orally-induced tolerance to proteins in irradiated and spleen-cell reconstituted mice. Adv Exp Med Biol 1987; 216A:733-738.

34. Peng HJ, Turner MW, Strobel S. Failure to induce oral tolerance to protein antigens in neonatal mice can be corrected by transfer of adult spleen cells. Pediatric Research 1989; 26:486-490.

35. Mowat AM, Parrot DM. Immunological responses to fed protein antigens in mice. IV. Effects of stimulating the reticuloendotelial system on oral tolerance and intestinal immunity to ovalbumin. Immunology 1983; 50:547-554.

36. Lamont AG, Gordon M, Ferguson A. Oral tolerance in protein-deprived mice. I. Profound antibody tolerance but impaired DTH tolerance after antigen feeding. Immunology 1987; 61:333-337.

37. Melamed D, Friedman A. In vivo tolerization of Th1 lymphocytes following a single feeding with ovalbumin: anergy in the absence of suppression. Eur J Immunol. 1994; 24:1974-1981.

38. Melamed D, Fishman-Lovell J, Uni Z et al. Peripheral tolerance of Th2 lymphocytes induced by continuous feeding of ovalbumin. Int Immunol 1996; 8:717-724.

39. Gregerson DS, Obritsch WF, Donoso LA. Oral tolerance in experimental autoimmune uveoretinitis. Distinct mechanisms of resistance are induced by low dose vs high dose feeding protocols. J Immunol 1993; 151:5751-5761.

40. Mowat AM, Steel M, Worthy EA et al. Inactivation of Th1 and Th2 cells by feeding ovalbumin. Ann NY Acad Sci 1996; 778:122-132.

41. Saklayen MG, Pesce AJ, Pollak VE et al. Kinetics of oral tolerance: study of variables affecting tolerance induced by oral administration of antigen. Int Arch Allergy Appl Immunol 1984; 73:5-9.

42. Gautam SC, Chikkala NF, Battisto JR. Oral administration of the contact sensitizer trinitrochlorobenzene: Initial sensitization and subsequent appearance of a suppressor population. Cell Immunol 1990; 125:437-448.

43. Hoyne GF, Thomas WR. T-cell responses to orally administered antigens. Study of the kinetics of lymphokine production after single and multiple feeding. Immunology 1995; 84:304-309.

44. Marth T, Strober W, Kelsall BL. High dose oral tolerance in ovalbumin TCR-transgenic mice: Systemic neutralization of IL-12 augments TGF-β secretion and T-cell apoptosis. J Immunol 1996; 157:2348-2357.

45. Chen Y, Inobe J-i, Weiner HL. Inductive events in oral tolerance in the TCR transgenic adoptive transfer model. Cell Immunol 1997; 178:62-68.

46. McMenamin C, McKersey M, Kuhnlein P et al. gd T-cells down-regulate primary IgE responses in rats to inhaled soluble protein antigens. J Immunol 1995; 154:4390-4394.

47. Cauley LS, Cauley KA, Shub F et al. Transferable anergy: superantigen treatment induces CD4⁺ T-cell tolerance that is reversible and requires CD-CD8-cells and IFN-γ. J Exp Med 1997; 186:71-81.

48. Liu CC, Joag SV, Kwon BS et al. Induction of perforin and serine esterases in a murine cytotoxic T lymphocyte clone. J Immunol 1990; 144:1196-201.

49. Miller A, Lider O, Weiner HL. Antigen-driven bystander suppression following oral administration of antigens. J Exp Med 1991; 174:791-798.

50. Miller A, al-Sabbagh A, Santos L et al. Epitopes of myelin basic protein that trigger TGF-β release following oral tolerization are distinct from encephalitogenic epitopes and mediate epitope driven bystander suppression. J Immunol 1993; 151:7307-7315.

51. Al-Sabbagh A, Miller A, Santos LMB et al. Antigen-driven tissue-specific suppression following oral tolerance: orally administered myelin basic protein suppresses proteolipid induced experimental autoimmune encephalomyelitis in the SJL mouse. Eur J Immunol 1994; 24:2104-2109.

52. Racke MK, Lovett-Racke AE. Bystander suppression in experimental autoimmune encephalomyelitis: Where and how does it occur? Res Immunol 1998; 149:820-827.

53. Cross AH, Tuohy VK, Raine CS. Development of reactivity to new myelin antigens during chronic relapsing autoimmune demyelination. Cell Immunol 1993; 146:261-270.

54. Kerlero de Rosbo N, Milo R, Lees MB et al. Reactivity to myelin antigens in multiple sclerosis: peripheral blood lymphocytes respond predominantly to myelin oligodendrocyte glycoprotein. J Clin Invest 1993; 92:2602-2608.

55. Harrison LC. Islet cell antigens in insulin-dependent diabetes: Pandora's box revisited. Immunol Today 1992; 13:348-352.

56. Groux H, O'Garra A, Bigler M et al. A CD4⁺ T-cell subset inhibits antigen-specific T-cell responses and prevents colitis. Nature 1997; 389:737-742.

57. Yoshino S. Antigen-induced arthritis in rats is suppressed by the inducing antigen administered orally before, but not after immunization. Cell Immunol 1995; 163:55-58.

58. Zhang JZ, Lee CSY, Lider O et al. Suppression of adjuvant arthritis in Lewis rats by oral administration of type II collagen. J Immunol 1990; 145:2489-2493.

59. Chen Y, Hancock WW, Marks R et al. Mechanisms of recovery from experimental allergic encephalomyelitis: T-cell deletion and immune deviation in myelin basic protein T-cell receptor transgenic mice. J Neuroimmunol 1998; 82:149-159.

60. Von Herrath MG, Dyrberg T, Oldstone MBA. Oral insulin treatment suppresses virus-induced antigen-specific destruction of beta cells and prevents autoimmune diabetes in transgenic mice. J Clin Invest 1996; 98:1324-1331.

61. Falcone M, Bloom BR. A T helper cell 2 (Th2) immune response against non-self antigens modifies the cytokine profile of autoimmune T-cells and protects against experimental allergic encephalomyelitis. J Exp Med 1997; 185:901-907.

62. Pullerits T, Lundin S, Cui ZH et al. Bystander suppression of occupational hapten sensitization in rats made tolerant to ovalbumin. Eur Respir J 1998; 12:889-894.

63. Wildner G, Thurau SR. Orally induced bystander suppression in experimental autoimmune uveoretinitis occurs only in the periphery and not in the eye. Eur J Immunol 1995; 25:1292-1297.

64. Miossec P, van den Berg W. Th1/Th2 cytokine balance in arthritis. Arthritis Rheum 1997; 40:2105-2115.

65. Lundin BS, Dahlgren UIH, Hanson LA et al. Oral tolerization leads to active suppression and bystander tolerance in adult rats while anergy dominates in young rats. Scand J Immunol 1996; 43:56-63.

66. Becker KJ, McCarron RM, Ruetzler C et al. Immunologic tolerance to myelin basic protein decreases stroke size after transient focal cerebral ischemia. Proc Natl Acad Sci USA 1997; 94:10873-10878.

67. Teng Y, Gorczynski R, Hozumi N. The function of TGF-beta-mediated innocent bystander suppression associated with physiological self-tolerance in vivo. Cell Immunol 1998; 190:51-60.

68. Inobe J, Slavin AJ, Komagata Y et al. IL-4 is a differentiation factor for transforming growth factor-beta secreting Th3 cells and oral administration of IL-4 enhances oral tolerance in experimental allergic encephalomyelitis. Eur J Immunol 1998; 28:2780-2790.

69. Seder RA, Marth T, Sieve MC et al. Factors involved in the differentiation of TGF-β-producing cells from naive CD4⁺ T-cells: IL-4 and IFN-γ have opposing effects, while TGF-β positively regulates its own production. J Immunol 1998; 160:5719-5728.

70. Slavin AJ, Maron R, Garcia G et al. Oral administration of IL-4 and IL-10 enhance the induction of low dose oral tolerance. FASEB J 1998; II:A599.

71. Xiao BG, Bai XF, Zhang GX et al. Suppression of acute and protracted-relapsing experimental allergic encephalomyelitis by nasal administration of low-dose IL-10 in rats. J Neuroimmunol 1998; 84:230-237.

72. Zhang Z, Michael JG. Orally induced immune responsiveness is abrogated by IFN-g treatment. J Immunol 1990; 144:4163-4165.

73. Claessen AM, von Blomberg BM, De Groot J et al. Reversal of mucosal tolerance by subcutaneous administration of interleukin-12 at the site of attempted sensitization. Immunology 1996; 88:363-367.

74. Rizzo LV, Miller-Rivero NE, Chan C-C et al. Interleukin-2 treatment potentiates induction of oral tolerance in a murine model of autoimmunity. J Clin Invest 1994; 94:1668-1672.

75. Khoury SJ, Lider O, al-Sabbagh A et al. Suppression of experimental autoimmune encephalomyelitis by oral administration of myelin basic protein. III. Synergistic effect of lipopolysaccharide. Cell Immunol 1990; 131:302-310.

76. Nelson PA, Akselband Y, Dearborn SM et al. Effect of oral beta interferon on subsequent immune responsiveness. Ann NY Acad Sci 1996; 778:145-155.

77. Elson CO, Ealding W. Cholera toxin feeding did not induce oral tolerance in mice and abrogated oral tolerance to an unrelated protein antigen. J Immunol 1984; 133:2892-2897.

78. Sun J-B, Holmgren C, Czerkinsky C. Cholera toxin B subunit: An efficient transmucosal carrier-delivery system for induction of peripheral immunological tolerance. Proc Natl Acad Sci USA 1994; 91:10795-10799.

79. Ma D, Mellon J, Niederkorn JY. Oral administration as a strategy for enhancing corneal allograft survival. Br J Ophthalmol 1997; 81:778-784.

80. Karpus WJ, Kennedy KJ, Kunkel SL et al. Monocyte chemotactic protein 1 regulates oral tolerance induction by inhibition of T helper cell1-related cytokines. J Exp Med 1998; 187:733-741.

81. Elson CO, Tomasi M, Dertzbaugh MT et al. Oral antigen delivery by way of a multiple emulsion system enhances oral tolerance. Ann NY Acad Sci 1996; 778:156-162.

82. Ke Y, Pearce K, Lake JP et al. Gamma delta T lymphocytes regulate the induction and maintenance of oral tolerance. J Immunol 1997; 158:3610-8.

83. Mengel J, Cardillo F, Aroeira LS et al. Anti-γδ T-cell antibody blocks the induction and maintenance of oral tolerance to ovalbumin in mice. Immunolology Letters 1995; 48:97-102.

84. Spahn TW, Weiner HL. γδ T-cells are necessary for low dose but not high dose oral tolerance. FASEB J 1998; I2:A597, 3464.

85. Wolvers DA, Bakker JM, Bagchus WM et al. The steroid hormone dehydroepiandrosterone (DHEA) breaks intranasally induced tolerance, when administered at time of systemic immunization. J Immunol 1998; 89:19-25.

86. Yoshino S, Ohsawa M, Sagai M. Diesel exhaust particles block induction of oral tolerance in mice. J Pharmacol Exp Ther 1998; 287:679-683.

87. Thorbecke GJ, Schwarcz R, Leu J et al. Modulation by cytokines of induction of oral tolerance to type II collagen. Arthritis Rheum 1999; 42:110-118.

88. Kuper CF, Koornstra PJ, Hameleers DM et al. The role of nasopharyngeal lymphoid tissue. Immunol Today 1992; 13:219-224.

89. Hiroi T, Iwatani K, Iijima H et al. Nasal immune system: distinctive Th0 and Th1/Th2 type environments in murine nasal-associated lymphoid tissues and nasal passage, respectively. Eur J Immunol 1998; 28:3346-3353.

90. Holt PG, Sedgwick JD. Suppression of IgE responses following inhalation of antigen. Immunol Today 1987; 8:14-815.

91. Kaltreider HB. Expression of immune mechanisms in the lung. Am Rev Respir Dis 1976; 113:347-379.

92. Sedgwick JD, Holt PG. Induction of IgE-isotype specific tolerance by passive antigenic stimulation of the respiratory mucosa. Immunology 1983; 50:625-630.

93. Lowrey JA, Savage NDL, Palliser D et al. Induction of tolerance via the respiratory mucosa. Int Arch Allergy Immunol 1998; 116:93-102.

94. Holt PG, Batty JE, Turner KJ. Inhibition of specific IgE response in mice by pre-exposure to inhaled antigen. Immunology 1981; 42:409-417.

95. McMenamin C, Pimm C, McKersey M et al. Regulation of IgE responses to inhaled antigen in mice by antigen-specific γδ T-cells. Science 1994; 265:1869-1871.

96. Sedgwick JD, Holt PG. Induction of IgE-secreting cells and IgE isotype-specific suppressor T-cells in the respiratory lymph nodes of rats in response to antigen inhalation. Cell Immunol 1985; 94:182-194.

97. Renz H, Bradley K, Saloga J et al. T-cells expressing specific V beta elements regulate immunoglobulin E production and airways responsiveness in vivo. J Exp Med 1993; 177:1175-1180.

98. Renz H, Lack G, Saloga J et al. Inhibition of IgE production and normalization of airways responsiveness by sensitized CD8 T-cells in a mouse model of allergen-induced sensitization. J Immunol 1994; 152:351-360.

99. Seymour BWP, Gershwin LJ, Coffman RL. Aerosol-induced immunoglobulin (Ig)-E unresponsiveness to ovalbumin does not require CD8' or T-cell receptor (TCR)-gamma/delta+ T-cells or interferon (IFN)-gamma in a murine model of allergen sensitization. J Exp Med 1998; 187:721-731.

100. Wolvers DA, van der Cammen MJ, Kraal G. Mucosal tolerance is associated with, but independent of, up-regulation Th2 responses. Immunology 1997; 92:328-33.

101. Daniel D, Wegmann DR. Intranasal administration of insulin peptide B: 9-23 protects NOD mice from diabetes. Ann NY Acad Sci 1996; 778:371-372.

102. Tian J, Atkinson MA, Clare-Salzler M et al. Nasal administration of glutamate decarboxylase (GAD65) peptides induces Th2 responses and prevents murine insulin-dependent diabetes. J Exp Med 1996; 183:1561-1567.

103. Harrison LC, Dempsey-Collier M, Kramer DR et al. Aerosol insulin induces regulatory CD8 γδ T-cells that prevent murine insulin-dependent diabetes. J Exp Med 1996; 184:2167-2174.
104. Myers LK, Seyer JM, Stuart JM et al. Suppression of murine collagen-induced arthritis by nasal administration of collagen. Immunology 1997; 90:161-164.
105. Staines NA, Harper N, Ward FJ et al. Mucosal tolerance and suppression of collagen-induced arthritis (CIA) induced by nasal inhalation of synthetic peptide 184-198 of bovine type II collagen (CII) expressing a dominant T-cell epitope. Clin Exp Immunol 1996; 103:368-375.
106. Lu S, Holmdahl R. Different therapeutic and bystander effects by intranasal administration of homologous type II and type IX collagens on the collagen-induced arthritis and pristance-induced arthritis in rats. Clin Immunol 1999; 90:119-127.
107. Garcia G, Komagata Y, Slavin AJ et al. Suppression of collagen-induced arthritis by oral or nasal administration of type II collagen. J Autoimmun 1999; 13:315-324.
108. Metzler B, Wraith DC. Inhibition of experimental autoimmune encephalomyelitis by inhalation but not oral administration of the encephalitogenic peptide: Influence of MHC binding affinity. Int Immunol 1993; 5:1159-1165.
109. Liu JQ, Bai XF, Shi FD et al. Inhibition of experimental autoimmune encephalomyelitis in Lewis rats by nasal administration of encephalitogenic MBP peptides: Synergistic effects of MBP 68-86 and 87-99. Int Immunol 1998; 10:1139-1148.
110. Zhang G-X, Shi F-D, Zhu J et al. Synthetic peptides fail to induce nasal tolerance to experimental autoimmune myasthenia gravis. J Neuroimmunol 1998; 85:96-101.
111. Li HL, Liu JQ, Bai XF et al. Dose-dependent mechanisms relate to nasal tolerance induction and protection against experimental autoimmune encephalomyelitis in Lewis rats. Immunology 1998; 94:431-437.
112. Shi FD, Bai XF, Li HL et al. Nasal tolerance in experimental autoimmune myasthenia gravis (EAMG): Induction of protective tolerance in primed animals. Clin Exp Immunol 1998; 111:506-512.
113. Xiao BG, Zhang GX, Shi FD et al. Decrease of LFA-1 is associated with upregulation of TGF-β in CD4(+) T-cell clones derived from rats nasally tolerized against experimental autoimmune myasthenia gravis. Clin Immunol Immunopathol 1998; 89:196-204.
114. Imaoka K, Miller CJ, Kubota M et al. Nasal immunization of nonhuman primates with simian immunodeficiency virus p55gag and cholera toxin adjuvant induces Th1/Th2 help for virus-specific immune responses in reproductive tissues. J Immunol 1998; 161:5952-5958.
115. Hoyne GF, O'Hehir RE, Wraith DC et al. Inhibition of T-cell and antibody responses to house dust mite allergen by inhalation of the dominant T-cell epitope in naive and sensitized mice. J Exp Med 1993; 178:1783-1788.
116. Hoyne GF, Jarnicki AG, Thomas WR et al. Characterization of the specificity and duration of T-cell tolerance to intranasally administered peptides in mice: A role for intramolecular epitope suppression. Int Immunol 1997; 9:1165-1173.
117. Hoyne GF, Askinas BA, Hetzel C et al. Regulation of house dust mite responses by intranasally administered peptide: transient activation of CD4+ T-cells precedes the development of tolerance in vivo. Int Immunol 1996; 8:335-342.
118. Javed NH, Gienapp IE, Cox KL et al. Exquisite peptide specificity of oral tolerance in experimental autoimmune encephalomyelitis. J Immunol 1995; 155:1599-1605.
119. Miller A, Zhang ZJ, Sobel RA et al. Suppression of experimental autoimmune encephalomyelitis by oral administration of myelin basic protein. VI. Suppression of adoptively transferred disease and differential effects of oral vs. intravenous tolerization. J Neuroimmunol 1993; 46:73-82.
120. Khoury SJ, Hancock WW, Weiner HL. Oral tolerance to myelin basic protein and natural recovery from experimental autoimmune encephalomyelitis as associated with downregulation of inflammatory cytokines and differential upregulation of transforming growth factor β, interleukin 4, and prostaglandin E expression in the brain. J Exp Med 1992; 176:1355-1364.
121. Brod SA, al-Sabbagh A, Sobel RA et al. Suppression of experimental autoimmune encephalomyelitis by oral administration of myelin antigens: IV. Suppression of chronic relapsing disease in the Lewis rat and strain 13 guinea pig. Ann Neuro 1991; 29:615-622.
122. Meyer A, Gienapp I, Cox K et al. Oral tolerance in myelin basic protein TCR transgenic mice. Ann NY Acad Sci 1996; 778:412-413.

123. al-Sabbagh A, Nelson PA, Akselband Y et al. Antigen-driven peripheral immune tolerance: Suppression of experimental autoimmmune encephalomyelitis and collagen-induced arthritis by aerosol administration of myelin basic protein or type II collagen. Cell Immunol 1996; 171:111-119.
124. Teitelbaum D, Arnon R, Sela M. Immunomodulation of experimental autoimmune encephalomyelitis by oral administration of copolymer 1. Proc Natl Acad Sci USA 1999; 96:3842-3847.
125. Maron R, Slavin A, Hoffmann E et al. Oral tolerance to copolymer 1 in myelin basic protein (MBP) TCR transgenic mice: cross-reactivity with MBP-specific TCR and differential induction of anti-inflammatory cytokines. Int Immunol 2002; 14(2).
126. Weiner HL. Oral tolerance with Copolymer 1 for the treatment of multiple sclerosis. Proc Natl Acad Sci USA 1999; 96:3333-3335.
127. Courtenay JS, Dallman MS, Dayan AD et al. Immunization against heterologous type II collagen induces arthritis in mice. Nature 1980; 283:666-668.
128. Trentham DE, Townes AS, Kang AS. Autoimmunity to type II collagen: an experimental model of arthritis. J Exp Med 1977; 146:857-868.
129. Khare SD, Krco CJ, Griffiths MM et al. Oral administration of an immunodominant human collagen peptide modulates collagen-induced arthritis. J Immunol 1995; 155:3653-3659.
130. Myers LK, Brand DD, Ye XJ et al. Characterization of recombinant type II collagen: Arthritogenicity and tolerogenicity in DBA/1 mice. Immunology 1998; 95:631-639.
131. al-Sabbagh AM, Goad EP, Weiner HL et al. Decreased CNS inflammation and absence of clinical exacerbation of disease after six months oral administration of bovine myelin in diseased SJL/J mice with chronic relapsing experimental autoimmune encephalomyelitis. J Neurosci Res 1996; 45:424-429.
132. Feldman M, Brennan FM, Maini RN. Role of cytokines in rheumatoid arthritis. Annu Rev Immunol 1996; 14:397-440.
133. Yoshino S. Treatment with an anti-IL-4 antibody blocks suppression of collagen-induced arthritis in mice by oral administration of type II collagen. J Immunol 1998; 160:3067-3071.
134. van Eden W, Thole JE, van der Zee R et al. Cloning of the mycobacterial epitope recognized by T lymphocytes in adjuvant arthritis. Nature 1988; 331:171-173.
135. Haque MA, Yoshino S, Inada S et al. Suppression of adjuvant arthritis in rats by induction of oral tolerance to mycobacterial 65-kDa heat shock protein. Eur J Immunol 1996; 26:2650-2656.
136. Prakken BJ, van der Zee R, Anderton SM et al. Peptide-induced nasal tolerance for a mycobacterial heat shock protein 60 T-cell epitope in rats suppresses both adjuvant arthritis and nonmicrobially induced experimental arthritis. Proc Natl Acad Sci USA 1997; 94:3284-3289.
137. Thompson SJ, Thompson HSG, Harper N et al. Prevention of pristane-induced arthritis by the oral administration of type II collagen. Immunology 1993; 79:152-157.
138. Inada S, Yoshino S, Haque MA et al. Clonal anergy is a potent mechanism of oral tolerance in the suppression of acute antigen-induced arthritis in rats by oral administration of the inducing antigen. Cell Immunol 1997; 175:67-75.
139. Yoshimoto T, Takeda K, Tanaka T et al. IL-12 up-regulates IL-18 receptor expression on T cells, Th1 cells, and B cells: synergism with IL-18 for IFN-gamma production. J Immunol 1998; 161:3400-3407.
140. Chen W, Jin W, Cook M et al. Oral delivery of group A streptococcal cell walls augments circulating TGF-beta and suppresses streptococcal cell wall arthritis. J Immunol 1998; 161:6297-6304.
141. Yoshino S, Quattrocchi E, Weiner HL. Oral administration of type II collagen suppresses antigen-induced arthritis in Lewis rats. Arthritis Rheum 1995; 38:1092-1096.
142. al-Sabbagh AM, Garcia G, Slavin AJ et al. Combination therapy with oral myelin basic protein and oral methotrexate enhances suppression of experimental autoimmune encephalomyelitis. Neurology 1997; 48:A421.
143. Weiner HL, Komagata Y. Oral tolerance and the treatment of rheumatoid arthritis. Springer Semin Immunopathol 1998; 20:289-308.
144. Zhang JZ, Davidson L, Eisenbarth G et al. Suppression of diabetes in NOD mice by oral administration of porcine insulin. Proc Natl Acad Sci USA 1991; 88:10252-10256.
145. Bergerot I, Arreaza GA, Cameron MJ et al. Insulin B-chain reactive CD4+ regulatory T-cells induced by oral insulin treatment protect from type 1 diabetes by blocking the cytokine secretion and pancreatic infiltration of diabetogenic effector T-cells. Diabetes 1999; 48:1720-1729.

146. Hancock WW, Polanski M, Zhang ZJ et al. Suppression of insulitis in NOD mice by oral insulin administration is associated with selective expression of IL-4, IL-10, TGF-β and prostaglandin-E. Am J Pathol 1995; 147:1193-1199.

147. King C, Davies J, Mueller R et al. TGF-β-1 alters APC preference, polarizing islet antigen responses toward a Th2 phenotype. Immunity 1998; 8:601-613.

148. Polanski M, Melican NS, Zhang J et al. Oral administration of the immunodominant B-chain of insulin reduces diabetes in a co-transfer model of diabetes in the NOD mouse and is associated with a switch from Th1 to Th2 cytokines. J Autoimmun 1997; 10:339-346.

149. Bellmann K, Kolb H, Hartmann B et al. Intervention in autoimmune diabetes by targeting the gut immune system. Int J Immunopharmacol 1997; 19:573-577.

150. Ma SW, Zhao DL, Yin ZQ et al. Transgenic plants expressing autoantigens fed to mice to induce oral immune tolerance. Nature Med 1997; 3:793-796.

151. Arakawa T, Yu J, Chong DK et al. A plant-based cholera toxin B subunit-insulin fusion protein protects against the development of autoimmune diabetes. Nat Biotechnol 1998; 16:934-938.

152. Mordes JP, Schirf B, Roipko D et al. Oral insulin does not prevent insulin-dependent diabetes mellitus in BB rats. Ann NY Acad Sci 1996; 778:418-421.

153. Bellmann K, Kolb H, Rastegar S et al. Potential risk of oral insulin with adjuvant for the prevention of Type I diabetes: a protocol effective in NOD mice may exacerbate disease in BB rats. Diabetologia 1998; 41:844-847.

154. Herbelin A, Gombert JM, Lepault F et al. Mature mainstream TCR alpha beta+CD4⁺ thymocytes expressing L-selectin mediate active tolerance in the nonobese diabetic mouse. J Immunol 1998; 161:2620-2628.

155. Blanas E, Carbone FR, Allison J et al. Induction of autoimmune diabetes by oral administration of autoantigen. Science 1996; 274:1707-1709.

156. Nussenblatt RB, Caspi RR, Mahdi R et al. Inhibition of S-antigen induced experimental autoimmune uveoretinitis by oral induction of tolerance with S-antigen. J Immunol 1990; 144:1689-1695.

157. Wildner G, Thurau SR. Cross-reactivity between an HLA-B27-derived peptide and a retinal autoantigen peptide: a clue to major histocompatibility complex association with autoimmune disease. Eur J Immunol 1994; 24:2579-2585.

158. Thurau SR, Caspi RR, Chan CC et al. Immunological suppression of experimental autoimmune uveitis. Fortschr Ophthalmol 1991; 88:404-407.

159. Thurau SR, Chan CC, Nussenblatt RB et al. Oral tolerance in a murine model of relapsing experimental autoimmune uveoretinitis (EAU): induction of protective tolerance in primed animals. Clin Exp Immunol 1997; 109:370-376.

160. Thurau SR, Diedrichs-Mohring M, Fricke H et al. Molecular mimicry as a therapeutic approach for an autoimmune disease: oral treatment of uveitis-patients with an MHC-peptide crossreactive with autoantigenófirst results. Immunol Lett 1997; 57:193-201.

161. Torseth JW, Gregerson DS. Oral tolerance in experimental autoimmune uveoretinitis: feeding after disease induction is less protective than prefeeding. Clin Immunol Immunopathol 1998; 88:297-304.

162. Ma D, Mellon J, Niederkorn JY. Conditions affecting enhanced corneal allograft survival by oral immunization. Invest. Ophthalmol Vis Sci 1998; 39:1835-1846.

163. Ma C-G, Zhang G-X, Xiao B-G et al. Suppression of experimental autoimmune myasthenia gravis by nasal administration of acetylcholine receptor. J Neuroimmunol 1995; 58:51-60.

164. Wang ZY, Qiao J, Link H. Suppression of experimental autoimmune myasthenia gravis by oral administration of acetylcholine receptor. J Neuroimmunol 1993; 44:209-214.

165. Okumura S, McIntosh K, Drachman DB. Oral administration of acetylcholine receptor: Effects on experimental myasthenia gravis. Ann Neurol 1994; 36:704-713.

166. Ma CG, Zhang GX, Xiao BG et al. Cellular mRNA expression of interferon-gamma (IFN-γ), IL-4 and transforming growth factor-beta (TGF-β) in rats nasally tolerized against experimental autoimmune myasthenia gravis (EAMG). Clin Exp Immunol 1996; 104:509-516.

167. Karachunski PI, Ostlie NS, Okita DK et al. Prevention of experimental myasthenia gravis by nasal administration of synthetic acetylcholine receptor T epitope sequences. J Clin Invest 1997; 100:3027-3035.

168. van Halteren AG, van der Cammen MJ, Cooper D et al. Regulation of antigen-specific IgE, IgG1, and mast cell responses to ingested allergen by mucosal tolerance induction. J Immunol 1997; 159:3009-3015.

169. Aramaki Y, Fujii Y, Suda H et al. Induction of oral tolerance after feeding of ragweed pollen extract in mice. Immunol Lett 1994; 40:21-25.

170. Sato MN, Carvalho AF, Silva AO et al. Oral tolerance induced to house dust mite extract in naive and sensitized mice: evaluation of immunoglobulin G anti-immunoglobulin G anti-immunoglobulin E autoantibodies and IgC-IgE comlexes. Immunology 1998; 95:193-199.

171. Hoyne GF, Lamb JR. Regulation of T-cell function in mucosal tolerance. Immunol Cell Biol 1997; 75:197-201.

172. Blank M, George J, Barak V et al. Oral tolerance to low dose B2-Glycoprotein I: Immunomodulation of experimental antiphospholipid syndrome. J Immunol 1998; 161:5303-5312.

173. Neurath MF, Fuss I, Kelsall BL et al. Experimental granulomatous colitis in mice is abrogated by induction of TGF-β-mediated oral tolerance. J Exp Med 1996; 183:2605-2616.

174. Gaupp S, Hartung HP, Toyka K et al. Modulation of experimental autoimmune neuritis in Lewis rats by oral application of myelin antigens. J Neuroimmunol 1997; 79:129-37.

175. Zou L-P, Zhu J, Deng G-M et al. Treatment with P2 protein peptide 57-81 by nasal route is effective in Lewis rat experimental autoimmune neuritis. J Neuroimmunol 1998; 85:137-145.

176. Browning MJ, Parrott DM. Protection from chronic immune complex nephritis by a single dose of antigen administered by the intragastric route. Adv Exp Med Biol 1987; 216B:1619-1625.

177. Devey ME, Bleasdale K. Antigen feeding modifies the course of antigen-induced immune complex disease. Clin Exp Immunol 1984; 56:637-644.

178. Gesualdo L, Lamm ME, Emancipator SN. Defective oral tolerance promotes nephritogenesis in experimental IgA nephropathy induced by oral immunization. J Immunol 1990; 145:3684-3691.

179. Wang Z-Y, He B, Qiao J et al. Suppression of experimental autoimmune myasthenia gravis and experimental allergic encephalomyelitis by oral administration of acetylcholine receptor and myelin basic protein: double tolerance. J Neuroimmunol 1995; 63:79-86.

180. van Hoogstraten IM, Boden D, von Blomberg ME et al. Persistent immune tolerance to nickel and chromium by oral administration prior to cutaneous sensitization. J Invest Dermatol 1992; 99:608-616.

181. van Hoogstraten IM, Boos C, Boden D et al. Oral induction of tolerance to nickel sensitization in mice. J Invest Dermatol 1993; 101:26-31.

182. Guimaraes VC, Quintans J, Fisfalen M-E et al. Suppression of experimental autoimmune thyroiditis by oral administration of thyroglobulin. Endocrinology 1995; 136:3353-3359.

183. Peterson KE, Braley-Mullen H. Suppression of murine experimental autoimmune thyroiditis by oral administration of porcine thyroglobulin. Cell Immunol 1995; 166:123-130.

184. Guimaraes VC, Quintans J, Fisfalen ME et al. Immunosuppression of thyroiditis. Endocrinology 1996; 137:2199-2204.

185. Zhang W, Kong YC. Noninvolvement of IL-4 and IL-10 in tolerance induction to experimental autoimmune thyroiditis. Cell Immunol 1998; 187:95-102.

186. Nakao A, Kasai M, Kumano K et al. High-dose oral tolerance prevents antigen-induced eosinophil recruitment into the mouse airways. Int Immunol 1998; 10:387-394.

187. Russo M, Jancar S, Siqueira ALP et al. Prevention of lung eosinophilic inflammation by oral tolerance. Immunol Letters 1998; 61:15-23.

188. Haneda K, Sano K, Tamura G et al. TGF-β induced by oral tolerance ameliorates experimental tracheal eosinophilia. J Immunol 1997; 159:4484-4490.

189. Sayegh MH, Zhang ZJ, Hancock WW et al. Down-regulation of the immune response to histocompatibility antigen and prevention of sensitization by skin allografts by orally administered alloantigen. Transplantion 1992; 53:163-166.

190. Hancock W, Sayegh M, Kwok C et al. Oral but not intravenous, alloantigen prevents accelerated allograft rejection by selective intragraft Th2 cell activation. Transplantion 1993; 55:1112-1118.

191. Ilan Y, Prakash R, Davidson A et al. Oral tolerization to adenoviral antigens permits long-term gene expression using recombinant adenoviral vectors. J Clin Invest 1997; 99:1098-1106.

192. Hachimura S, Fujikawa Y, Enomoto A et al. Differential inhibition of T and B cell responses to individual antigenic determinants in orally tolerized mice. Int Immunol 1994; 6:1791-1797.

193. Kim SM, Enomoto A, Hachimura S et al. Serum antibody response elicited by a casein diet is directed to only limited determinants of alpha s1-casein. Int Arch Allergy Immunol 1993; 101:260-265.

194. Maron R, Sukhova GK, Faria AM et al. Mucosal administration of HSP 65 decreases atherosclerosis and inflammation in the aortic arch of LDL receptor deficient mice. FASEB J 2000; A1199.

195. Weiner HL, Lemere CA, Maron R et al. Nasal administration of amyloid-beta peptide decreases cerebral amyloid burden in a mouse model of Alzheimer's disease. Ann Neurol 2000; 48:567-579.

196. Miller A, Lider O, Abramsky O et al. Orally administered myelin basic protein in neonates primes for immune responses and enhances experimental autoimmune encephalomyelitis in adult animals. Eur J Immunol 1994; 24:1026-1032.

197. Maron R, Guerau-de-Arellano M, Zhang X et al. Oral administration of insulin to neonates suppresses spontaneous and cyclophosphamide induced diabetes in the NOD mouse. J Autoimmun 2001; 16:21-28.

198. Meyer AL, Benson JM, Gienapp IE et al. Suppression of murine chronic relapsing experimental autoimmune encephalomyelitis by the oral administration of myelin basic protein. J Immunol 1996; 157:4230-4238.

199. Bai XF, Li HL, Shi FD et al. Complexities of applying nasal tolerance induction as a therapy for ongoing relapsing experimental autoimmune encephalomyelitis (EAE) in DA rats. Clin Exp Immunol 1998; 111:205-210.

200. Coutant R, Zeidler A, Rappaport R et al. Oral insulin therapy in newly-diagnosed immune mediated (type I) diabetes. Preliminary analysis of a randomized double blind placebo controlled study. Diabetes 1998; 47(Suppl 1):A97.

201. Terato K, Xiu JY, Miyahara H et al. Induction by chronic autoimmune arthritis in DBA/1 mice by oral administration of type II collagen and Escherichia coli lipopolysaccharide. Br J Rheumatol 1996; 35:828-838.

202. Hu W, Hasan A, Wilson A et al. Experimental mucosal induction of uveitis with the 60-kDa heat shock protein-derived peptide 336ñ351. J Immunol 1998; 28:2444-2455.

203. al-Sabbagh A, Miller A, Santos L et al. Antigen-driven tissue-specific suppression following oral tolerance: Orally administered myelin basic protein suppresses proteolipid induced experimental autoimmune encephalomyelitis in the SJL mouse. Eur J Immunol 1994; 24:2104-2109.

204. Karpus W, Kennedy K, Smith W et al. Inhibition of relapsing experimental autoimmune encephalomyelitis in SJL mice by feeding the immunodominant PLP139-151 peptide. J Neurosci Res 1996; 45:410-423.

205. Sieper J, Kary S, Sörensen H et al. Oral type II collagen treatment in early rheumatoid arthritis. Arthritis Rheum 1996; 39:41-51.

206. Nussenblatt RB, Gery I, Weiner HL et al. Treatment of uveitis by oral administration of retinal antigens: Results of a phase I/II randomized masked trial. Am J Ophthalmol 1997; 123:583-592.

207. Taudorf E, Laursen LC, Lanner A et al. Oral immunotherapy in birch pollen hay fever. J Allergy Clin Immunol 1987; 80:153-161.

208. Scadding GK, Brostoff J. Low dose sublingual therapy in patients with allergic rhinitis due to house dust mite. Clin Allergy 1986; 16:483-491.

209. Litwin A, Flanagan M, Entis G et al. Immunologic effects of encapsulated short ragweed extract: a potent new agent for oral immunotherapy. Ann Allergy Asthma Immunol 1996; 77:132-138.

210. Litwin A, Flanagan M, Entis G et al. Oral immunotherapy with short ragweed extract in a novel encapsulated preparation: a double-blind study. J Allergy Clin Immunol 1997; 100:30-38.

211. Ariano R, Panzani RC, Augeri G. Efficacy and safety of oral immunotherapy in respiratory allergy to Parietaria judaica pollen. A double-blind study. J Inv Allergol Clin Immunol 1998; 8:155-160.

212. Lowney ED. Tolerance of a contact sensitizer in man. Lancet 1968; 1:1377.

213. Krischer J, Ten S, Marker J et al. Endogenous insulin retention by oral insulin in newly diagnosed antibody positive type-1 diabetes. Diabetes 2001; 50:A44.

214. Chaillous L, Lefevre H, Thivolet C et al. Oral insulin administration and residual beta-cell function in recent-onset type 1 diabetes: A multicentre randomised controlled trial. Diabete Insuline Orale Group. Lancet 2000; 356:545-549.

215. Matsui M, Hafler DA, Weiner HL. Pilot study of oral tolerance to keyhole limpet hemocyanin in humans: down-regulation of KLH-reactive precursor-cell frequency. Ann NY Acad Sci 1996; 778:398-404.

216. Waldo FB, Van Den Wall Bake AWL, Mestecky J et al. Suppression of the immune response by nasal immunization. Clin Immunol Immunopathol 1994; 72:30-34.

217. Campbell DA, Jr., Lorber MI, Sweeton JC et al. Breast feeding and maternal-donor renal allografts. Possibly the original donor-specific transfusion. Transplantion 1984; 37:340-344.

218. Josien R, Douillard P, Guillot C et al. A critical role for transforming growth factor-β in donor transfusion-induced allograft tolerance. J Clin Invest 1998; 102:1920-1926.

219. Fukaura H, Kent SC, Pietrusewicz MJ et al. Induction of circulating myelin basic protein and proteolipid protein-specific transforming growth factor-beta1-secreting Th3 T-cells by oral administration of myelin in multiple sclerosis patients. J Clin Invest 1996; 98:70-77.

220. Benson JM, Stuckman SS, Cox KL et al. Oral administration of myelin basic protein is superior to myelin in suppressing established relapsing experimental autoimmune encephalomyelitis. J Immunol 1999; 152(10):6247-54.

221. Bagot M, Charue D, Flechet ML et al. Oral desensitization in nickel allergy induces a decrease in nickel-specific T-cells. Eur J Dermatol 1995; 5:614-617.

222. Morris DL. Intradermal testing and sublingual desensitization for nickel. Cutis 1998; 61:129-132.

223. van Hoogstraten IM, von Blomberg BM, Boden D et al. Effects of oral exposure to nickel or chromium on cutaneous sensitization. Curr Probl Dermatol 1991; 20:237-241.

224. Barnett ML, Kremer JM, St. Clair EW et al. Treatment of rheumatoid arthritis with oral type II collagen: Results of a multicenter, double-blind, placebo-controlled trial. Arthritis Rheum 1998; 41:290-297.

225. Barnett ML, Combitchi D, Trentham DE. A pilot trial of oral type II collagen in the treatment of juvenile rheumatoid arthritis. Arthritis Rheum 1996; 39:623-628.

226. Trentham D, Dynesius-Trentham R, Orav E et al. Effects of oral administration of type II collagen on rheumatoid arthritis. Science 1993; 261:1727-1730.

227. Choy E, Scott D, Kingsley G et al. Control of Rheumatoid Arthritis by Oral Tolerance. Arthritis Rheum 2001; 44:1993-1997.

228. Myers LK, Higgins GC, Finkel TH et al. Juvenile arthritis and autoimmunity to type II collagen. Arthritis Rheum 2001; 44:1775-1781.

229. Postlethwaite AE. Can we induce tolerance in rheumatoid arthritis? Curr Rheumatol Rep 2001; 3:64-69.

230. Lee S, Scherberg N, De Groot LJ. Induction of oral tolerance in human autoimmune thyroid disease. Thyroid 1998; 8:229-234.

231. McKown KM, Carbone LD, Bustillo J et al. Open trial of oral type I collagen in patients with systemic sclerosis. Arthritis Rheum 1997; 40:S100.

232. McKown KM, Carbone LD, Bustillo J et al. Induction of immune tolerance to human type I collagen in patients with systemic sclerosis by oral administration of bovine type I collagen. Arthritis Rheum 2000; 43:1054-1061.

233. Husby S, Jensenius JC, Svehag S-E. Passage of undergraded dietary antigen into the blood of healthy adults. Further characterization of the kinetics of uptake and the size distribution of the antigen. Scand J Immunol 1986; 24:447-452.

234. Biancone L, Paganelli R, Fais S et al. Peripheral and intestinal lymphocyte activation after in vitro exposure to cow's milk antigens in normal subjects and in patients with Crohn's disease. Clin Immunol Immunopathol 1987; 45:491-498.

235. Quinti I, Paganelli R, Scala E et al. Humoral response to food antigens. Allergy 1989; 44:59-64.

236. Lippard VW, Schloss OM, Johnson PA. Immune reactions induced in infants by intestinal absorption of incompletely digested cow's milk protein. Am J Dis Child 1936; 52:462-474.

237. Lown KS, Bailey DG, Fontana RJ et al. Grapefruit juice increases felodipine oral availability in humans by decreasing intestinal CYP3A protein expression. J Clin Invest 1997; 99:2545-2553.

238. Miller A, Zhang AJ, Prabdu-Das M et al. Active suppression vs. clonal anergy following oral or IV administration of MBP in actively and passively induced EAE. Neurology 1992; 42 (suppl. 3):301.

239. Fuller KA, Pearl D, Whitacre CC. Oral tolerance in experimental autoimmune encephalomyelitis: serum and salivary antibody responses. J Neuroimmunol 1990; 28:15-26.

240. Whitacre CC, Gienapp IE, Orosz CG et al. Oral tolerance in experimental autoimmune encephalomyelitis. III. Evidence for clonal anergy. J Immunol 1991; 147:2155-2163.

241. Miller A, Lider O, al-Sabbagh A et al. Suppression of experimental autoimmune encephalomyelitis by oral administration of myelin basic protein. V. Hierarchy of suppression by myelin basic protein from different species. J Neuroimmunol 1992; 39:243-250.

242. Miller A, Lider O, Roberts AB et al. Suppressor T-cells generated by oral tolerization to myelin basic protein suppress both in vitro and in vivo immune responses by the release of TGF-β following antigen specific triggering. Proc Natl Acad Sci USA 1992; 89:421-425.

243. Kelly KA, Whitacre CC. Oral tolerance in EAE: reversal of tolerance by T helper cell cytokines. J Neuroimmunol 1996; 66:77-84.

244. Popovich PG, Yu JY, Whitacre CC. Spinal cord neuropathology in rat experimental autoimmune encephalomyelitis: modulation by oral administration of myelin basic protein. J Neuropathol Exp Neurol 1997; 56:1323-1338.

245. Goldman-Brezinski S, Brezinski K, Zhang XM et al. Effects of oral tolerance induction by myelin basic protein on Vbeta8+ Lewis rat T-cells. J Neurosci Res 1998; 51:67-75.

246. Sun JB, Xiao BG, Lindblad M et al. Oral administration of cholera toxin B subunit conjugated to myelin basic protein protects against experimental autoimmune encephalomyelitis by inducing transforming growth factor-beta-secreting cells and suppressing chemokine expression. Int Immunol 2000; 12:1449-1457.

247. Sun JB, Rask C, Olsson T et al. Treatment of experimental autoimmune encephalomyelitis by feeding myelin basic protein conjugated to cholera toxin B subunit. Proc Natl Acad Sci USA 1996; 93:7196-7201.

248. Xu LY, Yang JS, Huang YM et al. Combined nasal administration of encephalitogenic myelin basic protein peptide 68-86 and IL-10 suppressed incipient experimental allergic encephalomyelitis in Lewis rats. Clin Immunol 2000; 96:205-211.

249. Oettinger HF, al-Sabbagh A, Jingwu Z et al. Biological activity of recombinant human myelin basic protein. J Neuroimmunol 1993; 44:157-162.

250. Santos LMB, al-Sabbagh A, Londono A et al. Oral tolerance to myelin basic protein induces regulatory TGF-β-secreting T-cells in Peyer's patches of SJL mice. Cell Immunol 1994; 157:439-447.

251. Chen Y, Kuchroo VK, Inobe J-I et al. Regulatory T-cell clones induced by oral tolerance: suppression of autoimmune encephalomyelitis. Science 1994; 265:1237-1240.

252. Chen Y, Inobe J, Weiner HL. Induction of oral tolerance to myelin basic protein in CD8-depleted mice: both CD4⁺ and CD8⁺ cells mediate active suppression. J Immunol 1995; 155:910-916.

253. Slavin AJ, Maron R, Weiner HL. Mucosal administration of IL-10 enhances oral tolerance in autoimmune encephalomyelitis and diabetes. Int Immunol 2001; 13:825-833.

254. Bebo BF, Jr., Adlard K, Schuster JC et al. Gender differences in protection from EAE induced by oral tolerance with a peptide analogue of MBP-Ac1-11. J Neurosci Res 1999; 55:432-440.

255. Chen Y, Inobe J, Kuchroo VK et al. Oral tolerance in myelin basic protein T-cell receptor transgenic mice: suppression of autoimmune encephalomyelitis and dose-dependent induction of regulatory cells. Proc Natl Acad Sci USA 1996; 93:388-391.

256. Meyer AL, Benson J, Song F et al. Rapid depletion of peripheral antigen-specific T cells in TCR-transgenic mice after oral administration of myelin basic protein. J Immunol 2001; 166:5773-5781.

257. Karpus WJ, Lukacs NW. The role of chemokines in oral tolerance: abrogation of nonresponsiveness by treatment with antimonocyte chemotactic protein-1. Ann NY Acad Sci 1996; 778:133-144.

258. Bai XF, Shi FD, Xiao BG et al. Nasal administration of myelin basic protein prevents relapsing experimental autoimmune encephalomyelitis in DA rats by activating regulatory cells expressing IL-4 and TGF-β mRNA. J Neuroimmunol 1997; 80:65-75.

259. Anderton S, Wraith D. Hierarchy in the ability of T-cell epitopes to induce peripheral tolerance to antigens from myelin. Eur J Immunol 1998; 28:1251-2161.

260. Pietropaolo M, Olson CD, Reiseter BS et al. Intratracheal administration to the lung enhances therapeutic benefit of an MBP peptide in the treatment of murine experimental autoimmune encephalomyelitis. Clin Immunol 2000; 95:104-116.

261. Brod SA, al-Sabbagh A, Sobel RA et al. Suppression of experimental autoimmune encephalomyelitis by oral administration of myelin antigens. IV. Suppression of chronic relapsing disease in the Lewis rat and strain 13 guinea pig. Ann Neurol 1991; 29:615-622.

262. Benson JM, Stuckman SS, Cox KL et al. Oral administration of myelin basic protein is superior to myelin in suppressing established relapsing experimental autoimmune encephalomyelitis. J Immunol 1999; 162:6247-6254.

263. Teitelbaum D, Arnon R, Sela M. Immunomodulation of experimental allergic encephalomyelitis by oral administration of copolymer 1 (Copaxone®). J Neuroimmunol 1998; 90:85.

264. Thompson HSG, Harper N, Bevan DJ et al. Suppression of collagen induced arthritis by oral administration of type II collagen: Changes in immune and arthritic responses mediated by active peripheral suppression. Autoimmunity 1993; 16:189-199.

265. Derry CJ, Harper N, Davies DH et al. Importance of dose of type II collagen in suppression of collagen-induced arthritis by nasal tolerance. Arthritis Rheum 2001; 44:1917-1927.

266. van Tienhoven EA, Broeren CP, Noordzij A et al. Nasal application of a naturally processed and presented T cell epitope derived from TCR AV11 protects against adjuvant arthritis. Int Immunol 2000; 12:1715-1721.

267. Yoshino S. Downregulation of silicone-induced chronic arthritis by gastric administration of type II collagen. Immunopharm 1995; 31:103-108.

268. Bergerot J, Fabien N, Maguer V et al. Oral administration of human insulin to NOD mice generates CD4⁺ T-cells that suppress adoptive transfer of diabetes. J Autoimmun 1994; 7:655-663.

269. Hancock WW, Khoury SJ, Carpenter CB et al. Differential effects of oral versus intrathymic administration of polymorphic major histocompatibility complex class II peptides on mononuclear and endothelial cell activation and cytokine expression during a delayed-type hypersensitivity response. Am J Pathol 1994; 144:1149-1158.

270. Bergerot I, Fabien N, Mayer A et al. Active suppression of diabetes after oral administration of insulin is determined by antigen dosage. Ann NY Acad Sci 1996; 778:362-367.

271. Sai P, Rivereau AS. Prevention of diabetes in the nonobese diabetic mouse by oral immunological treatments. Comparative efficiency of human insulin and two bacterial antigens, lipopolysacharide from Escherichia coli and glycoprotein extract from Klebsiella pneumoniae. Diabetes Metab 1996; 22:341-348.

272. Bergerot I, Fioix C, Peterson J et al. A cholera toxoid-insulin conjugate as an oral vaccine against spontaneous autoimmune diabetes. Proc Natl Acad Sci USA 1997; 94:4610-4614.

273. Hartmann B, Bellman K, Ghiea I et al. Oral insulin for diabetes prevention in NOD mice: Potentiation by enhancing Th2 cytokine expression in the gut through bacterial adjuvant. Diabetol 1997; 40:902-909.

274. Ploix C, Bergerot I, Fabien N et al. Protection against autoimmune diabetes with oral insulin is associated with the homing of IL-4 T helper type 2 cells to the pancreas and pancreatic lymph nodes. Diabetes 1998; 47:39-44.

275. Daniel D, Wegmann DR. Protection of nonobese diabetic mice from diabetics by intranasal or subcutaneous administration of insulin peptide B-(9-23). Proc Natl Acad Sci USA 1996; 93:956-960.

276. Thurau SR, Chan CC, Suh E et al. Induction of oral tolerance to S-antigen induced experimental autoimmune uveitis by a uveitogenic 20mer peptide. J Autoimmun 1991; 4:507-516.

277. Singh VK, Kalra HK, Yamaki K et al. Suppression of experimental autoimmune uveitis in rats by the oral administration of the uveitopathogenic S-antigen fragment and a cross-reactive homologous peptide. Cell Immunol 1992; 139:81-90.

278. Vrabec TR, Gregerson DS, Dua HS et al. Inhibition of experimental autoimmune uveoretinitis by oral administration of S-antigen and synthetic peptides. Autoimmunity 1992; 12:175-184.

279. Suh ED, Vistica BP, Chan C-C et al. Splenectomy abrogates the induction of oral tolerance in experimental autoimmune uveoretinitis. Curr Eye Res 1993; 12:833-839.

280. Singh VK, Anand R, Sharma K et al. Suppression of experimental autoimmune uveitis in Lewis rats by oral administration of recombinant Escherichia coli expressing retinal S-antigen. Cell Immunol 1996; 172:158-162.

281. Vistica BP, Chanaud NPr, Felix N et al. CD8 T-cells are not essential for the induction of "low-dose" oral tolerance. Clin Immunol Immunopathol 1996; 78:196-202.

282. Thurau SR, Diedrichs-Mohring M, Fricke H et al. Oral tolerance with an HLA-peptide mimicking retinal autoantigen as a treatment of autoimmune uveitis. Immunol Lett 1999; 68:205-212.

283. Wildner G, Hunig T, Thurau SR. Orally induced, peptide-specific g/d TCR+ cells suppress experimental autoimmune uveitis. Eur J Immunol 1996; 26:2140-2148.

284. Wang ZY, Qiao J, Melms A et al. T-cell reactivity to acetylcholine receptor in rats orally tolerized against experimental autoimmune myasthenia gravis. Cell Immunol 1993; 152:394-404.
285. Wang ZY, Link H, Ljungdahl A et al. Induction of interferon-γ, interleukin-4, and transforming growth factor-β in rats orally tolerized against experimental autoimmune myasthenia gravis. Cell Immunol 1994; 157:353-368.
286. Wang ZY, Huang J, Olsson T et al. B cell responses to acetylcholine receptor in rats orally tolerized against experimental autoimmune myasthenia gravis. J Neurol Sci 1995; 128:167-174.
287. Antozzi C, Baggi F, Andreetta F et al. Oral administration of an immunodominant TAChR epitope modulates antigen-specific T-cell responses in mice. Ann NY Acad Sci 1998; 841:568-571.
288. Im SH, Barchan D, Souroujon MC et al. Role of tolerogen conformation in induction of oral tolerance in experimental autoimmune myasthenia gravis. J Immunol 2000; 165:3599-3605.
289. Im SH, Barchan D, Fuchs S et al. Suppression of ongoing experimental myasthenia by oral treatment with an acetylcholine receptor recombinant fragment. J Clin Invest 1999; 104:1723-1730.
290. Baggi F, Andreetta F, Caspani E et al. Oral administration of an immunodominant T-cell epitope downregulates Th1/Th2 cytokines and prevents experimental myasthenia gravis. J Clin Invest 1999; 104:1287-1295.
291. Li HL, Shi FD, Bai XF et al. Nasal tolerance to experimental autoimmune myasthenia gravis: Tolerance reversal by nasal administration of minute amounts of interferon-gamma. Clin Immunol Immunopathol 1998; 87:15-22.
292. Holt PG, Vines J, Britten D. Sublingual allergen administration. I. selective suppression of IgE production in rats by high allergen doses. Clin Allergy 1988; 18:229-234.
293. Hoyne GF, Callow MG, Kuo MC et al. Differences in epitopes recognized by T-cells during oral tolerance and priming. Immunol. Cell Biol 1994; 72:29-33.
294. Astori M, von Garnier C, Kettner A et al. Inducing tolerance by intranasal administration of long peptides in naive and primed CBA/J mice. J Immunol 2000; 165:3497-505.
295. Rask C, Holmgren J, Fredriksson M et al. Prolonged oral treatment with low doses of allergen conjugated to cholera toxin B subunit suppresses immunoglobulin E antibody responses in sensitized mice. Clin Exp Allergy 2000; 30:1024-1032.
296. Dasgupta A, Kesari KV, Ramaswamy KK et al. Oral administration of unmodified colonic but not small intestinal antigens protects rats from hapten-induced colitis. Clin Exp Immunol 2001; 125:41-47.
297. Jung S, Gaupp S, Hartung HP et al. Oral tolerance in experimental autoimmune neuritis (EAN) of the Lewis rat. II. Adjuvant effects and bystander suppression in P2 peptide-induced EAN J Neuroimmunol 2001; 116:21-28.
298. Sayegh MH, Khoury SJ, Hancock WH et al. Induction of immunity and oral tolerance with polymorphic class II major histocompatability complex allopeptides in the rat. Proc Natl Acad Sci USA 1992; 89:7762-7766.
299. He YG, Mellon J, Niederkorn JY. The effect of oral immunization on corneal allograft survival. Transplantion 1996; 61:920-926.
300. Sun JB, Li BL, Czerkinsky C et al. Enhanced immunological tolerance against allograft rejection by oral administration of allogeneic antigen linked to cholera toxin B subunit. Clin Immunol 2000; 97:130-139.
301. Yasufuku K, Heidler KM, O'Donnell PW et al. Oral tolerance induction by type V collagen downregulates lung allograft rejection. Am J Respir Cell Mol Biol 2001; 25:26-34.
302. Niimi M, Witzke O, Bushell A et al. Nondepleting anti-CD4 monoclonal antibody enhances the ability of oral alloantigen delivery to induce indefinite survival of cardiac allografts: oral tolerance to alloantigen. Transplantion 2000; 70:1524-1528.
303. Broug-Holub E, Persoons JH, Schornagel K et al. Changes in cytokine and nitric oxide secretion by rat alveolar macrophages after oral administration of bacterial extracts. Clin Exp Immunol 1995; 101:302-307.
304. Enomoto A, Konishi M, Hachimura S et al. Milk whey protein fed as a constituent of the diet induced both oral tolerance and a systemic humoral response, while heat-denatured whey protein induced only oral tolerance. Clin Immunol Immunopathol 1993; 66:136-142.
305. Russo M, Nahori MA, Lefort J et al. Suppression of asthma-like responses in different mouse strains by oral tolerance. Am J Respir Cell Mol Biol 2001; 24:518-526.

306. Gotsman I, Beinart R, Alper R et al. Induction of oral tolerance towards hepatitis B envelope antigens in a murine model. Antiviral Res 2000; 48:17-26.

307. Ilan Y, Gotsman I, Pines M et al. Induction of oral tolerance in splenocyte recipients toward pretransplant antigens ameliorates chronic graft versus host disease in a murine model. Blood 2000; 95:3613-3619.

308. Nagler A, Pines M, Abadi U et al. Oral tolerization ameliorates liver disorders associated with chronic graft versus host disease in mice. Hepatology 2000; 31:641-648.

309. Taudorf E. Oral immunotherapy of adults with allergic rhinoconjunctivitis: clinical effects in birch and grass pollinosis. Dan Med Bull 1992; 39:542-560.

310. Kalanadhabhatta V, Muppidi D, Sahni H et al. Successful oral desensitization to trimethoprim-sulfamethoxazole in acquired immune deficiency syndrome. Ann Allergy Asthma Immunol 1996; 77:394-400.

311. Lowney ED. Immunologic unresponsiveness to a contact sensitizer in man. J Invest Dermatol 1968; 51:411-417.

312. Lowney ED. Tolerance of dinitrochlorobenzene, a contact sensitizer, in man. J Allergy Clin Immunol 1971; 48:28-35.

313. Lowney ED. Suppression of contact sensitization in man by prior feeding of antigen. J Invest Dermatol 1973; 61:90-93.

314. Lowney ED. A single-step procedure for inducing partial tolerance of DNCB in human subjects. J Invest Dermatol 1974; 63:260-261.

315. van Hoogstraten IM, Andersen KE, von Blomberg BM et al. Reduced frequency of nickel allergy upon oral nickel contact at an early age. Clin Exp Immunol 1991; 85:441-445.

316. Korenblatt PE, Rothberg RM, Minden P et al. Immune responses of human adults after oral and parenteral exposure to bovine serum albumin. J Allergy Clin Immunol 1968; 41:226-235.

317. Gold WR, Jr., Queenan JT, Woody J et al. Oral desensitization in Rh disease. Am J Obstet Gynecol 1983; 146:980-981.

318. Shenker BJ, Listgarten MA, Taichman NS. Suppression of human lymphocyte responses by oral spirochetes: A monocyte-dependent phenomenon. J Immunol 1934; 132:2039-2045.

319. Czerkinsky C, Prince SJ, Michalek SM et al. IgA antibody-producing cells in peripheral blood after antigen ingestion: Evidence for a common mucosal immune system in humans. Proc Natl Acad Sci USA 1987; 84:2449-2453.

Index

Made in the USA
Middletown, DE
27 August 2018